Dedication

Richard Johanson 1957–2002

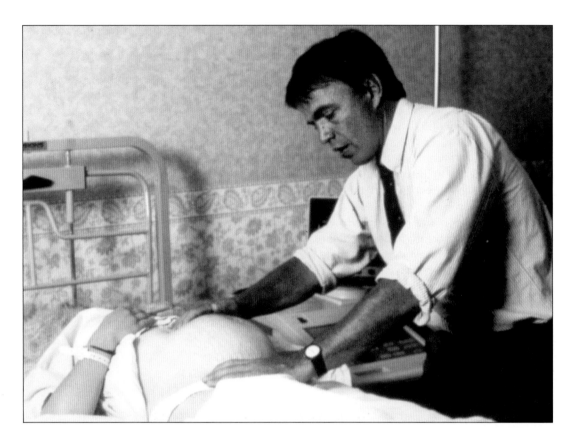

This book is dedicated to the memory of Richard Johanson, who died on 20 February 2002, before he could see this work come to fruition.

"It's never too late to be what you might have been"

George Eliot

This quotation had meaning for Richard – it was posted on his study wall.

Richard had two major aims in obstetrics – to avoid unnecessary intervention but to apply urgent skilled intervention when needed and he had a gift for both. He wanted interventions to be based on the best evidence available and for there to be good audit to check that the correct processes were being followed. His experience in Stoke and overseas had given him the skills to achieve these aims. His drive was for simple emergency protocols to save the lives of mothers and babies. This led to his leadership in practice and education in labour ward emergencies.

Initially he organised structured training for life-threatening obstetric emergencies in the West Midlands and in 1997 he and Charles Cox were the inspiration for developing the 'Managing

Obstetric Emergencies and Trauma' (MOET) course, aimed at senior obstetricians and anaesthetists. A modified MOET course was taken overseas where he introduced ideas and protocols with tact and efficiency.

He worked closely with midwives in research and in the implementation of labour ward guidelines. He organised national meetings dealing with childbirth and worked with the National Childbirth Trust and Baby Lifeline, again to promote safer childbirth without over-medicalisation. The foundation of his research charity 'Childbirth without Fear' aims to continue to improve the care of women during childbirth.

Richard will be remembered by many, particularly by his trainees. His boundless enthusiasm and generosity with his time, ideas and academic work meant that there was a queue to work with him. The publication problem would be solved and the trainee would have a nationally respected mentor who continued to take an interest in their career.

Perhaps instinctively feeling that time was precious led him to achieve so much so quickly. Much of it was due to the intellectual sparking between him and his anaesthetist wife, Charlotte. They demonstrated the teamwork that is part of the philosophy of MOET.

"To see a human being reveal really exceptional qualities one must be able to observe his activities over many years. If these activities are completely unselfish; if the idea motivating them is unique in its magnanimity; if it is quite certain that they have never looked for any reward; and if in addition they have left visible traces on the world – then one may say, without fear of error, that one is in the presence of an unforgettable character."

[Jean Giono, from a short story called *The Man Who Planted Trees*]

THE MOET COURSE MANUAL

Managing Obstetric Emergencies and Trauma

Benjamin Black

Second Edition

EDITED BY

Kate Grady

Charlotte Howell

Charles Cox

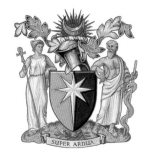

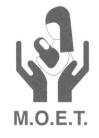

M.O.E.T.

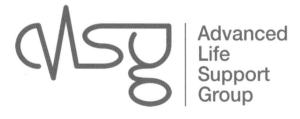

Contents

Working Group

Kathy Boardman,	ALSG, Manchester
Charles Cox,	Obstetrics and Gynaecology, Wolverhampton
Diana Fothergill,	Obstetrics and Gynaecology, Sheffield
Kate Grady,	Anaesthetics, Manchester
Kim Hinshaw,	Obstetrics and Gynaecology, Sunderland
Charlotte Howell,	Anaesthetics, Stoke-on-Trent
Shirin Irani,	Obstetrics and Gynaecology, Birmingham
Geraldine Masson,	Obstetrics, Stoke-on-Trent
Sara Paterson-Brown,	Obstetrics and Gynaecology, London
BGR Prasad,	Anaesthetics, Birmingham
Susan Wieteska,	ALSG, Manchester

About the authors

Contributors to the second edition

Charles Cox	Consultant Obstetrician and Gynaecologist, Wolverhampton
James Drife	Professor of Obstetrics and Gynaecology, Leeds
John Elton	Consultant Anaesthetist, Coventry
Diana Fothergill	Consultant Obstetrician and Gynaecologist, Sheffield
Kavita Goswami	Consultant Obstetrician and Gynaecologist, Coventry
Kate Grady	Consultant Anaesthetist, Manchester
Kim Hinshaw	Consultant Obstetrician and Gynaecologist, Sunderland
Charlotte Howell	Consultant Anaesthetist, Stoke-on-Trent
Shirin Irani	Consultant Obstetrician and Gynaecologist, Birmingham
Geraldine Masson	Consultant Obstetrician, Stoke-on-Trent
Elaine Metcalfe	ALSG, Manchester
Margaret Oates	Consultant Perinatal Psychiatrist, Nottingham
Sara Paterson-Brown	Consultant Obstetrician and Gynaecologist, London
Felicity Plaat	Consultant Anaesthetist, London
Poonam Pradhan	Consultant Obstetrician and Gynaecologist, Birmingham
BGR Prasad	Consultant Anaesthetist, Birmingham
Abdul Sultan	Consultant Obstetrician and Gynaecologist, Croydon
Gargeswari Sunanda	Consultant Obstetrician and Gynaecologist, Birmingham
Ranee Thaker	Consultant Obstetrician and Gynaecologist, Croydon
Derek Tuffnell	Consultant Obstetrician and Gynaecologist, Bradford
Sarah Vause	Consultant Obstetrician and Gynaecologist, Manchester
Steve Walkinshaw	Consultant in Fetomaternal Medicine, Liverpool
Sue Wieteska	ALSG, Manchester
Catherine Wykes	Consultant Obstetrician and Gynaecologist, Brighton

Additional contributors to the first edition

The late Professor Richard Johanson

Nick Coleman	Consultant Anaesthetist, Stoke-on-Trent
Mona Khadra	Specialist Registrar in Obstetrics, Oxford
David Griffiths	Consultant Obstetrician and Gynaecologist, Swindon
Harmini Sidhu	Consultant Obstetrician and Gynaecologist, Craigavon
Peter Young	Consultant Obstetrician and Gynaecologist, Stoke on Trent

Contact details and website information

ALSG: www.alsg.org
BestBETS: www.bestbets.org
For details on ALSG courses visit the Web site or contact:
Advanced Life Support Group
ALSG Centre for Training & Development
29–31 Ellesmere Street
Swinton, Manchester
M27 0LA

Tel: +44 (0) 161 794 1999
Fax: +44 (0) 161 794 9111
Email: enquiries@alsg.org

Updates

The material contained within this book is updated on a 5-yearly cycle following the recommendations of CEMACH. However, practice may change in the interim period. We will post any changes on the ALSG website, so we advise you to visit the website regularly to check for updates (www.alsg.org/updates). The website will provide you with a new page to download and replace the existing page in your book.

Online feedback

It is important to ALSG that the contact with our providers continues after a course is completed. We now contact everyone 6 months after the course has taken place, asking for online feedback. This information is then used whenever the course is updated to ensure that MOET provides optimum training to its participants.

Abbreviations

ABG	arterial blood gas
ACLS	Advanced Cardiac Life Support
AED	automated external defibrillator
AFP	alphafetoprotein
ALS	Advanced Life Support
ALSO	Advanced Life Support in Obstetrics
ALT	alanine aminotranferase
APCR	activated protein C resistance
APLS	Advanced Paediatric Life Support
APTT	activated partial thromboplastin time
ARDS	acute respiratory distress syndrome
ATLS	Advanced Trauma Life Support
BMI	body mass index
BP	blood pressure
CEMACH	Confidential Enquiry into Maternal and Child Health
CEMD	Confidential Enquiry into Maternal Deaths
CNS	central nervous system
CPP	cerebral perfusion pressure
CPR	cardiopulmonary resuscitation
CSF	cerebral spinal fluid
CT	computed tomography
CTG	cardiotocography
CVA	cerebrovascular accident
CVP	central venous pressure
CXR	chest X-ray
DIC	disseminated intravascular coagulation
DVT	deep vein thrombosis
EACA	epsilon-aminocaproic acid
ECG	electrocardiograph
ECMO	extracorporeal membrane oxygenation
EDTA	ethylenediamine tetraacetic acid
EMD	electromechanical dissociation
FAST	focused assessment by sonography for trauma
FBC	full blood count
FDP	fibrin degradation products
FFP	fresh frozen plasma
FHR	fetal heart rate
GTN	glyceryl trinitrate
HDU	high dependency unit

HOCM	hypertrophic obstructive cardiomyopathy
HPA	Health Protection Agency
ICP	intracranial pressure
ICU	intensive care unit
INR	international normalised ratio
IQR	interquartile range
ITU	intensive therapy unit
IV	intravenous
LDH	lactate dehydrogenase
LFTs	liver function tests
LMWH	Low-molecular-weight heparin
LVF	left ventricular function
MAP	mean arterial pressure
$MgSO_4$	magnesium sulphate
MOET	Managing Obstetric Emergencies and Trauma
MRI	magnetic resonance imaging
MSSU	midstream sample of urine
ONS	Office for National Statistics
PE	pulmonary embolus
PEA	pulseless electrical activity
PEEP	positive end expiratory pressure
PIOPED	Prospective Investigation of Pulmonary Embolism Diagnosis study
PV	per vaginum
RCOG	Royal College of Obstetricians and Gynaecologists
SAG-M	saline-adenine-glucose-mannitol
U&E	urea and electrolytes
UKOSS	UK Obstetric Surveillance System
UTI	urinary tract infection
VF	ventricular fibrillation
VT	ventricular tachycardia
VTE	venous thromboembolism

Preface to the second edition

The Managing Obstetric Emergencies and Trauma (MOET) courses have been running now for 9 years and, in that time, the growth and the increase in strength of the organisation has been dramatic. The course has developed nationally and internationally. At the time of this manual going to press, within the UK, there are now 14 centres and approximately 25 courses are run each year. MOET is fully established in the Netherlands, where six courses are run annually and full courses have been taken to Eire, Barbados and Abu Dhabi. 'MOET-like' courses have been taken to Armenia, Bangladesh, Russia, Estonia and, with the support of the British Military and the Leonard Cheshire Centre for Conflict Recovery, three times to Iraq. It is estimated that some 1000 doctors have been 'MOET trained', worldwide. MOET has formed the basis of the Emergencies in Maternal and Child Health course, which is being exported to other developing nations.

The second edition of the MOET manual closely follows the findings and recommendations of the Confidential Enquiry into Maternal and Child Health (CEMACH) 2000–2002. We are delighted to have the contribution and insight of Professor James Drife. The manual has been reworked to include a new chapter on caesarean section, the most common obstetric emergency. Other chapters have been revised and updated. Chapters on cardiac disease and mental illness have been introduced, as these health problems have been identified as being significant contributors to maternal mortality by CEMACH. Two important topics (consent and perineal trauma) are included in an appendix, as they will not be formally taught during the course but form a source of reference.

The need for MOET continues and has been emphasised by Clinical Negligence Scheme for Trusts' emergency obstetric training requirements. It has become recognised as a desirable postgraduate training acquisition.

As MOET has developed, attention has been given to the quality of the learning provision and instructors are now all formally trained in teaching and educational methods through the Generic Instructor Course of the Advanced Life Support Group. A cohort of MOET instructors teach on this course.

This, the second edition of the MOET manual has been followed by a revision of the MOET course material and the introduction of competency-based assessment to the courses.

To ensure that the reader is able to update this book with any evidence-based changes to practice as they evolve, new pages will be available to download from the ALSG website and inserted in the current text.

The official nonproprietary names of some medicines changed during 2005; international nonproprietary names are used in this text. Readers should note that, as adrenaline and nor-adrenaline are the names established in the European Pharmacopoeia and are recommended within the European states, these names are used in this text. The international name will appear in parentheses.

Since its inception, a large number of experts have contributed to the development of MOET and we extend our thanks both to them and to those instructors who have provide helpful feedback.

Kate Grady
Charlotte Howell
Charles Cox

Preface to the first edition

This book is the core text for the Managing Obstetric Emergencies and Trauma (MOET) course. It is also useful as a stand-alone text.

Obstetricians should be able to advise on and be prepared to be involved with the care of all pregnant women, including those who have suffered trauma, either accidental or deliberate.

In the good (bad) old days trainee obstetricians were likely to have been exposed to a range of emergencies through working in accident and emergency, surgery and even anaesthetics. Those days are long gone!

Wide experience in a variety of specialties now invites the accusation of 'lack of focus' and indecisiveness.

It is unrealistic to expect trainees to have recent first-hand experience of uncommon emergencies such as cardiac arrest or trauma and even in their own specialty it is unlikely that they will have personally managed all of the major obstetric emergencies, despite the requirement to complete a logbook of experience.

Other disciplines have recognised that one way to achieve confidence and competence in dealing with the less common life-threatening emergencies is to run 'skills and drills' courses. Perhaps the most well known of these courses is the Advanced Trauma Life Support (ATLS) course, sponsored by the American College of Surgeons.

It is worth remembering how this course came into being. In February 1976, a Nebraskan orthopaedic surgeon crashed in his plane, with his wife and four children aboard. His wife was killed, three children sustained critical injuries, the other child had minor injuries and he sustained serious injuries. The care he received at the primary healthcare centre led him to state 'When I can provide better care in the field with limited resources than what my children and I received at the primary care facility, there is something wrong with the system and the system has to be changed'.

From this tragedy developed Advanced Trauma Life Support, which was intended for all medical practitioners to enable them to supply supportive treatment for the first hour after injury – 'the golden hour'.

In the United Kingdom, the Military introduced a course called Battlefield Advanced Trauma Life Support BATLS in advance of The College of Surgeons of England introducing ATLS to this country.

These principles of trauma life support included in BATLS are now taught to all members of the Defence Medical Services including doctors, nurses, veterinary surgeons, physiotherapists and combat medical technicians.

Charles Cox teaches on these courses, Kate Grady directs ATLS courses and instructs on the instructor course, while Richard Johanson and Charlotte Howell have run courses on the management of obstetric emergencies for a number of years.

It was suggested that a course merging the broader concepts of advanced life support and managing obstetric emergencies should be developed as part of Calman implementation for obstetricians. So the Managing Obstetric Emergencies and Trauma courses came to be. The course is interactive and aims to consolidate and share old knowledge and hopefully gain new insights from one's colleagues and very occasionally from the instructors!

Early on in the development of MOET, there was interaction with those leading the Advanced Life Support in Obstetrics (ALSO) programme. From the curricula and experiences of trainees, these two courses complement each other. MOET is aimed at the senior trainee and established specialist.

The anaesthetist, as a universal emergency person, is part of every emergency medical drill team known to hospital practice and outside. The concept of 'skills and drills' courses is not unfamiliar to the anaesthetist. Advanced Life Support courses (ALS — cardiopulmonary resuscitation) are 'core' in many region's training and anaesthetists train as ATLS, APLS (Advanced Paediatric Life Support) and ALSO or MOET providers at their own choice according to their subspecialty interests. Anaesthetists are aware of the universal demand for their resuscitation skills but equally aware that supportive resuscitation measures must be backed by definitive treatment of a medical and, more frequently in an emergency setting, a surgical nature. They are aware, from their day-to-day practice, their experience of medical emergencies and their experience of drill-style courses, that they are part of a team and that the team requires surgical input. It is a principle of 'skills and drills' courses that every team member, regardless of specialty, should be able to provide immediate life support, to a life-saving level, and that every team member recognises the role of the specialist and when the specialist skills are required.

The realisation that life threats to the heavily pregnant patient, both obstetric and non-obstetric, require specific management has attracted anaesthetists to ALSO and MOET courses. With this in mind, MOET has developed an anaesthetic slant to its course and guarantees that a proportion of the faculty on each course will be anaesthetists.

Alongside this natural development of the team, an unsolicited interest has developed among accident and emergency doctors, who are most welcome to our organisation as they are likely to be the first to see obstetric patients who have suffered major trauma and cardiorespiratory arrest outside hospital.

The course comprises a first day devoted to basic trauma life support and basic cardiopulmonary life support (CPR). This includes what the self-respecting first-aider should be able to achieve and should be immediately familiar to devotees of *ER* and *Casualty!* This part of the course is didactic and teaches an approach that is familiar to the emergency services around the world and may come in useful at rugby matches, equestrian events, on aeroplanes and by the side of the road. The philosophy is to develop an approach to the ill or traumatised patient that will carry over to the assessment and management of the pregnant patient.

The second day is not so didactic and deals with emergency obstetric conditions, both common and not so common, including conditions unfamiliar in countries with developed health systems.

The course is supported by midwife 'observers' who attend lectures and undertake skills training alongside their medical colleagues. Their presence and input is valued, not least for the emphasis towards a team approach. The course has been successfully evaluated. Further follow-up studies are being undertaken. Modified versions of MOET have been run in Bangladesh and Armenia under the auspices of UNICEF and the Family Care charity, and in Russia and Estonia.

Richard Johanson
Charlotte Howell
Charles Cox
Kate Grady

Acknowledgements

A great many people have put a lot of hard work into the production of this book and the accompanying course. The editors would like to thank all the contributors for their efforts and all the MOET providers and instructors who took the time to send their comments during the development of the text and the course.

We would also like to thank the Advanced Life Support Group (ALSG), who gave permission for the reproduction of some of the material used in this text in particular from the books *Advanced Paediatric Life Support: The Practical Approach* (Blackwell Publishing), *Safe Transfer and Retrieval: The Practical Approach* (Blackwell Publishing) and *Major Incident Medical Management and Support: The Practical Approach in the Hospital* (Blackwell Publishing). We would also like to thank Bios Scientific Publishers for permission to reproduce material from the book *Managing Obstetric Emergencies*.

Chapter 21 Shoulder Dystocia was derived from the chapter on shoulder dystocia written by Onsy Louca and Richard Johanson for the *Yearbook of Obstetrics and Gynaecology* Volume 6. We acknowledge comments from Barbara Franks.

The chapters on resuscitation have been informed by the new international guidelines produced by an evidence-based process from the collaboration of many international experts under the umbrella of the International Liaison Committee on Resuscitation (ILCOR).

We acknowledge and sincerely thank Elaine Metcalfe for her hard work in the preparation of the manuscript. Our grateful appreciation goes to Jane Moody at the Royal College of Obstetrics and Gynaecology Publishing.

We would like to thank Helen Carruthers and Kate Wieteska for their work on many of the line drawings within the text.

We would like to thank and acknowledge Celia Kendrick and Neil Hipkiss for their advice on log-rolling technique included in the appendix and Paul Wade from the Jehovah's Witness group for his advice and provision of information.

Finally, we would like to thank, in advance, those of you who will attend the Managing Obstetric Emergencies and Trauma (MOET) course; no doubt you will have much constructive critique to offer.

Foreword

**"If only I had done...
if only I had taught her how to...
if only I had used him...
if only I had listened...
if only I had attended...
if only I had seen it once before...
if only..."**

All of us who have been present either by accident or design at the birth of a baby are aware that there is nothing as normal in the world as normal child birth and there is nothing as abnormal as abnormal child birth – and nothing that goes devastatingly so fast from one to the other.

Real, instant first aid, properly instituted, can really save lives. Worldwide, we need an army of healthcare workers with the skills to deal with these emergencies when they arrive. It may be that many of the skills required and acquired may never be needed but wouldn't it be great if they were and that they came to us as second nature?

All those who want to live with their conscience must consolidate their knowledge, achieve understanding and regularly practise their skills and drills, so that life saving skills are second nature, even first time round. The MOET (Managing Obstetric Emergency Trauma) course provides that knowledge and understanding so that, at its conclusion, the participants know what they are doing, why they are doing it and what are the likely outcomes.

There are many life saving skills courses available. Each has its own area of maximum affect. MOET can take those workers whose participants supply a comprehensive obstetric care in their own setting and elevate them to new heights and so to brand them as leaders and motivators.

How much better to feel the glow of contentment that you have done your best, rather than inwardly suffer the 'if only'.

Professor Jim Dornan FRCOG
Senior Vice President, Royal College of Obstetricians and Gynaecologists

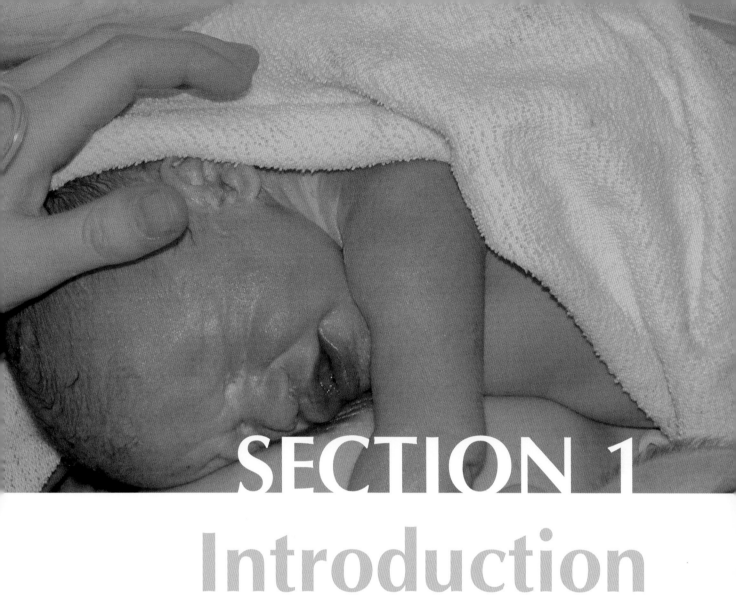

SECTION 1
Introduction

Chapter 1

Introduction

Throughout both the developed and the developing world, maternal mortality continues to present a serious challenge. Globally, there is estimated to be one maternal death every minute. This course will provide you with a system for managing the seriously ill and seriously injured. The system is designed to be simple and easy to remember when life-threatening emergencies arise. The system is known as the structured approach. The structured approach is the ABC of resuscitation and is practised throughout all walks of medicine and the emergency services. It is familiar to the lay person and known even to schoolchildren. The structured approach has led to the development of courses that attend to the needs of all patients, from neonates to children, adults and now for those with the altered physiology and anatomy of pregnancy.

This course (and the manual) is divided into sections that provide a structured revision in resuscitation, trauma, life support and obstetric emergencies for obstetricians, anaesthetists, emergency physicians and midwives. The structured approach is applied to resuscitation and is taught didactically as a drill. Subsequently, what has been learned is applied to the seriously ill and injured patient. The management of the seriously injured patient follows the same principles as the management of a seriously ill patient. The seriously injured patient is a good model to teach these principles – providing hooks to which the practice can be applied.

Trauma management is not widely taught to obstetricians but trauma happens to their patients and those in other specialties will consider them the experts.

The physiological adjustments of pregnancy affect the response of the mother to illness and injury. These changes mean that resuscitation should be tailored to the pregnant patient. This course teaches the application of resuscitation and trauma management to pregnancy.

The third section allows sound principles as learned in the foregoing two sections to be applied to life-threatening problems in obstetrics. This allows the doctor caring for the pregnant patient to practise the management of both common and rare emergencies until confidence has been achieved.

Chapter 2

Why mothers die

Introduction

Much of the wisdom in this book has been learned the hard way, some of it in the hardest way of all. When a woman dies as a result of an obstetric complication, the only good thing that can come out of the tragedy is that appropriate lessons are learned. For over 50 years, England and Wales have had a system in place to analyse all maternal deaths, identify the causes and highlight avoidable factors.

The Confidential Enquiries into Maternal Deaths (CEMD) have become so familiar to UK obstetricians and midwives that we can hardly imagine life without them. The UK, however, is one of only a few countries with a national system in which experienced clinicians scrutinise cases in detail to work out how death could be prevented when a similar emergency happens again.

CEMD recommendations carry considerable weight at both political and clinical levels. This chapter will describe the system that produces these recommendations and will then focus on lessons relevant to emergencies and trauma – including those learned in the early years of the Enquiry, which are all too easily forgotten.

How the Enquiries work

The CEMD for England and Wales began collecting data in 1952 and has published reports every 3 years since 1957. Similar enquiries began in Northern Ireland in 1956 and in Scotland in 1965. Since 1985, the CEMD has covered the whole of the UK and in 2003 it became part of the Confidential Enquiry into Maternal and Child Health (CEMACH).

From the outset, confidentiality was recognised to be essential if staff were to give an honest account of events without fear of litigation or disciplinary action. In this and in other essentials, the approach initiated in the 1950s is still used today. The process summarised here applies to England but is similar in the other UK countries.

Regional reporting

When a maternal death occurs, a form is sent to all the professionals involved to obtain factual information and reflective comments. This is now coordinated by the CEMACH Regional Manager, who anonymises the completed form. The anonymised form is reviewed by Regional Assessors in obstetrics, midwifery, anaesthetics and pathology, who add further comments. Regional Assessors are senior clinicians who have the respect of local clinical colleagues.

Central assessment

The form is sent to a named doctor at the Department of Health (since 1995, Dr Gwyneth Lewis), who keeps it under lock and key. All cases (still anonymised) are reviewed by Central Assessors, who are senior clinicians in the above disciplines and in medicine, intensive care and psychiatry. They look for emerging patterns and lessons for clinical colleagues, managers and politicians.

Public health messages are particularly important and denominator data are obtained from the Office for National Statistics (ONS).

The triennial reports

Chapters are drafted by the Central Assessors of the four countries and discussed by the whole editorial panel, which includes epidemiologists. Individual chapters may be reviewed by outside experts. Once the final manuscript of the report is sent to the printers, the individual forms are destroyed. The published report is put on sale to the public, a fact that surprises doctors in countries which have a less open approach.

A challenge for any report is to ensure that people read it. The last three CEMD reports have been called *Why Mothers Die*, given an emotive cover picture and launched with a press conference. They are bestsellers in the Royal College of Obstetricians and Gynaecologists (RCOG) bookshop, partly because examination candidates know that they are essential reading. Their messages also need to be heard by other specialties, however, and this is more difficult to achieve.

Lessons from the past

Effective intervention

Before the CEMD started, maternal mortality had fallen dramatically in the UK, from 400/100 000 in 1935 to 66/100 000 in 1952–55. It dropped rapidly during the Second World War, contradicting the idea that social conditions are the major factor determining the safety of pregnancy. The reasons for the fall were the introduction of effective treatments as follows:

- Antibiotics: puerperal sepsis was the leading cause of maternal death in the 1930s, despite the widespread use of asepsis. When sulphonamides were introduced in 1937 the effect on death rates was spectacular.

- Blood transfusion became safe during the 1940s.

- Ergometrine, for the treatment and prevention of postpartum haemorrhage, was introduced in the 1940s.

In the 1930s, Britain had a well-developed medical infrastructure, so that when effective treatment became available its effects were rapidly felt.

Obstetric injury

In the first CEMD report, covering 1952–54, obstetric injury was the second cause of death after hypertensive disease (Table 2.1). It did not, however, warrant its own chapter and Table 2.1 is drawn from the Appendix to the report.

Nowadays we can hardly imagine a woman dying of prolonged labour and we can only guess at what the terms 'other trauma' and 'other complications' conceal (Table 2.1). In the 1950s, the caesarean section rate was less than 3% and maternity care was very different from that of today. The 1955–57 report included 33 deaths from ruptured uterus, mostly due to intrauterine manipulations. In 1958–60, there were 43 deaths from obstructed labour, 'of whom 18 were delivered in the patient's own home and 14 in a general practitioner Maternity Home'. These reports are a useful corrective to the idea that the 1950s were a golden age of non-medicalised childbirth.

Table 2.1. Number of obstetric deaths from obstetric injury, 1952–54

Cause	Deaths (n)
Prolonged labour	63
Disproportion or malposition of the fetus	23
Other trauma	55
Other complications of childbirth	66
Total	197

Obstetric injury today

In 2000–02, there was one death from genital tract trauma, which was due to a uterine tear. The improvement is due to high standards of obstetric practice and to caesarean section becoming a safer option. There is a downside, however: such cases are now rare and therefore consultants have limited experience of dealing with them. This should be recognised by the increased use of practice drills and by a greater readiness to call for help from colleagues when problems arise.

Recent lessons

Who is at risk?

Using ONS denominator data, the CEMD identifies social as well as medical factors.

Age

There is a five-fold increase in maternal mortality between the ages of 20 years and 40 years. The average age at childbearing in the UK has risen and 18% of pregnant women are now aged 35 years or over.

Obesity

In the 2000-02 CEMD report, 35% of the women were obese, with a body mass index (BMI) of 30 or more.

Social class

In 1999–2001, the maternal mortality rate among social class 9 – the unemployed and socially excluded – was over 135/100 000, compared with under 3/100 000 in social class 1. Attention should be focused on women who book late or are poor attenders for antenatal care, particularly travellers and asylum seekers.

Ethnicity

Black women have higher maternal mortality rates than white women in all countries for which data are available. In the UK, ethnic minority women have three times the risk of white women and for black African women the risk is increased seven-fold. The figures raise disturbing questions about communication between ethnic minority women and the maternity services (Table 2.2).

Table 2.2. Maternal mortality rates by ethnic group, UK 2000–02

Ethnic group	Deaths (*n*)	Rate/100 000	Relative risk
Black African	30	72.1	6.7
Black Caribbean	13	25.8	2.4
Pakistani	10	12.3	1.2
Indian	7	15.5	1.4
Bangladeshi	8	22.5	2.1
Asian and others	4	5.7	0.5
Total non-white	72	31.0	2.9
White	151	10.7	1.0

Direct deaths

Hypertensive disease

Deaths from pre-eclampsia and eclampsia have fallen steadily to only 14 in 2000–02, the lowest-ever total and a far cry from the 246 deaths in 1952–54 (Table 2.3). Nevertheless, in seven of these 14 cases there was substandard care, such as unnecessary delay in delivery and inappropriate fluid management.

The main recommendations of the 2000–02 report for hypertensive patients were that:

▓ clear protocols are essential to guide treatment of hypertensive disease in hospital

▓ high systolic blood pressure must be treated. Nine of the 14 deaths in 2000–02 were due to intracranial haemorrhage

▓ in severe cases there is a need for early involvement of consultant obstetricians and intensive care specialists.

Previous reports highlighted fluid balance problems (death was often caused by pulmonary oedema) and the need to warn women to report symptoms such as headache and abdominal pain.

Table 2.3. The changes in direct deaths reported to the CEMD

Cause	1952–54 (England & Wales)	2000–02 (UK)
Hypertensive disease	246	14
Obstetric injury	197	1
Haemorrhage	188	17
Abortion	153	4
Thromboembolism	138	30
Anaesthesia	49	6
Sepsis	42	13

Haemorrhage

Deaths from haemorrhage increased sharply from seven in 1997–99 to 22 in 2000–02. Some occurred because women failed to seek care or refused blood. The 2000–02 report included guidelines for the management of women who decline blood transfusion.

The report also commented that 'Recent changes in medical training may be relevant to the increased numbers of deaths from haemorrhage'. Reduction in the duration of training and increasing subspecialisation may mean that obstetricians now have reduced surgical skills. This further underlines the need for regular 'skills drills'.

Deaths from haemorrhage seem to rise and fall with peaks and troughs occurring at approximately 15-year intervals (Table 2.4).

This apparently regular pattern may be due to chance but it may represent relaxation and tightening of standards. For example, the peak in 1988–90 (Table 2.4) included cases in which doctors had ignored the recommendation that caesarean section for placenta praevia should be carried out by a consultant.

Thromboembolism

Thromboembolism is still the leading direct cause in the UK but there are grounds for optimism. Deaths have almost halved since 1994–96, despite increases in risk factors such as maternal age and obesity and a rising caesarean section rate. The keys to further reduction are:

- All women should be assessed early in pregnancy for risk factors for venous thromboembolism (VTE).
- Women with a past history of VTE should be tested from thrombophilia to guide thromboprophylaxis.
- Acute symptoms suggestive of VTE in women who are at risk are an emergency and treatment should precede confirmation of the diagnosis.

RCOG guidelines on thromboprophylaxis should be followed. These have been updated and now apply to all women, not just those undergoing caesarean section.

Unfortunately, women still die after presenting to a general practitioner, casualty officer or physician with classic symptoms that are not taken seriously enough, despite obvious risk factors in some cases. Lessons from the CEMD need to get across to other specialties.

Table 2.4. Deaths from haemorrhage reported in CEMD reports, 1976–78 to 2000–02

Year	Deaths from haemorrhage (*n*)
1976–78	24
1979–81	14
1982–84	9
1985–97	10
1988–90	22
1991–93	15
1994–96	12
1997–99	7
2000–02	22

Ectopic pregnancy

The same applies to ectopic pregnancy, which shows no sign of a reduction in numbers of deaths. Atypical presentation is common and the CEMD has drawn attention to gastrointestinal symptoms, which may mimic food poisoning. The 2000–02 report recommended that all pregnant women presenting with abdominal pain to accident and emergency departments should be reviewed by staff from the obstetrics and gynaecology department.

Abortion

The Abortion Act of 1967 eliminated deaths from criminal abortion, which in the 1950s caused about 30 deaths a year but, in 2000–02, five deaths followed legal abortion. Delay was a major factor, including one case where termination was urgently needed because of serious cardiac disease. RCOG guidelines state that no woman should wait more than 3 weeks from referral to termination.

Amnniotic fluid embolism

The number of deaths from amniotic fluid embolism has fallen during the last 40 years but we do not know why. In an attempt to gain more information about effective treatment, a register of non-fatal cases is maintained and the 2000–02 report asks clinicians to report all cases, whether fatal or not, to UK Obstetric Surveillance System (UKOSS) at the National Perinatal Epidemiology Unit in Oxford.

Sepsis

In 1982–84, there was not a single death from puerperal sepsis but unfortunately the streptococcus has reappeared and in 2000–02 sepsis caused 13 deaths, two of which occurred after home delivery. Because puerperal sepsis is now rare, midwives and doctors may not recognise the seriousness of its early signs until the woman is gravely ill.

Other direct deaths

An emerging concern is bowel perforation after caesarean section, which caused four direct deaths and one late death in 2000–02. Postoperative care on postnatal wards is often lax, with midwives who lack surgical training and inadequate involvement of consultant obstetricians.

Anaesthesia

Deaths from anaesthesia fell from 10/year to 15/year in the 1970s to a single death in 1994–96. This improvement, in the face of a rising caesarean section rate, was due to a move to regional anaesthesia and better training of anaesthetists. Unfortunately, deaths rose again to six in 2000–02, all of them associated with general anaesthesia. There is now concern over the lack of experience of some anaesthetists when general anaesthesia is required.

Indirect deaths

Indirect deaths now outnumber direct deaths in the UK (Table 2.5). This is only partly due to improved ascertainment.

Cardiac disease

Cardiac disease is now the leading cause of maternal death in the UK, with 44 cases in 2000–02. Women with congenital heart disease are surviving and embarking on pregnancy in spite of the risks. Most of the deaths are from acquired disease and the recent sharp rise is related mainly to myocardial infarction and cardiomyopathy.

Table 2.5. The rise in indirect deaths: maternal deaths notified to the CEMD 1991–2002

	1991–93	**1994–96** (+linkage*)	**1997–99** (+ linkage*)	**2000–02** (CEMACH**)
Direct	129	134	106	106
Indirect	100	134	136	155
Total	229	268	242	261

* 'Linkage' refers to the linking by ONS of birth and death registrations, which led to improved ascertainment;

** 'CEMACH' refers to the involvement of CEMACH Regional Managers in collecting data; this has also improved ascertainment

Psychiatric disease

Most psychiatric deaths occur after pregnancy. If late deaths are included, psychiatric disease becomes the leading cause of pregnancy-associated death. Unlike most causes, it shows no social class gradient. Suicide is usually by violent means, such as hanging or jumping from a height. Awareness of the early signs of disease can prevent these tragedies. Skilled help in mother and baby units is essential.

Other indirect deaths

Of the many causes of indirect death, the leading category is central nervous system disease, including 13 deaths from epilepsy. Medical diseases in pregnancy may be inadequately supervised because responsibility falls between the obstetrician, midwife, GP and physician. Good communication is essential.

Coincidental deaths

The most common cause of coincidental death is not road traffic accidents but murder. Eleven women were killed in 2000–02, in each case by her male partner. The Enquiries are encouraging maternity hospitals to develop ways of offering help to women affected by domestic violence.

Substandard care

Standards are rising all the time and the proportion of cases with substandard care tends to remain the same from one report to another. In 2000–02, care was substandard in 67% of direct and 36% of indirect deaths. Aspects highlighted were:

- failure of obstetric and midwifery staff to recognise medical conditions outside their immediate experience
- failure of accident and emergency staff to ask for obstetric or midwifery assessment
- failure of GPs and other medical specialists to pass information to maternity staff.

The underlying message is that communication between specialties must be improved.

The international dimension

The World Health Organization has calculated that, across the world, there are over 600 000 maternal deaths annually, most of which occur in developing countries. The leading causes are shown in Table 2.6.

Table 2.6. Estimated numbers of maternal deaths worldwide (Source: WHO)

Causes of maternal death	Estimated deaths worldwide/year	
	(n)	*(%)*
Haemorrhage	132 000	28
Sepsis	79 000	16
Unsafe abortion	69 000	15
Pre-eclampsia/Eclampsia	63 000	13
Obstructed labour	42 000	9

The underlying problems include lack of access to contraception, lack of primary care or transport facilities and inadequate equipment and staffing in district hospitals. Only 55% of deliveries in the developing world have a trained attendant and only 37% occur within health facilities.

The CEMD Director and Assessors are assisting increasing numbers of countries in setting up confidential enquiries adapted from the UK model. Examples include the *Saving Mothers* reports in South Africa and initiatives in former Soviet countries of Eastern Europe and Central Asia.

Summary

The common assumption that safe childbirth is a side effect of national prosperity is incorrect. Complications such as haemorrhage, pre-eclampsia or malpresentation cannot be prevented but they can be treated promptly and effectively. It is often forgotten that women's lives are routinely saved on a daily basis throughout the UK. When a death does occur, the public expects exhaustive analysis. This may reinforce old lessons but, often, new lessons emerge. One conclusion is clear from reviewing CEMD reports over the years: when vigilance is relaxed, people die.

Chapter 3

Structured approach to emergencies in the obstetric patient

Objectives

On successfully completing this topic, you will be able to:

■ identify the correct sequence to be followed in assessing and managing seriously ill or seriously injured patients

■ understand the concept of primary and secondary survey.

The structured approach refers to the ABCDE approach to lifesaving. The aim of the structured approach is to provide a system of assessment and management that is effective and simple to remember in the heat of an emergency. It can be applied to any patient with threat to life, be that from illness or injury. Assessment is divided into primary survey and secondary survey.

The approach is the same for all: adults, children, elderly, pregnant women

Primary survey

The system follows a simple 'ABC' approach, with resuscitation taking place as problems are identified i.e. a process of simultaneous evaluation and resuscitation.

A B C D E

Airway (with cervical spine control if appropriate)

Manoeuvres to secure the patient's airway should not cause harm or further harm to the cervical spine. Therefore, if an injury to the cervical spine is suspected, in caring for the airway, the cervical spine must be immobilised.

Breathing and ventilation

Circulation with volume replacement and haemorrhage control

Disability or neurological status

Exposure and environmental control (adequately expose the patient to make a full assessment, taking care to avoid cooling and potential hypothermia)

The primary survey uncovers immediately life-threatening problems by priority, i.e. in the order in which they will most quickly kill.

The medical logic in the ABC approach is that an Airway problem will kill the patient more quickly than a Breathing (ventilation) problem, which in turn will kill a patient more quickly than a Circulation (bleeding) problem, which in turn will kill a patient more quickly than a Disability (neurological) problem.

Resuscitation

- The resuscitation phase is carried out at the same time as the primary survey.

- Life-threatening conditions are managed as they are identified. Do not move on to the next stage of the primary survey until a problem found has been corrected.

- If a patient's condition seems unsatisfactory, go back and reassess, starting again with ABC.

Secondary survey

The secondary survey is a comprehensive assessment, which takes place after life-threatening problems have been found and treated (primary survey) and uncovers problems that are not as immediately threatening.

The secondary survey is performed once the patient is stable. The secondary survey might not take place until after surgery, if surgery has been necessary as part of the resuscitation phase.

This is a top-to-toe process, as follows:

- scalp and vault of skull

- face and base of skull

- neck and cervical spine

- chest

- abdomen

- pelvis

- remainder of spine and limbs

- neurological examination

- rectal and vaginal examinations, if indicated

- examination of holes caused by injury.

If the Glasgow Coma Score has not been evaluated in the primary survey it should be done during the secondary survey (see Chapter 12).

Management of collapsed person using ABC approach

First, speak loudly to the patient: "Hello, how are you Mrs Tilt?"

The response gives you several pieces of clinical information. To be able to respond verbally, the patient must:

- have circulating oxygenated blood (i.e. has not had a cardiopulmonary arrest)

- have a reasonably patent airway

- have a reasonable tidal volume to phonate

- have reasonable cerebral perfusion to comprehend and answer.

Management of the apparently lifeless person

The approach to an apparently lifeless person is the cardiopulmonary resuscitation (CPR) drill, which starts with a swift assessment of airway and breathing, to define whether there is a cardiac output (circulation), and action as necessary (Chapter 4).

Management of the seriously injured person

In the seriously injured person who has signs of life, the following approach is taken.

Seek as much history as possible (from person and/or witnesses), including:

- history of the acute illness
- mechanism, speed, height of fall if injury
- pre-existing medical problems, medications
- details of pregnancy where appropriate.

Consider their management in three phases:

1. Primary survey and resuscitation: identify life-threatening problems and deal with these problems as they are identified.

2. Secondary survey: top to toe, back to front examination.

3. Definitive care: specific management.

Management of the pregnant woman

In the pregnant woman, the sequence should be as follows:

1. Primary survey and resuscitation: identify life-threatening problems and deal with these problems as they are identified.

2. Assess fetal wellbeing and viability: may require delivery.

3. Secondary survey: top to toe, back to front examination.

4. Definitive care: specific management.

Continuous re-evaluation is very important to identify new life-threatening problems as they arise.

Monitoring (applied during primary survey)

- Pulse oximetry: use to detect inadequate SaO_2 (saturation of haemoglobin with oxygen) secondary to airway, breathing or circulation problems. It works on the principle of differential absorption of light of a particular wavelength by oxygenated and deoxygenated haemoglobin. Depending upon the absorption levels, a ratio of oxygenated to deoxygenated blood is determined. The pulse oximeter's limitations are that the patient must be well perfused to get a reading and ambient light and dyes such as nail polish or methaemoglobin in the blood cause erroneous readings. A fall in oxygen saturation is a late sign of an airway, breathing or even a circulation problem.

- Heart rate/ECG.

- Blood pressure: non-invasive or invasive.

- Respiratory rate.

- F_ECO_2: (end tidal CO_2) monitoring may be appropriate in an intubated patient.

- Urine output: as a measure of adequate perfusion and fluid resuscitation.

- Fetal heart monitoring where appropriate.

Assess fetal wellbeing and viability

▓ Ultrasound: use ultrasound to:

☐ detect fetal heart and check rate

☐ ascertain the number of babies and their positions

☐ locate the position of the placenta and the amount of liquor

☐ look for retroplacental bleeding and haematoma

☐ detect an abnormal position of the fetus and free fluid in the abdominal cavity suggesting rupture of the uterus

☐ detect damage to other structures

☐ check for free fluid and blood in the abdominal cavity.

Adequately resuscitating the mother will improve the outcome for the baby.

Adjuncts to assessment

▓ Urinary catheter.

▓ Nasogastric tube: contraindicated if there is a suspected fracture of the base of the skull.

▓ Essential X-rays during the primary survey and resuscitation are chest, pelvis and lateral cervical spine. Other X-rays are taken if they are a guide to the assessment and management of life-threatening injuries, such as major long-bone fractures.

Definitive care

Definitive care takes place under the supervision of relevant specialists. It is of utmost importance to the patient's continued quality of life.

The mismanaged minor injury may be the only residual effect of a life-threatening series of injuries but it is that with which the patient has to live for the rest of her life.

Summary

Primary survey	Identify life-threatening problems (A B C D E)
	▓ **A**irway with cervical spine control
	▓ **B**reathing and ventilation
	▓ **C**irculation with volume replacement and haemorrhage control
	▓ **D**isability or neurological status
	▓ **E**xposure and environmental control
Resuscitation	Deal with these problems as you find them
Assess fetal wellbeing and viability	May require delivery
Secondary survey	Top-to-toe, back-to-front examination
Definitive care	Specific management

Continuous re-evaluation

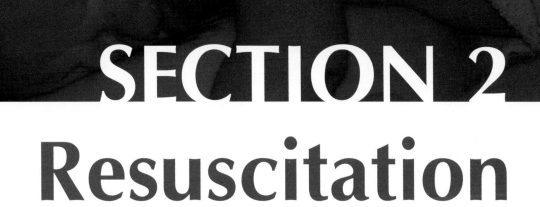

SECTION 2
Resuscitation

Algorithm 4.1 **Basic life support: pregnant patient**

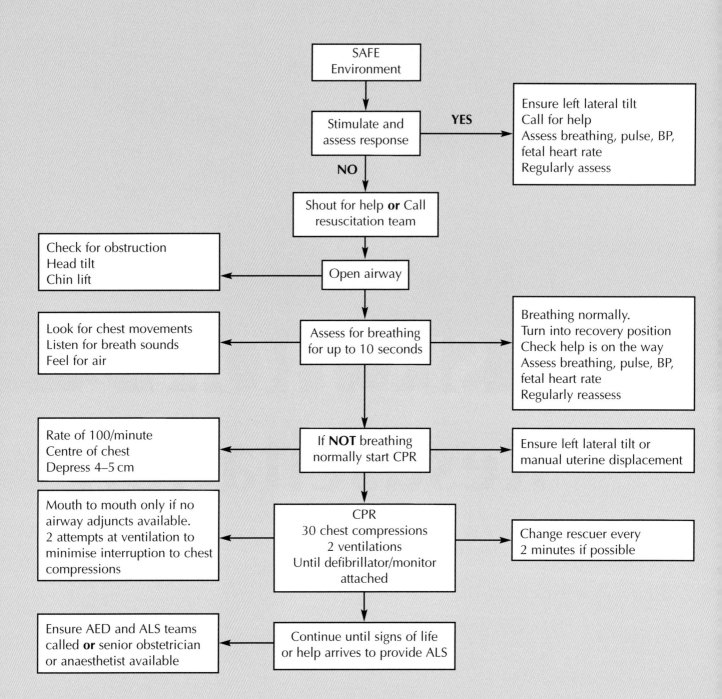

SAFE Environment

→ **Stimulate and assess response**

YES → Ensure left lateral tilt
Call for help
Assess breathing, pulse, BP, fetal heart rate
Regularly assess

NO ↓

Shout for help or Call resuscitation team

↓

Check for obstruction
Head tilt
Chin lift
← **Open airway**

↓

Look for chest movements
Listen for breath sounds
Feel for air
← **Assess for breathing for up to 10 seconds** →
Breathing normally.
Turn into recovery position
Check help is on the way
Assess breathing, pulse, BP, fetal heart rate
Regularly reassess

↓

Rate of 100/minute
Centre of chest
Depress 4–5 cm
← **If NOT breathing normally start CPR** →
Ensure left lateral tilt or manual uterine displacement

↓

Mouth to mouth only if no airway adjuncts available.
2 attempts at ventilation to minimise interruption to chest compressions
← **CPR**
30 chest compressions
2 ventilations
Until defibrillator/monitor attached
→ Change rescuer every 2 minutes if possible

↓

Ensure AED and ALS teams called **or** senior obstetrician or anaesthetist available
← **Continue until signs of life or help arrives to provide ALS**

Algorithm 4.2 **Automated external defibrilator (AED)**

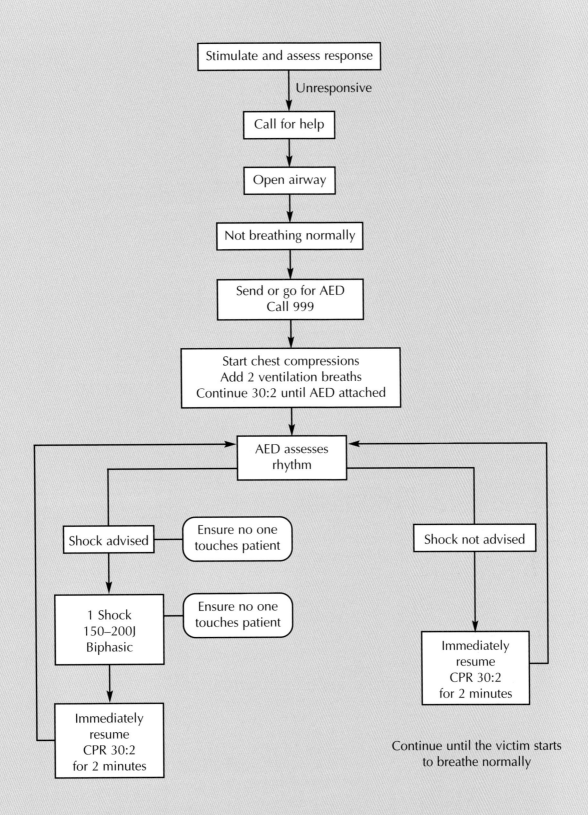

Stimulate and assess response

Unresponsive

Call for help

Open airway

Not breathing normally

Send or go for AED
Call 999

Start chest compressions
Add 2 ventilation breaths
Continue 30:2 until AED attached

AED assesses rhythm

Shock advised

Ensure no one touches patient

Shock not advised

1 Shock
150–200J
Biphasic

Ensure no one touches patient

Immediately resume
CPR 30:2
for 2 minutes

Immediately resume
CPR 30:2
for 2 minutes

Continue until the victim starts to breathe normally

Algorithm 4.3 **Advanced life support (ALS)**

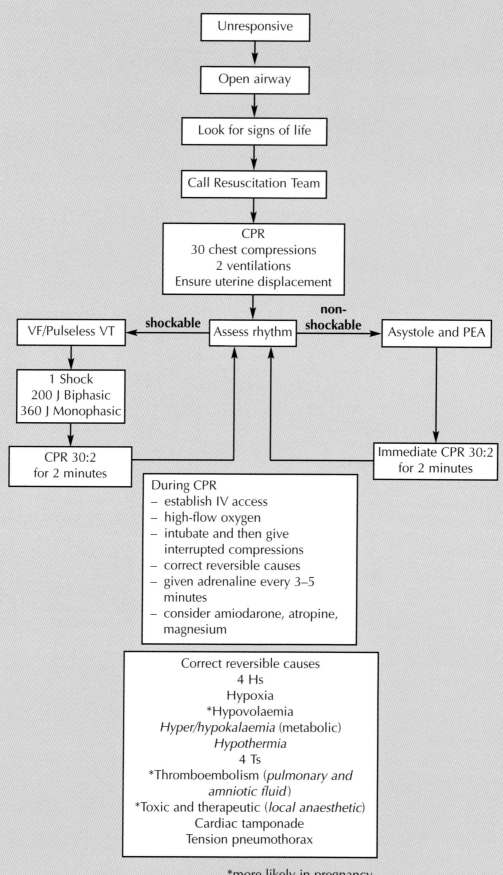

Unresponsive

Open airway

Look for signs of life

Call Resuscitation Team

CPR
30 chest compressions
2 ventilations
Ensure uterine displacement

VF/Pulseless VT   **shockable** ← Assess rhythm → **non-shockable**   Asystole and PEA

1 Shock
200 J Biphasic
360 J Monophasic

CPR 30:2
for 2 minutes

Immediate CPR 30:2
for 2 minutes

During CPR
– establish IV access
– high-flow oxygen
– intubate and then give
  interrupted compressions
– correct reversible causes
– given adrenaline every 3–5
  minutes
– consider amiodarone, atropine,
  magnesium

Correct reversible causes
4 Hs
Hypoxia
*Hypovolaemia
Hyper/hypokalaemia (metabolic)
Hypothermia
4 Ts
*Thromboembolism (*pulmonary and
amniotic fluid*)
*Toxic and therapeutic (*local anaesthetic*)
Cardiac tamponade
Tension pneumothorax

*more likely in pregnancy

Chapter 4

Cardiopulmonary resuscitation in the nonpregnant and pregnant woman

Objectives

On successfully completing this topic, you will be able to:

■ understand and perform basic and advanced life support

■ understand the importance of early defibrillation where appropriate

■ understand the adaptations of CPR in the pregnant woman.

Introduction and incidence

Although cardiac arrest is fortunately a rare event in pregnancy, it is estimated to occur in every 30 000 deliveries. The Confidential Enquiry into Maternal and Child Health reports a common direct cause of maternal death is thromboembolism, which will present usually as a sudden collapse. It is important that the healthcare teams know the appropriate actions to take in such an event, to promote positive outcomes for both the mother and the child.

Basic life support describes the procedures that a trained lay person could be expected to provide. These include:

■ recognising an absence of breathing or other signs of life

■ provision of chest compressions and mouth-to-mouth or pocket mask breathing

■ the use of automated external defibrillators.

Advanced life support describes the procedures that a trained healthcare professional could be expected to provide. This includes all of the above, and in addition:

■ the use of other airway adjuncts to provide more effective ventilation

■ the insertion of intravenous cannulae to give drugs

■ the use of semi-automated or manual defibrillators.

It should not be necessary to perform mouth-to-mouth ventilation in a hospital, as airway adjuncts should be close to hand.

In a hospital setting, the distinction between basic and advanced life support is arbitrary. The clinical team should be able to provide cardiopulmonary resuscitation, the main components of which are:

■ early recognition of cardiopulmonary collapse

■ calling for help using a standard procedure/number

■ starting cardiopulmonary resuscitation using appropriate adjuncts

■ early defibrillation if possible within 3 minutes.

Emphasis in the 2005 guidelines is on the need for early commencement of effective chest compressions as opposed to taking time to establish rescue breathing in the context of a cardiac arrest.

Management

The rescuer must ensure a safe environment, shake the woman and shout. If no response, call for help and then return to the woman.

If the woman appears to have collapsed but there are still signs of life then urgent medical attention should be called, and further assessment and appropriate treatment should be administered.

In the event of few signs of life, the following instructions may be carried out almost simultaneously by multiple helpers but of necessity are described in an appropriate order for one person.

1. Turn the woman on to her back with left lateral tilt.

In a noticeably pregnant woman, i.e. one with a significant intra-abdominal mass (usually by 20 weeks) it is important to obtain a left lateral tilt of the pelvis (Figure 4.1) at the earliest opportunity to minimise the risk of aortocaval compression.

Figure 4.1 Left lateral tilt

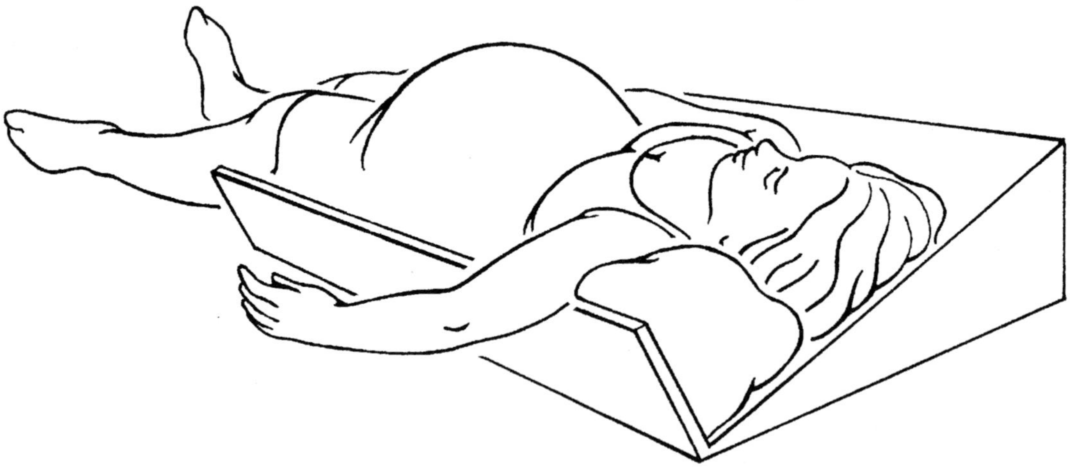

2. Open the airway.

Check in the mouth for foreign body or material. Use suction if required or remove foreign body with care and use of forceps. To open the airway, place your hand on the woman's forehead and gently tilt head back. At the same time, with your fingertips under the point of the woman's chin, lift the chin to open the airway. A jaw thrust may be required to open the airway. Do this by placing fingers behind the angle of the jaw and moving jaw anteriorly to displace tongue from the pharynx.

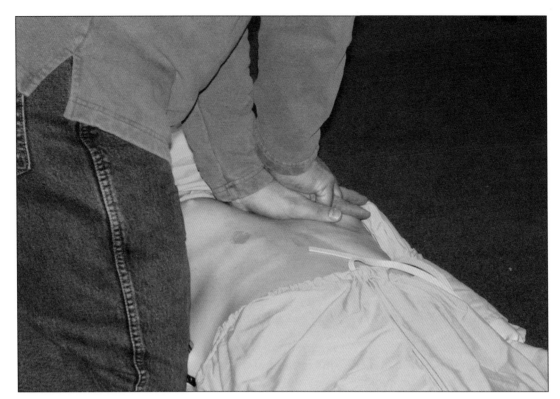

Figure 4.2 Place heel of one hand on sternum, other on top and interlock fingers

If injury to the neck is suspected, use manual in line stabilisation, avoid head tilt and use mainly jaw thrust to open the airway.

3. Assess breathing (and circulation).

Assess breathing for no more than ten seconds by looking for chest movements, listening for breath sounds and feeling for the movement of air. Absence of breathing in the presence of a clear airway is now used as a marker of absence of circulation. Experienced staff may want to check the carotid pulse for no more than 10 seconds at the same time as assessing breathing.

Gasping or agonal breathing may be seen in the immediate time after cardiac arrest and should not be taken as a sign of life – it is a sign of dying and CPR should commence immediately.

4. Start CPR.

If no circulation (or you are at all unsure) give 30 chest compressions followed by two ventilations.

a. The position for chest compressions should be the middle of the lower half of the sternum. Place the heel of one hand there, with the other hand on top of the first. Interlock the fingers of both hands and lift the fingers to ensure that pressure is not applied over the woman's ribs (Figure 4.2). Keep in the midline at all times. Do not apply any pressure over the top of the abdomen or bottom tip of the sternum.

Position yourself above the woman's chest and, with your arms straight, press down on the sternum to depress it 4–5 cm at a rate of 100 beats/minute (Figure 4.1). Change the person doing chest compressions about every 2 minutes to maintain efficiency but avoid any delays in the changeover.

b. Ventilation breaths. Keep an open airway and provide ventilation with appropriate adjuncts. This might be a pocket mask, oral airway or self-inflating bag with mask. Oxygen in high flow should be added as soon as possible.

c. Each ventilatory breath should last about 1 second and should make the chest rise as if a normal breath. Tracheal intubation is the most effective way of providing adequate ventilation and should be performed as soon as a trained member of staff is available.

d. Once the woman is intubated, ventilation should continue at 10 breaths/minute but does not need to be synchronised with chest compressions. These should then be uninterrupted.

e. Mouth-to-mouth breathing (not usually required).

Ensuring head tilt and chin lift. Close the soft part of the woman's nose with your thumb and index finger. Open her mouth a little but maintain chin lift. Take a breath and place your lips around her mouth, making sure that you have a good seal. Blow steadily into her mouth over 1 second, watching for her chest to rise. Maintaining head tilt and chin lift, take your mouth away from the woman and watch for her chest to fall as the air comes out. Take another breath and repeat the sequence to give another effective breath. Return to chest compressions quickly.

If circulation present but no breathing (respiratory arrest) continue rescue breathing at a rate of ten breaths/minute.

Recheck the circulation every ten breaths, taking no more than 10 seconds each time. If the woman starts to breathe on her own but remains unconscious, turn her into the recovery position and apply oxygen 15 litres/minute. Check her condition and be ready to turn her back to start rescue breathing if she stops breathing.

5. Use defibrillator.

As soon as possible, attach the defibrillator and pause briefly to assess the rhythm. The use of adhesive pads or using the paddles held over the gel pads may be quicker than attaching the ECG stickers. Follow the automated external defibrillator (AED) voice prompts or use manual defibrillation as appropriate (see Algorithm 4.3).

Automated external defibrillator

If automatic external defibrillator (AED) is available, attach, analyse rhythm and defibrillate as indicated in Algorithm 4.2.

The most frequent initial rhythm in the context of sudden collapse (i.e. not preceded by gradual deterioration or illness) is ventricular fibrillation (VF). The chances of successful defibrillation diminish with time. The AED allows for early defibrillation by less well-trained personnel, as it performs rhythm analysis, gives information by voice or visual display and the delivery of the shock is then delivered automatically.

Attach AED pads (or position gel pads for manual defibrillator)

Expose the chest and place the adhesive defibrillator pads on patient's chest, one to the right of the sternum below the right clavicle and one in the mid-axillary line taking care to avoid breast tissue. Keep the axillary electrode vertical to maximise efficiency.

After each shock, restart CPR for 2 minutes when there will be a further prompt for a rhythm analysis. If defibrillation is not indicated, CPR should be continued for 2 minutes, at which stage the AED will prompt further analysis of rhythm.

Turn immediately to advanced life support algorithm (Algorithm 4.3).

When advanced life support arrives, the rhythm is assessed as a shockable rhythm or non-shockable rhythm and defibrillation is instituted if required. An airway is secured and intravenous access obtained.

Defibrillation sequence (Algorithm 4.2) and use of drugs (Algorithm 4.3) can be followed on the algorithms.

Shockable rhythms:

■ Shockable rhythms are treated with a single shock followed by immediate continuation of CPR without stopping for a rhythm or pulse check.

■ Every 2 minutes the rhythm should be assessed and if necessary a further shock delivered. The pulse is not checked unless there is organised electrical activity, i.e. something that looks as though it might produce an output.

■ The energy used for defibrillation depends on whether it is a monophasic or biphasic defibrillator. Most modern defibrillators are biphasic as this is the most efficient way of delivering energy. The charge needed is therefore lower than on the older monophasic machines.

■ Recommended energy levels will vary from manufacturer to manufacturer, as well as using fixed or escalating energy levels. It is recommended that the initial biphasic shock should be at least 150J. Should an operator not know the correct energy level for a biphasic device, 200J is the default energy to use. The recommended initial energy level when using a monophasic defibrillator is 360J.

■ On the shockable side of the algorithm, adrenaline (epinephrine) 1 mg is given intravenously immediately before the third and every subsequent alternate shock, i.e. approximately every 4 minutes. Amiodarone 300 mg is given intravenously before the fourth shock.

Non-shockable rhythms:

■ On the non-shockable side of the algorithm, i.e. pulseless electrical activity or asystole, adrenaline (epinephrine) 1 mg should be given as soon as intravenous access is available.

■ Atropine 3 mg may be given intravenously once for asystole or slow rate, i.e. less than 60 beats/minute. This will minimise any vagal tone if present.

Reversible causes of cardiac arrest are considered and treated as necessary. Those highlighted in bold type are most common causes of cardiac arrest or collapse in pregnancy.

Four Hs:

■ Hypoxia

■ **Hypovolaemia (haemorrhage or sepsis)**

■ Hyperkalaemia and other metabolic disorders

■ Hypothermia.

Four Ts:

■ **Thromboembolism**

■ **Toxicity (drugs associated with regional or general anaesthesia)**

■ Tension pneumothorax

■ Cardiac tamponade.

Doubt about the rhythm

If there is doubt about whether the rhythm is asystole or fine VF, CPR should be maintained and treat as for asystole.

Other drugs

Sodium bicarbonate: 50 mmol intravenously should only be given to patients if the arrest is associated with tricyclic antidepressant overdose or hyperkalaemia. Otherwise it should be given in response to the clinical condition of the patient, e.g. with severe acidosis pH less than 7.1, base excess greater than –10.

Magnesium sulphate: 8 mmol (4 ml 50% solution) may be used for refractory VF. Other use may be in possible hypomagnesaemia, *torsade de pointes* (a persistent VF) or digoxin toxicity. These are unlikely in pregnancy.

Calcium: 10 ml of 10% calcium chloride intravenously can be used if it is thought that pulseless electrical activity is caused by hyperkalaemia, hypocalcaemia, overdose of calcium channel-blocking drugs or overdose of magnesium (for treatment of pre-eclampsia). Calcium can be given as a bolus if the patient has no output, but not in the same IV line as sodium bicarbonate as this will precipitate.

Physiological changes in pregnancy affecting resuscitation

There are a number of reasons why the processes of cardiopulmonary resuscitation are more difficult to perform and may be less effective in the pregnant than in the nonpregnant population. When these changes occur is not precise, but gradually the presence of increasing mass in the abdomen compromises resuscitative efforts. This may be the case from 20 weeks but will be more marked as the mother approaches term.

Vena caval occlusion

At term, in a well woman, the vena cava is completely occluded in 90% of supine pregnant women and the stroke volume may be only 30% of that of a nonpregnant woman. As soon as the infant is delivered, the vena cava returns towards normal and adequate venous return and consequently cardiac output is restored.

During cardiac arrest, in order to minimise the effects of the gravid uterus on venous return and cardiac output, a maternal pelvic tilt to the left of greater than 15 degrees is recommended. The tilt needs to be less than 30 degrees for effective closed-chest compression to take place. An alternative, manual displacement of uterus to the left should be effective (Figure 4.3).

Delivery of the fetus during cardiac arrest will reduce the oxygen demands on the mother and also increase the venous return to the heart making it more possible that resuscitation will be successful.

Changes in lung function

Mothers become hypoxic more readily because of a 20% decrease in their functional residual capacity due to the pressure from the gravid uterus on the diaphragm and the lungs, i.e. there is less of a reservoir of oxygen in the lungs so they become hypoxic much more quickly. This is exacerbated by a 20% increase in their resting oxygen demand due to servicing the needs of the fetus and uterus. These changes make it difficult to provide enough oxygen delivery using CPR to resuscitate a near-term pregnant mother.

Effectiveness of ventilation

In the later part of pregnancy it becomes increasingly difficult to provide effective ventilation breaths during CPR due to the increased weight of the abdominal contents and the breasts. In addition, the oesophageal sphincter is more relaxed, so the ease of introducing air into the stomach is increased. Passive regurgitation of stomach contents is a very real concern as these are greater in volume and more acidic in pregnancy so more likely to lead to damaging acid aspiration into the lungs. It is imperative that experienced staff provide a protected airway and adequate ventilation via an endotracheal tube as quickly as possible following cardiac arrest.

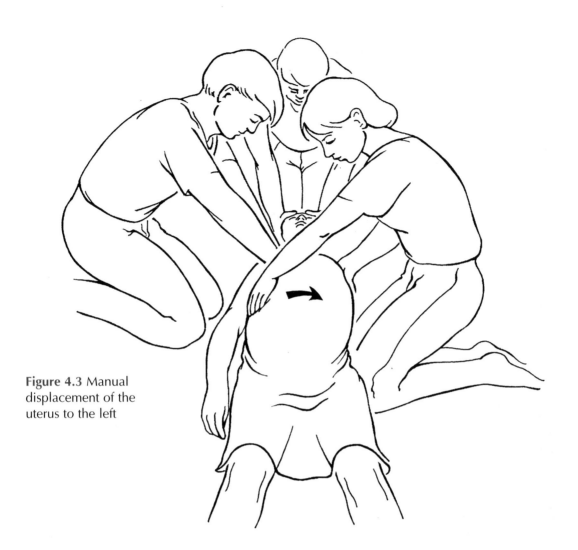

Figure 4.3 Manual displacement of the uterus to the left

Periarrest or perimortem caesarean section to improve chances of maternal survival

The Resuscitation Council (UK) has recommended that prompt caesarean delivery should be considered as a resuscitative procedure for cardiac arrest in near-term pregnancy. Delivery of the fetus will obviate the effects of aortocaval compression and significantly improve the chance for maternal resuscitation. This will reduce maternal oxygen consumption, increase venous return, make ventilation easier and allow CPR in the supine position.

When to do it

Evidence from literature and review of maternal and fetal physiology suggests that a caesarean delivery should begin within 4 minutes of cardiac arrest and delivery should be accomplished by 5 minutes. Pregnant women develop anoxia faster than nonpregnant women and can suffer irreversible brain damage within 4–6 minutes after cardiac arrest.

When a mother in the second half of her pregnancy suffers a cardiac arrest, immediate resuscitation should commence. Should immediate resuscitation fail, every attempt should be made to start the caesarean section by 4 minutes and deliver the infant by 5 minutes. CPR must be continued throughout the caesarean section and afterwards, as this increases the chances of a successful neonatal and maternal outcome.

Where to do it

Moving the mother to an operating theatre (e.g. from a labour room or accident and emergency department) is not necessary. Diathermy will not be needed initially, as there is little blood loss if no cardiac output. If the mother is successfully resuscitated, she can be moved to theatre to complete the operation.

How to do it

A limited amount of equipment is required in this situation. Sterile preparation and drapes are unlikely to improve survival. A surgical knife and forceps should be sufficient to effect delivery of the baby.

There are no recommendations regarding the surgical approach for caesarean section but there is no doubt that the classical approach is aided by the natural diastasis of recti abdomini that occurs in late pregnancy and a bloodless field in this clinical situation. It is accepted, however, that operators should use the technique with which they are most comfortable and in the current context most obstetricians can deliver a baby via a routine approach in less than 1 minute.

Consider open cardiac massage in the context of caesarean section when the abdomen is already open and the heart can be reached relatively easily through the diaphragm.

It is important that an anaesthetist is in attendance at the earliest opportunity. They should provide a protected airway, ensure continuity of effective chest compressions and adequate ventilation breaths as well as helping to determine and treat any underlying cause (4 Hs and 4 Ts).

Should resuscitation be successful and the mother regain a cardiac output, appropriate sedation or general anaesthesia needs to be administered to provide amnesia and pain relief. If resuscitation is successful the mother should be moved to a theatre to complete the operation.

Fetal outcome

Timing of delivery is also important for the survival of the infant and its normal neurological development. From discussion so far, there is no doubt that uterine evacuation is an important step during maternal resuscitation. However, there seems to be reluctance among obstetricians to perform peri-arrest caesarean sections. Concerns include worries about neurological damage to the delivered infant. In a comprehensive review of postmortem caesarean deliveries between 1900 and 1985, 70% (42/61) of infants delivered within 5 minutes survived and all developed normally. However, only 13% (8/61) of those delivered at 10 minutes and 12% (7/61) of infants delivered at 15 minutes survived. One infant in both of these groups of later survivors had neurological sequelae.

While the optimal interval from arrest to delivery is 5 minutes, there are case reports of intact infant survival after more than 20 minutes of maternal cardiac arrest. Review of postmortem caesarean section, as reported in Confidential Enquiries over the past 25 years, shows that there was no reported case where survival beyond the early neonatal period was accompanied by neurological disability. Evidence suggests that if the fetus survives the neonatal period then the chances of normal development are good.

Make decision to abandon CPR if unsuccessful

Do not abandon CPR if rhythm continues as VF/VT. A decision to abandon CPR should only be made after discussion with the consultant obstetrician and senior clinicians.

Medico-legal issues

No doctor has been found liable for performing a postmortem caesarean section. Theoretically, liability may concern either criminal or civil wrongdoing. Operating without consent may be argued as battery if the mother is successfully resuscitated. However, the doctrine of emergency exception would be applied because a delay in treatment could cause harm. The second criminal offence could be 'mutilation of corpse'. An operation performed to save the infant would not be wrongful, because there would be no criminal intent. The unanimous consensus of the literature is that a civil suit for performing perimortem caesarean is very unlikely to succeed.

Communication and teamwork

Wherever possible, have senior input from the obstetric, anaesthetic and midwifery professions. Ensure that the family is looked after and kept informed. Document timings and interventions accurately. If the mother dies, you will need to inform the coroner and the GP.

Logistics

Recruit as many staff as possible. You will need an individual responsible for each of the following:

- recording events and management
- communication
- runner/porter/transport.

Suggested further reading

Katz VL, Dotters DJ, Droegemueller W. Perimortem cesarean delivery. *Obstet Gynecol* 1986;68:571–6.

Algorithm 5.1 **Amniotic fluid embolism**

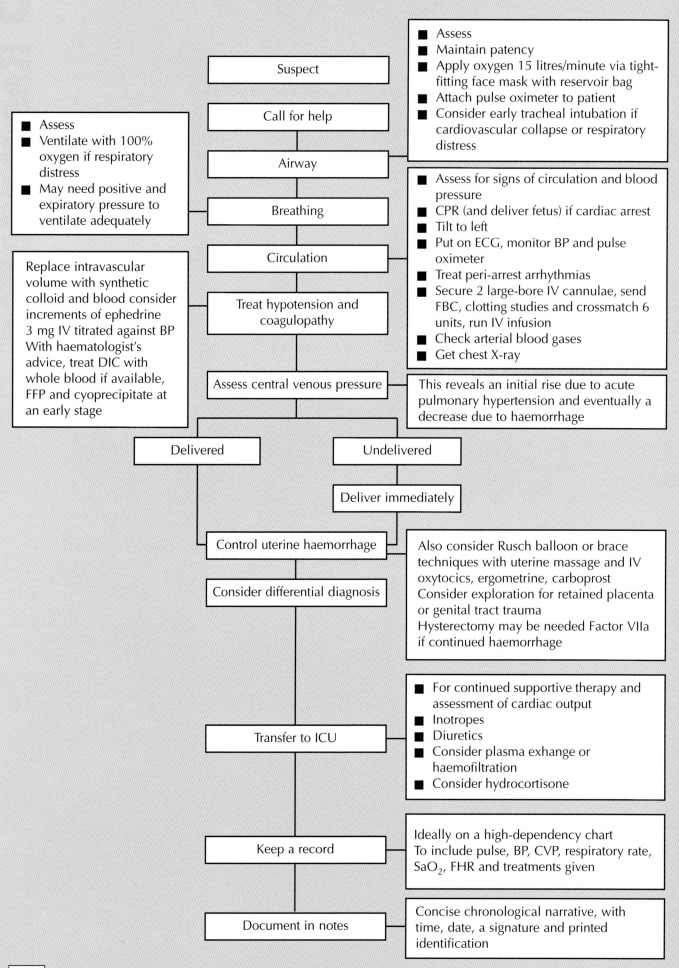

Suspect

Call for help

- Assess
- Maintain patency
- Apply oxygen 15 litres/minute via tight-fitting face mask with reservoir bag
- Attach pulse oximeter to patient
- Consider early tracheal intubation if cardiovascular collapse or respiratory distress

Airway

- Assess
- Ventilate with 100% oxygen if respiratory distress
- May need positive and expiratory pressure to ventilate adequately

Breathing

- Assess for signs of circulation and blood pressure
- CPR (and deliver fetus) if cardiac arrest
- Tilt to left
- Put on ECG, monitor BP and pulse oximeter
- Treat peri-arrest arrhythmias
- Secure 2 large-bore IV cannulae, send FBC, clotting studies and crossmatch 6 units, run IV infusion
- Check arterial blood gases
- Get chest X-ray

Circulation

Replace intravascular volume with synthetic colloid and blood consider increments of ephedrine 3 mg IV titrated against BP With haematologist's advice, treat DIC with whole blood if available, FFP and cyoprecipitate at an early stage

Treat hypotension and coagulopathy

Assess central venous pressure

This reveals an initial rise due to acute pulmonary hypertension and eventually a decrease due to haemorrhage

Delivered   **Undelivered**

Deliver immediately

Control uterine haemorrhage

Also consider Rusch balloon or brace techniques with uterine massage and IV oxytocics, ergometrine, carboprost
Consider exploration for retained placenta or genital tract trauma
Hysterectomy may be needed Factor VIIa if continued haemorrhage

Consider differential diagnosis

- For continued supportive therapy and assessment of cardiac output
- Inotropes
- Diuretics
- Consider plasma exhange or haemofiltration
- Consider hydrocortisone

Transfer to ICU

Keep a record

Ideally on a high-dependency chart
To include pulse, BP, CVP, respiratory rate, SaO$_2$, FHR and treatments given

Document in notes

Concise chronological narrative, with time, date, a signature and printed identification

Chapter 5

Amniotic fluid embolism

Objectives

On successfully completing this topic you will be able to:

■ successfully consider amniotic fluid embolism when appropriate, so making an early diagnosis

■ describe the immediate treatment of a suspected amniotic fluid embolism

■ describe the options in treatment following initial assessment and resuscitation.

Introduction

The dramatic nature of amniotic fluid embolism and the poor outcome with which it is associated mean that, although it is rare, prompt and appropriate management will be needed if a satisfactory outcome is to be achieved. The evidence upon which this guidance is based comes from retrospective series from the USA and information from the United Kingdom Amniotic Fluid Embolism Register. The Confidential Enquiry into Maternal Deaths in the UK also gives information about women who have died. All of this evidence is observational and it is improbable that any higher-quality evidence will be available. The treatments are largely reported in individual cases and so we can only establish general principles and options to be considered in any individual case.

Incidence

Amniotic fluid embolism is estimated to occur in between 1/8000 and 1/80 000 pregnancies but because it is difficult to confirm the diagnosis there is no certainty about these figures. A population-based study suggested a frequency of 1/20 646 deliveries. The 2000–2002 Confidential Enquiries into Maternal Deaths in the UK showed a drop in cases over each of the last two triennia and amniotic fluid embolism was the seventh leading cause of death. However, over the last six triennia it has been responsible for 60 deaths, which is 8% of direct deaths.

In France, 13% of deaths are caused by amniotic fluid embolism, the third highest cause. In Singapore, a study of postmortem examinations found that over 30% of direct maternal deaths were caused by amniotic fluid embolism, the most common cause. In the USA and Australia, it is responsible for 7.5–10.0% of maternal deaths. However, there is increasing evidence that the gloomy outlook for women with amniotic fluid embolism may no longer be appropriate. A review from 1979 suggested a mortality rate of 86% and the national registry from the USA in 1995 suggested a mortality of 61% but only 15% survived neurologically intact. However, population-based surveys suggest mortality of under 30% and the UK register of cases had a mortality of 30% for reported cases. This changing mortality is probably as a result of both better intensive care and recognition of the fact that 'milder' cases do occur.

Clinical manifestations

Effects of amniotic fluid in the circulation

Steiner and Luschbaugh demonstrated that rabbits and dogs could be killed by the infusion of human amniotic fluid and meconium. Clark considered studies up to 1990 but noted that the amniotic fluid infused was more particulate than encountered in human clinical practice, even when the amniotic fluid was thick. Clark felt that the over-reliance of investigators on animal models had led to an incorrect belief that the pathophysiology of amniotic fluid embolism principally involved pulmonary hypertension secondary to occlusion or vasospastic changes in the pulmonary vasculature.

Studies by Clark and Girard in humans showed only mild to moderate elevations in pulmonary artery pressure but evidence of left ventricular dysfunction or failure. There is also *in vitro* evidence of decreased myometrial contractility in the presence of amniotic fluid. This may affect the myocardium and possibly the myometrium. Clark reconciled these two findings of both pulmonary hypertension and left ventricular failure by suggesting a biphasic model. Some patients would have a profound acute pulmonary hypertension and this could cause neurological damage and early fatalities but this was not a sustained feature. The survivors would resolve the pulmonary hypertension and go on to develop left ventricular failure.

The myocardial depressant effect of amniotic fluid may come from its constituents, such as endothelin. This is a powerful bronchoconstrictor and causes constriction of the coronary and pulmonary arteries. Leukotrienes, which may be generated from amniotic fluid surfactant, are produced in response to amniotic fluid in the circulation. Leukotrienes and prostaglandins could cause the haemodynamic changes in amniotic fluid embolism. Inhibitors of leukotriene synthesis have been shown to prevent the fatal haemodynamic collapse of amniotic fluid embolism in experimental studies.

The development of coagulopathy with amniotic fluid embolism may be linked to amniotic fluid and meconium. Tissue factor has been shown to have a direct factor X activating property and thromboplastin-like effect and levels of these increase in amniotic fluid with gestational age. They may also cause pulmonary vasoconstriction. Their direct effect on clotting is enhanced by the presence of meconium with reductions in platelet count, prolonged prothrombin index and reduced fibrinogen.

Clark, reviewing the national registry, suggested that 'The syndrome of peripartum cardiovascular collapse and coagulopathy is, from a clinical, haemodynamic and haematologic standpoint, similar to anaphylaxis and septic shock and suggests the possibility of a common underlying pathophysiologic mechanism.' It was suggested that, while material may pass from fetus to mother, it was a predisposition to react that created the clinical syndrome. The response to the stimulus of fetal material in the maternal circulation is dependent upon the nature and quantity of the material and also the susceptibility of the mother. It is plausible that the effect is sometimes occlusive, sometimes a direct 'toxic' effect and sometimes a trigger to a cascade reaction. In some women, events may progress through each element. This suggests that clinical management will be aimed at supportive therapy with an understanding that the patient will pass through different phases of the clinical presentation.

The issue of amniotic fluid in the circulation is important if one is going to consider intra-operative autologous blood transfusion. This has been considered in relation to cell salvage and leucocyte depletion filtering seems to reduce particulate contaminants to the level equivalent to maternal venous blood. The safety of intraoperative autologous blood collection has been examined in a cohort study of 139 women and no demonstrable increase in complications was found.

Other clinical manifestations

In order to suspect an amniotic fluid embolism, we have to be aware of the features of the condition. The following were described by Clark in the USA registry as requirements for the condition and the same features were used in the UK register. To make a diagnosis there should be:

■ acute hypotension or cardiac arrest

■ acute hypoxia (dyspnoea, cyanosis or respiratory arrest)

■ coagulopathy (laboratory evidence of intravascular coagulation or severe haemorrhage)

■ onset of all of the above during labour or within 30 minutes of delivery

■ no other clinical conditions or potential explanations for the symptoms and signs.

It is important to note that the coagulopathy may not develop if there is a rapid deterioration and the woman dies. It will be present or develop if the woman survives the initial collapse.

Symptoms and signs

The following symptoms and signs were noted in the Registers from the USA. Comparative data from the UK, where available, are included (Table 5.1).

The UK register describes several initial patterns of presentation:

■ maternal hypotension, shortness of breath, fetal bradycardia then delivery (14%)

■ maternal loss of consciousness or seizure then delivery (35%)

■ maternal collapse after delivery of baby at caesarean section (14%)

■ fetal distress and then maternal collapse (23%)

■ immediately following delivery loss of consciousness or seizures (14%).

In each case, coagulation difficulties usually with profuse haemorrhage followed. In the US Registry cases 70% occurred in labour (72% UK), 11% after vaginal delivery (14% UK) and 19% at caesarean section (14% UK).

It becomes apparent that the condition presents with either an acute fetal or maternal collapse characterised by circulatory problems and profound hypoxia, often with seizures, and then the development of coagulation failure.

Suspecting an amniotic fluid embolism

Amniotic fluid embolism should be part of the differential diagnosis of women who present with any of the following during labour or after delivery:

■ respiratory distress

■ seizures

■ cardiovascular collapse

■ disseminated intravascular coagulation with or without revealed haemorrhage

■ cyanosis

■ profound fetal distress, with any maternal symptoms.

Table 5.1. Symptoms and signs of amniotic fluid embolism and their rate of occurrence, in USA and UK (where available)

Symptom/sign	USA (%)	UK (%)
Hypotension	100	100
Fetal distress*	100	
Baby had severe hypoxia ischaemia*		56
Pulmonary oedema or acute respiratory distress syndrome	93	
Cardiopulmonary arrest	87	57
Cyanosis	83	
Coagulopathy	83	100
Dyspnoea	49	
Seizure	48	47
Uterine atony	23	23
Bronchospasm	15	
Transient hypertension	11	
Cough	7	
Headache	7	
Chest pain	2	

* Of those *in utero* at the time

Awareness of the condition is also important around miscarriage or evacuation of the uterus, as there have been isolated reports. Premonitory signs such as restlessness, numbness and tingling have also been reported.

Diagnosis

The diagnosis is a clinical one. Absolute confirmation is only possible following death, with fetal squames in the maternal pulmonary circulation. However, other clinical features still need to be present to confirm the diagnosis. This is because fetal squames have been found in central venous blood in other conditions, and even in the nonpregnant woman. In the living, fetal squames or lanugo on central venous samples cannot be taken as indicative of the diagnosis without a compatible clinical presentation.

The differential diagnosis involves considering an exhaustive list of the causes of maternal collapse in the peripartum period:

- postpartum haemorrhage (uterine atony)
- placental abruption
- uterine rupture
- pre-eclampsia or eclampsia
- septic shock
- thrombotic embolus
- air embolus
- acute myocardial infarction
- peripartum cardiomyopathy

- local anaesthetic toxicity

- anaphylaxis

- transfusion reactions

- aspiration of gastric contents.

Only after exclusion of all the other causes can a diagnosis be confirmed clinically.

A clotting screen is often very abnormal even before haemorrhage becomes apparent and will exclude a large number of other diagnoses. When haemorrhage is already present, abnormal clotting could be secondary to the haemorrhage but normally considerable blood loss with blood replacement needs to have occurred in the case of haemodilutional coagulopathy.

An ECG is helpful, to look for signs of myocardial damage. In amniotic fluid embolism, often bizarre cardiac rhythms can be present making interpretation difficult.

Arterial blood gases and a pulse oximeter may aid management but will not differentiate causes.

A ventilation perfusion scan of the lungs may demonstrate defects with either pulmonary embolism or amniotic fluid embolism.

Zinc coproporphyrin levels are increased to a mean of 97 nmol/l (range 38–240 nmol/l) in amniotic fluid embolism with normal women having a mean of 26 nmol/l after delivery. A cut off of 35 nmol/l has been suggested for diagnosis. Although in theory rapidly available, it is not likely to be routinely available.

Tryptase levels have also been looked at because of the suggestion that amniotic fluid embolism may be anaphylactoid but differing results have been found. Other studies have found high fetal antigen levels and abnormally low levels of complement suggesting a role for complement activation rather than anaphylaxis.

Management

The management of amniotic fluid embolism is supportive rather than specific with current knowledge. Multidisciplinary treatment with early involvement of senior, experienced staff is essential. Obstetricians, anaesthetists, intensivists and haematologists are mandatory to give the best prospect of survival.

As collapse is the predominant presentation the initial management is basic resuscitation to maintain vital organ perfusion.

Airway/breathing:

- High flow oxygen with early intubation and mechanical ventilation.

Circulation:

- Cardiac arrhythmias or cardiac arrest may occur.

- Inotropic support is likely to be needed.

- Following cardiac arrest, rapid delivery, within 5 minutes, aids resuscitation.

- Coagulopathy and haemorrhage are likely.

- Cardiac output measurement may guide therapy. Ensure that fluid overload does not occur as this can lead to worsening pulmonary oedema and subsequent acute respiratory distress syndrome. This is particularly when the coagulopathy and haemorrhage develops, in what has been described as the 'secondary' phase of the condition, when there are high filling pressures reflecting a failing left ventricle.

In this secondary phase, when coagulopathy and haemorrhage develop, prompt transfusion of fluids will be necessary to replace blood loss. This occurs at a variable point after initial presentation. Vasopressors such as phenylephrine or ephedrine may be useful in restoring aortic perfusion pressure. The early consideration of clotting factor replacement with fresh frozen plasma, cryoprecipitate and platelets is important if there are signs of coagulopathy, such as haematuria or bleeding from the gums, even before massive blood loss is apparent. It is appropriate to commence this before receiving the laboratory confirmation of coagulopathy.

Cryoprecipitate may be of intrinsic value beyond its clotting factor components as it contains fibronectin, which aids the reticuloendothelial system in the filtration of antigenic and toxic particulate matter. The haemorrhage that occurs is usually as a result of uterine atony, which may be exacerbated by hypoxia and the coagulopathy. Hence, cryoprecipitate, by removing fibrin degradation products, may assist in the treatment of the uterine atony. Aggressive treatment of uterine atony with medical (oxytocics, ergometrine and prostaglandin) and adjunctive techniques (packing, tamponade, Rusch balloons) should be used though early recourse to hysterectomy may be life saving.

The presentation of amniotic fluid embolism can sometimes be acute fetal collapse, which is followed a little time after by maternal deterioration. Checking coagulation studies and monitoring pulse oximetry in women who have a sudden deterioration in fetal condition and the baby is unexpectedly severely acidotic may identify abnormalities providing the opportunity for earlier invasive monitoring.

The literature contains a number of reports of specific treatments:

- extracorporeal membrane oxygenation (ECMO)
- prostacyclin
- nitric oxide plasma exchange
- haemofiltration
- cardiopulmonary bypass
- ligation of the infundibulopelvic ligament and uterine arteries
- factor VIIa.

As each is an individual report it is difficult to come to a definitive view. As there is a theoretical view that the condition is anaphylactoid, Clark suggested that high-dose hydrocortisone, 500 mg 6-hourly, might be appropriate but no studies have examined this. A number of the treatments aim to filter or 'cleanse' the circulating blood volume and these may be effective in more rapidly reversing coagulation abnormalities. This, in effect, would be similar to the use of cryoprecipitate described above.

Risk of recurrence

Further pregnancies have been reported in women with a successful outcome after amniotic fluid embolism. There are a total of six cases, all with good fetal and maternal outcome.

Maternal morbidity and neonatal outcome

In the US Register, 11 of 18 women (61%) who survived had neurological impairment whereas in the UK Register only two women (7%) who survived had neurological impairment. In the UK, 39% of survivors had a cardiac arrest, 23% required hysterectomy and 7% had further laparotomies. One woman developed subglottic stenosis consequent to a tracheostomy; 24 of the 31 (77%) survivors were admitted to intensive care units and had a median length of stay of 3 days (IQR 1.5–6.0 days). In those women surviving long enough to receive blood, the number of units of blood products ranged from 12–106 units, with units of blood ranging from 2–37 units.

In the US registry cases, 22 of 28 fetuses (79%) alive and *in utero* at the time of collapse survived but only 11 (50% of survivors) were neurologically intact. In the UK series, six fetuses of the 13 women who died survived. Four of these were acidotic, one had hypoxic ischaemic encephalopathy and went on to develop cerebral palsy. The outcome of the other three acidotic babies seemed initially uneventful. Three of the babies did well after immediate delivery. Five babies were either a neonatal death, surviving up to 11 days or a fresh stillbirth. One was an intrauterine death before presentation. In the 18 surviving women with a fetus alive and *in utero* at the time of the maternal collapse, four died, four had hypoxic ischaemic encephalopathy, with one developing cerebral palsy, and two others had low cord pH.

Summary

■ Amniotic fluid embolism is rare and often devastating for both the woman and her baby.

■ Outcomes may be improving and prompt resuscitation, assessment and support may lead to a better chance of a good outcome.

■ Specific therapies have not been evaluated.

Suggested further reading

Clark SL. New concepts of amniotic fluid embolism: a review. *Obstet Gynecol Surv* 1990:45:360–8.

Clark SL, Hankins GD, Dudley DA, Dildy GA, Porter TF. Amniotic fluid embolism: analysis of the national registry. *Am J Obstet Gynecol* 1995;172:1158–67.

Davies S. Amniotic fluid embolus a review of the literature. *Can J Anaesth* 2001;48:88–98.

Gilbert WM, Danielsen B. Amniotic fluid embolism: decreased mortality in a population-based study. *Obstet Gynecol* 1999;93:973–7.

Lewis G, editor. *Why Mothers Die. The Sixth Report of Confidential Enquiries into Maternal Deaths in the United Kingdom.* London: RCOG Press; 2004

Tuffnell DJ. Amniotic fluid embolism. In: MacLean AB, Neilson JP, editors. *Maternal Mortality and Morbidity.* London: RCOG Press; 2002. p. 190–200.

Tuffnell DJ. United Kingdom amniotic fluid embolism register. *BJOG* 2005;112:1625–9.

Algorithm 6.1 Pulmonary embolism (PE)

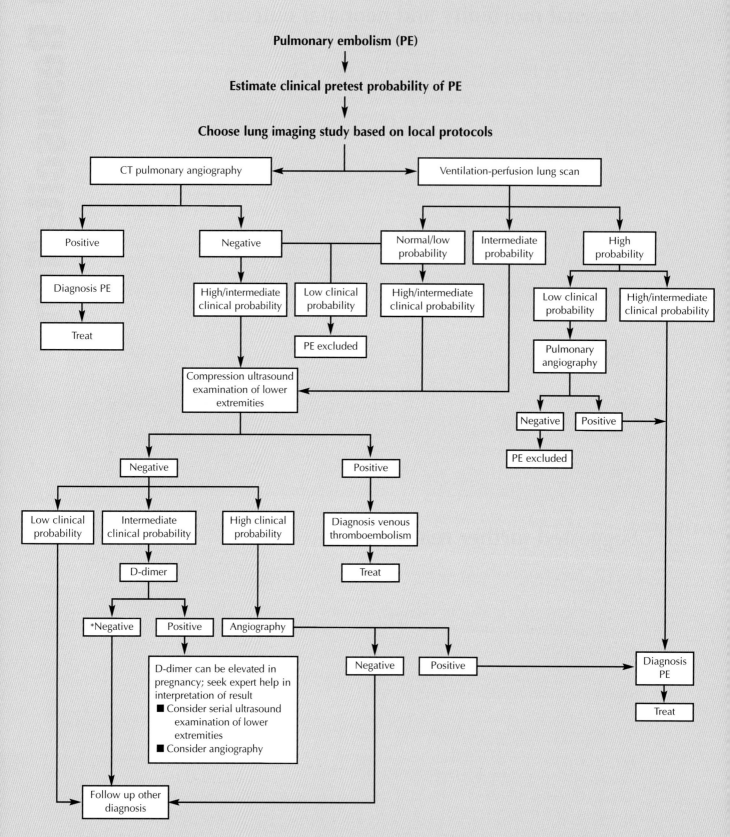

Pulmonary embolism (PE)

↓

Estimate clinical pretest probability of PE

↓

Choose lung imaging study based on local protocols

CT pulmonary angiography ←→ Ventilation-perfusion lung scan

CT pulmonary angiography branch:
- Positive → Diagnosis PE → Treat
- Negative →
  - High/intermediate clinical probability → Compression ultrasound examination of lower extremities
  - Low clinical probability → PE excluded

Ventilation-perfusion lung scan branch:
- Normal/low probability →
  - High/intermediate clinical probability → Compression ultrasound examination of lower extremities
- Intermediate probability → Compression ultrasound examination of lower extremities
- High probability →
  - Low clinical probability → Pulmonary angiography
    - Negative → PE excluded
    - Positive →
  - High/intermediate clinical probability → Diagnosis PE → Treat

Compression ultrasound examination of lower extremities:
- Negative →
  - Low clinical probability → Follow up other diagnosis
  - Intermediate clinical probability → D-dimer
    - *Negative → Follow up other diagnosis
    - Positive → D-dimer can be elevated in pregnancy; seek expert help in interpretation of result
      - ■ Consider serial ultrasound examination of lower extremities
      - ■ Consider angiography
  - High clinical probability → Angiography
    - Negative → Follow up other diagnosis
    - Positive → Diagnosis PE → Treat
- Positive → Diagnosis venous thromboembolism → Treat

*Quantitative enzyme linked immunosorbent assay <500μg/l, negative semiquantitative latex or negative haemagglutination D-dimer test

Chapter 6

Pulmonary embolism

Objectives

On successfully completing this topic, you will be able to:

■ recognise the features of pulmonary embolism and suspect the diagnosis early

■ describe the treatment of suspected pulmonary embolism.

Introduction and incidence

The 2000–02 report on Confidential Enquiries into Maternal Deaths showed thrombosis and thromboembolism to be the leading cause of all direct maternal deaths. Of the 30 deaths from thrombosis and/or thromboembolism, 25 were due to pulmonary embolism; 17 deaths occurred in the postpartum period. Substandard care took the form of a failure to recognise risk factors, failure to appreciate the significance of signs and symptoms in the light of background risk factors, failure to act promptly enough in implementing either prophylaxis or treatment and inadequate dosage of thromboprophylaxis.

The incidence of pulmonary embolism in pregnancy varies between 1/1000 and 1/3000 deliveries. This depends upon whether deep venous thrombosis (DVT) has been treated adequately. Untreated, as many as 24% of patients with DVT will have pulmonary embolism, resulting in approximately 15% mortality. When patients are treated with anticoagulants, pulmonary embolism occurs in only 4.5% and mortality is reduced to less than 1%. The importance of timely diagnosis and treatment is therefore apparent.

This chapter addresses thrombotic venous thromboembolism, even though the term 'pulmonary embolism' encompasses embolism from many sources, including air, bone marrow, amniotic fluid, tumour and sepsis.

Pregnancy is a thrombogenic state with a five- to six-fold increase in the risk of DVT. The majority of DVT in pregnancy are ileofemoral, which are more likely to embolise.

Additional risk factors include:

■ operative delivery: caesarean section increases the risk of pulmonary embolism two- to eight-fold. The risk is greater after an emergency procedure. The risk is also increased after prolonged labour and instrumental vaginal delivery

■ age: mortality from pulmonary embolism is nearly 100 times greater in pregnant women aged over 40 years compared with those aged 20–25 years

■ increasing parity

■ obesity: the risk of pulmonary embolism is due to poor mobility and higher likelihood of venous stasis

■ congenital and acquired thrombophilia: patients with congenital thrombophilia (antithrombin-3 deficiency, protein C and S deficiency, activated protein C resistance, prothrombin gene variant) and acquired thrombophilia (lupus anticoagulant and antiphospholipid antibody) are at increased risk of pulmonary embolism. It is difficult to estimate the risk for each thrombophilia. Family or past history of thromboembolism should warrant a search for these factors.

■ surgical procedures in pregnancy or puerperium: surgical procedures such as postpartum sterilisation, ovarian cystectomy and caesarean hysterectomy further increase the risk of pulmonary embolism.

The other risk factors are restricted activity, hypertensive disease, hyperemesis, dehydration and excessive blood loss. Medical disorders such as homocysteinuria, sickle cell disease, inflammatory bowel disease, nephritic syndrome, certain cardiac diseases and myeloproliferative disorders also increase the risk of thromboembolism.

Pathophysiology

Hypercoagulability leads to the formation of thrombus in the leg veins, with proximal extension as the clot propagates. As thrombi form in the deep veins of the legs, pelvis or arms, they may dislodge and embolise to the pulmonary arteries, with potentially serious consequences.

Pulmonary arterial obstruction and the release by platelets of vasoactive agents, such as serotonin elevate pulmonary vascular resistance. The resulting increase in alveolar dead space and redistribution of blood flow impairs gas exchange.

As right ventricular afterload increases, tension rises in the right ventricular wall and may lead to dilatation, dysfunction and ischaemia of the right ventricle.

Stimulation of irritant receptors causes alveolar hyperventilation. Reflex bronchoconstriction augments airway resistance and lung oedema decreases pulmonary compliance.

Clinical presentation

For clinical purposes, pulmonary embolism can be classified into two main groups: massive and non-massive.

Massive pulmonary embolism consists of cyanosis, shock syncope and/or circulatory collapse with hypotension (defined as a systolic blood pressure less than 90 mmHg or a pressure drop of 40 mmHg for more than 15 minutes if not caused by new-onset arrhythmia, hypovolemia or sepsis). Otherwise, non-massive pulmonary embolism can be diagnosed (Table 6.1).

The clinical diagnosis of pulmonary embolism is unreliable, because the clinical features are poorly sensitive and poorly specific for the diagnosis. Tachycardia and a few atelectatic râles may be the only findings on physical examination. Massive pulmonary embolism may produce right-sided heart failure with jugular venous distension, an enlarged liver, a left parasternal heave and fixed splitting of the second heart sound. Clinical evidence of DVT including leg pain is rarely found in patients with pulmonary embolism. In the Prospective Investigation of Pulmonary Embolism Diagnosis (PIOPED) study, only 15% of patients with pulmonary embolism had clinical evidence of DVT.

False-negative diagnoses may arise because the symptoms of pulmonary embolism may mimic those of other common cardiopulmonary conditions. Because there are no absolute diagnostic clinical features of pulmonary embolism, the role of the clinical assessment is to formulate the patient's presenting symptoms and signs into an estimate of the pre-test probability of pulmonary embolism. Various models exist for arriving at a pre-test probability, which will guide the strategy for specialist investigations.

6

Resuscitation

Table 6.1. Signs and symptoms of pulmonary embolism (PE) (ACOG Educational Bulletin)

Findings in patients with proven PE	Occurrence (%)
Tachypnoea	89
Dyspnoea	81
Pleuritic pain	72
Apprehension	59
Cough	54
Tachycardia	43
Haemoptysis	34
Temperature > 37°C	34

In summary, symptoms and physical findings must be interpreted with caution during pregnancy, because dyspnoea, tachypnoea and leg discomfort occur commonly as pregnancy progresses.

Management

1. **Remember the risk factors for thromboembolism.**

2. **Suspect pulmonary embolism in all women presenting with sudden onset of shortness of breath, chest pain, unexplained tachycardia or cardiovascular collapse.**

3. **Involve the senior obstetrician, anaesthetist and medical team.**

4. **Assess and ensure adequate airway, breathing and circulation. Commence cardiopulmonary resuscitation if the woman is in cardiac arrest.**

5. **Transfer the woman to the high-dependency area when appropriate and commence monitoring: non-invasive blood pressure, pulse oximetry, ECG, urine output.**

6. **Send full blood count, clotting studies, urea and electrolytes, liver function tests and thrombophilia screen.**

7. **Request ECG, arterial blood gas and chest X-ray.**

These investigations do not confirm or refute the diagnosis of pulmonary embolism.

ECG

ECG is non-specific for diagnosis of pulmonary embolism. The changes in electrical axis that occur in normal pregnancy make the ECG findings in pulmonary embolism even less specific. Sinus tachycardia is the most common abnormality. Right-axis deviation and right-ventricular strain pattern may be present with a large pulmonary embolism. S waves in lead 1, Q wave in lead 3 and inverted T waves in lead 3 (S1Q3T3) pattern are very rare.

Chest X-ray

Chest X-ray will help to exclude pneumothorax and pneumonia. The non-specific radiological changes in pulmonary embolism include segmental collapse, a raised hemidiaphragm, consolidation and unilateral pleural effusion. Wedge-shaped infarction is a rare finding. Chest X-ray is necessary for the accurate interpretation of ventilation/perfusion scans. The radiation exposure to the fetus is small (less than 10 µGy) and therefore should not be withheld.

Arterial blood gases

Arterial blood gases should be monitored in the upright position to avoid a false low PaO_2. Arterial blood gases in pulmonary embolism may reveal a reduced PaO_2 and a normal or low $PaCO_2$. With smaller emboli, normal values may be found. If the patient is unstable, radial artery cannulation is of benefit both for repeated arterial blood gases and haemodynamic monitoring.

Commence anticoagulation

Treat clinically suspected pulmonary embolism while awaiting confirmation from objective tests. The aim of treatment is to prevent further thromboembolic complications and extension of the existing thrombus. Prompt anticoagulation reduces mortality from thromboembolism by 75%.

Intravenous unfractionated heparin used to be the mainstay of treatment. Low molecular weight heparin is as effective, easy to administer, requires less monitoring and has lesser risk of haemorrhagic complications.

Perform ventilation/perfusion (V/Q) scan and duplex Doppler leg ultrasound scan

V/Q scanning is the most useful initial test in patients with suspected pulmonary embolism and should be organised urgently (Table 6.2). V/Q scans are interpreted using standardised criteria (PIOPED). Based on the extent of ventilation–perfusion mismatches, the scan is interpreted as normal, low probability, intermediate probability or high probability for pulmonary embolism. A normal scan reliably excludes pulmonary embolism and a high-probability V/Q scan is considered sufficient evidence for diagnosing pulmonary embolism in a patient with a high clinical suspicion. The low and intermediate scans are considered non-diagnostic and further investigations are necessary to confirm or refute the diagnosis. The radiation dose from V/Q scan is considered to pose negligible risk to the fetus. Perfusion scan alone can be performed with a ventilation scan being performed only if the perfusion scan is abnormal.

Bilateral Doppler ultrasound leg studies should be performed in all cases of suspected pulmonary embolism. A positive scan study for DVT is considered sufficient to justify the use of anticoagulation therapy.

Perform pulmonary angiography

Pulmonary angiography is the gold standard for diagnosing pulmonary embolism. It is indicated following an intermediate or low probability result on V/Q scan with a high clinical suspicion of pulmonary embolism, even if Doppler ultrasound of the legs is negative. It should also be considered if cardiovascular collapse or hypotension is present and where other investigations have failed to give a firm diagnosis. This is an invasive test with high radiation exposure. It may be associated with reactions to intravenous contrast agents.

Table 6.2. Probability of pulmonary thromboembolism based on V/Q scan report

Scan category	Probability (%)
High probability	87
Intermediate probability	30
Low probability	14
Normal	4

Additional tests

Non-invasive imaging techniques such as spiral computed tomography (CT) and magnetic resonance imaging (MRI) have been used for diagnosing pulmonary embolism. These modalities allow direct visualisation of the thrombus within the pulmonary artery. These techniques have not been fully evaluated in pregnancy.

Spiral CT

Spiral CT after contrast injection permits excellent visualisation of the pulmonary arteries and direct visualisation of pulmonary arterial clots in larger vessels – all during a single breath hold. Sensitivity and specificity of spiral CT appear to be quite good for a proximal clot in the main, lobular or segmental pulmonary arteries. The procedure also provides images of mediastinal and chest wall structures such as lymph nodes, lung parenchyma, the pleura and pericardium. By visualising abnormalities other than pulmonary embolism that may be causing or contributing to the symptoms, spiral CT offers an important advantage over V/Q scanning. In fact, in one study on nonpregnant women an alternative diagnosis to pulmonary embolism was established by spiral CT in 31% of women without pulmonary embolism. Spiral CT does have some limitations, including poor visualisation of the peripheral areas of the upper and lower lobes (subsegmental arteries).

Magnetic resonance imaging

MRI avoids the use of radiation and nephrotoxic contrast agents, is comparable to venography for the diagnosis of DVT and offers excellent resolution of the inferior vena cava and pelvic veins. Therefore, MRI could rule out pulmonary embolism, DVT and pelvic vein clots in a single test. Its current limitations include expense, lack of universal availability, and the specialised expertise required for interpretation. It can be difficult for a pregnant woman to lie supine in the MRI scanner and provision may be needed for left lateral tilt to avoid supine hypotension syndrome.

Echocardiography

Experience with use of echocardiography in pregnancy is limited. It can show well-defined abnormalities with a large central pulmonary embolus. It may also help to eliminate other causes of central chest pain, collapse and hypotension such as myocardial infarction, pericardial tamponade and aortic dissection. Its usefulness lies in the fact that it is a bedside test and can be done in patients who are unstable to be transported for pulmonary angiography.

D-dimer

In pregnancy, D-dimer levels are elevated due to alterations in the physiology and particularly if there is a concomitant problem such as pre-eclampsia. Hence a 'positive' D-dimer test in pregnancy is not diagnostic of a venous thromboembolism and further investigations are required. However, a low-level D-dimer suggests an absence of venous thromboembolism and further testing is not required.

Additional options for patients in shock

Additional options for patients in shock include thrombolytic therapy, pulmonary embolectomy and transvenous catheter fragmentation of the clot. Expert advice from intensivists, cardiothoracic surgeons, and interventional radiologists should be sought, where appropriate.

Patients in shock should be managed on the intensive care unit. These patients will need arterial blood pressure and central venous pressure monitoring. They will also need haemodynamic support with adequate fluid management and inotropic agents in order to ensure maximal right-heart filling. They may need intubation and ventilation, measurement of pulmonary artery pressure, wedge pressure and cardiac output using pulmonary artery floatation catheters.

Anticoagulation

Anticoagulation following pulmonary embolism should be continued throughout pregnancy and at least 6 weeks postpartum or until a 3-month course of anticoagulation therapy is completed.

Heparin is the anticoagulant of choice in pregnancy, since it does not cross the placenta. There are no randomised controlled studies for the treatment of pulmonary embolism in pregnancy. However, rapid and prolonged anticoagulation prevents extension of the thrombus and its recurrence. If unfractionated heparin is being used, initiate treatment with an intravenous bolus of 5000 iu heparin given over 5 minutes. Follow this with heparin infusion of 1000–2000 iu/hour and adjust the dose to maintain activated partial thromboplastin time (APTT) at 1.5–2.5 times the patient's control. Repeat APTT every 6 hours during the first 24 hours of therapy. Thereafter, monitor the APTT daily unless outside the therapeutic range.

Treatment thereafter may be continued with subcutaneous heparin in a dose of 10 000 iu twice daily. Maintaining mid-interval APTT in the therapeutic range (1.5–2.5 times the control) following subcutaneous heparin may be problematic and lead to under or over anticoagulation. Assessment of anti-Xa level may then be helpful in preventing such complications.

Complications of heparin therapy are allergy, thrombocytopenia and osteoporosis. Platelet count should be monitored on a monthly basis in patients on long-term heparin therapy.

Low-molecular-weight heparins (LMWH) are being increasingly used in pregnancy. They have been shown to be effective, safe and associated with fewer adverse effects when compared with unfractionated heparin in nonpregnant women.

LMWH have higher bioavailability following subcutaneous administration (85% versus 10% for unfractionated heparin). The half-life is two to four times (18 hours) that of unfractionated heparin, allowing once daily administration. Anticoagulation using enoxaparin (Clexane®, Rhône-Poulenc Rorer) 1 mg/kg subcutaneously, based on the early pregnancy weight, every 12 hours is being used in the immediate treatment of DVT and pulmonary embolism in pregnancy. Frequent monitoring does not appear to be necessary. The platelet count should be rechecked 7–9 days after commencing treatment. Other options are dalteparin 90 units/kg 12-hourly or tinzaparin 90 units/kg 12-hourly.

Following acute therapy, the dose of LMWH could be reduced to prophylactic levels, i.e. 40 mg enoxaparin once a day or 5000 iu dalteparin once a day. Monitoring is by measuring anti-Xa activity, therapeutic range being 0.4–1.0 units/ml 3 hours post-injection. Enoxaparin is available in syringes of 40 mg, 60 mg, 80 mg and 100 mg. The dose closest to the patient's weight should be employed.

Warfarin crosses the placenta and is associated with a characteristic embryopathy in the first trimester. Major fetal central nervous system abnormalities, such as microcephaly and optic atrophy, are seen with warfarin use in the second and third trimesters. In addition, there is a higher risk of intracerebral bleeds from the trauma of delivery and a higher risk of bleeding complications during labour and delivery. For all these reasons, warfarin is not preferred in the antenatal period. However, warfarin can be initiated in the postpartum period and overlapped with heparin until INR is maintained at 2.0–3.0.

Vena caval filters are indicated when there is recurrent pulmonary embolism, despite adequate anticoagulation, contraindication to anticoagulation and complication of anticoagulation such as heparin-induced thrombocytopenia. Suprarenal placement is recommended in pregnancy.

Suggested further reading

American College of Obstetrics and Gynecology. Educational bulletin. Thromboembolism in pregnancy. *Int J Gynecol Obstet* 1997;57:209–18.

De Swiet M. Management of pulmonary embolism in pregnancy. *Eur Heart J* 1999;20:1378–85.

De Swiet M. Thromboembolism. In: de Swiet M, editor. *Medical Disorders in Obstetric Practice*. 3rd ed. Oxford: Blackwell Scientific; 1995. p. 116–42.

Garg K, Welsh CH, Feyerabend AJ, Subber SW, Russ PD, Johnston RJ, *et al*. Pulmonary embolism: diagnosis with spiral CT and ventilation-perfusion scanning-correlation with pulmonary angiography results and clinical outcome. *Radiology* 1998;208;201–8.

Ginsberg JS, Hirsh J, Rainbow AG, Coates G. risks to the fetus of radiological procedures used in the diagnosis of maternal venous thromboembolic disease. *Thromb Haemost* 1989;61:189–96.

Goldhaber SZ. Pulmonary embolism. *N Engl J Med* 1998; 339:93–104.

Greer IA. Thrombosis in pregnancy: maternal and fetal issues. *Lancet* 1999;353:1258–65.

Lewis G, editor. *Why Mothers Die. The Sixth Report of Confidential Enquiries into Maternal Deaths in the United Kingdom*. London: RCOG Press; 2004

Macklon NS. Diagnosis of deep venous thrombosis and pulmonary embolism in pregnancy. *Curr Opin Pulm Med* 1999;5:233–7.

PIOPED Investigators. Value of the ventilation/perfusion scan in acute PE. Results of a prospective investigation of the pulmonary embolism diagnosis. *JAMA* 1990;263:2753–9.

Royal College of Obstetricians and Gynaecologists. *Thromboembolic Disease in Pregnancy and the Puerperium: Acute Management*. Guideline No. 28. London: RCOG; 2001.

Royal College of Obstetricians and Gynaecologists. *Thromboprophylaxis During Pregnancy, Labour and after Vaginal Delivery*. Guideline No. 37. London: RCOG; 2004.

Task Force on Pulmonary Embolism, European Society of Cardiology. Guidelines on diagnosis and management of acute pulmonary embolism. *Eur Heart J* 2000; 21:1301–36.

Thomson AG, Greer IA. Non-haemorrhagic obstetric shock. *Balliere's Best Practice Res Clin Obstet Gynaecol* 2000;1491:19–41.

Toglia MR, Nolan TE. Venous thromboembolism during pregnancy: a current review of diagnosis and management. *Obstet Gynecol Surv* 1997;52:60–72.

Chapter 7

Airway management and ventilation

Objectives

On successfully completing this topic you will be able to:

- understand the importance of airway patency, maintenance and protection
- identify the circumstances in which airway compromise can occur
- be able to assess and manage the airway and ventilation.

Introduction

An obstructed airway or inadequate ventilation results in tissue hypoxia within minutes and this can lead to organ failure and death. Some organs are more sensitive to hypoxia than others. For example, cerebral hypoxia, even for a short period of time, will cause agitation, then a decreased level of consciousness and eventually, irreversible or fatal brain damage.

Management of the airway is of first concern because obstruction to the airway can quickly result in hypoxia, with damage or death. The next presenting threat to life results from inadequate ventilation (breathing) so attention to this is given next priority.

Supplementary oxygen must be administered to all seriously injured and ill patients through a tight-fitting facemask attached to a reservoir bag at a flow of 12–15 litres/minute (full on at the wall rotameter). The primary goal in providing supplementary oxygen is to maximise the delivery of oxygen to the cells. A pocket mask with an oxygen flow can deliver up to 55% oxygen when attached to high flow oxygen. A correctly fitting bag-valve-mask system with a reservoir can be used to deliver up to 100% oxygen to the lungs.

Carbon dioxide is produced by cellular metabolism and carried in the blood to the lungs to be exhaled. If there is airway obstruction, there is a build up of carbon dioxide in the blood (hypercarbia), which causes drowsiness, acidosis and a rise in intracranial pressure secondary to vasodilatation.

A before B before C before D

Importance of patency, maintenance and protection of airway

The airway must be open, maintained and protected if there is risk of regurgitation and aspiration (which there is in the heavily pregnant patient). The gold standard for doing this is intubation. If there is a B problem, ventilatory support may also be necessary once you have established a patent airway.

Circumstances in which an airway problem is likely to occur

Suspect an airway problem in:

- patient with decreased level of consciousness (because there is reduced muscle tone and the tongue is likely to slip back into the pharynx):
  - ☐ hypoxia
  - ☐ hypotension
  - ☐ eclampsia
  - ☐ poisoning
  - ☐ alcohol
  - ☐ intracranial pathology or injury.
- maxillofacial injuries:
  - ☐ mid-face fractures can move backwards and block the airway
  - ☐ mandibular fractures can allow the tongue to fall backwards
  - ☐ bleeding and secretions caused by these injuries can block or soil the airway.
- open injuries to the neck:
  - ☐ direct trauma to the larynx and supporting structures
  - ☐ bleeding inside the neck compressing the hypopharynx or trachea.
- burns to the face and neck: swelling of the upper and lower airway due to direct burns or inhaling hot smoke, gases or steam, will cause airway obstruction.

Airway problems may be:

- immediate (block the airway quickly) or
- delayed (come on after a time delay – minutes or hours) or
- deteriorate with time – this is often insidious because of its slow progression and is easily overlooked (as with burns to the upper airway; consider the potential for deterioration during transfer and if a risk secure a definitive airway before transfer).

An airway that has been cleared may obstruct again:

- if the support for keeping the airway patent is removed (e.g. chin lift)
- if the patient's level of consciousness decreases
- if there is further bleeding into the airway
- if there is increasing swelling in or around the airway.

Assessment of airway

Talk to the patient. Failure to respond implies an obstructed airway or a breathing problem, with inability to exhale enough air to phonate or an altered level of consciousness with the potential for airway compromise. A positive, appropriate reply in a normal voice indicates that the airway is patent, breathing normal and brain perfusion adequate.

Look to see if the patient is agitated, drowsy or cyanosed. The absence of cyanosis does not mean the patient is adequately oxygenated. Look for use of accessory muscles of respiration.

A patient who refuses to lie down quietly may be trying to sit up in an attempt to keep his airway open or his breathing adequate. The abusive patient may be hypoxic and should not be presumed to be merely aggressive or intoxicated.

Listen for abnormal sounds. Snoring, gurgling and gargling sounds are associated with partial obstruction of the pharynx. Hoarseness implies laryngeal injury. An absence of sound does not mean the airway is patent; if the airway is totally obstructed there may be total silence.

Feel for air movement on expiration and check if the trachea is in the midline.

Assessment of ventilation

To make the airway patent is the first step but only the first step. A patent airway allows oxygen to pass to the lungs but this will only happen with adequate ventilation. Ventilation may be compromised by airway obstruction, altered ventilatory mechanics or by central nervous system depression. If breathing is not improved by clearing the airway, attempt to ventilate by facemask. If ventilation is possible the airway is patent but there is a problem with spontaneous ventilation. If ventilation is not possible this would suggest that the airway continues to be obstructed. If there is a problem with spontaneous ventilation look for a cause within the chest or an intra-cranial or spinal injury as a cause and assist ventilation.

- **Inspect**
  Look for chest movement and obvious injuries.

- **Palpate**
  Palpate for chest movement and palpate the back of the patient's chest for injuries. Palpate the trachea, checking it is in the midline.

- **Percuss**
  Percussion should be resonant and equal bilaterally.

- **Auscultate**
  Air entry should be equal bilaterally.

Airway management

Management comprises:

- clearing the obstructed airway

- maintaining the intact airway

- recognising and protecting the airway at risk.

The airway is at risk from aspiration in any patient with reduced level of consciousness, but in the pregnant patient regurgitation is more likely so the potential for aspiration is increased.

Techniques for clearing, maintaining and protecting the airway need be modified in the trauma patient in whom cervical spine injury is suspected or present.

Cervical spine injury is suspected

Cervical spine immobilisation should be instituted wherever there is suspicion of injury either by manual in-line immobilisation or by semi-rigid cervical collar, head blocks and backboard and straps.

Clearing the obstructed airway

In the patient with suspected cervical spine injury, manual inline immobilisation of the cervical spine and airway clearance manoeuvres are carried out together. In a patient with an altered level of consciousness, the tongue falls backwards and obstructs the pharynx. This can be readily corrected by chin lift or jaw thrust manoeuvres and blood and debris cleared by suction.

Chin lift

■ Place the fingers of one hand under the chin and gently lift it upwards to bring the chin anteriorly.

■ This will open the upper airway in 70–80% of patients.

See Figure 7.1.

Do not hyperextend the neck if a cervical spine injury is suspected.

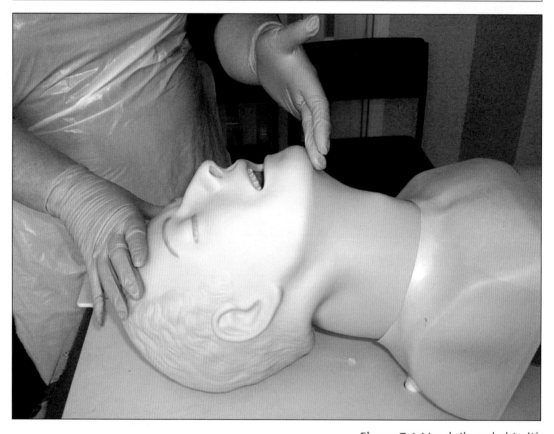

Figure 7.1 Head tilt and chin lift

Jaw thrust

Grasp the angles of the mandible, one hand on each side, and move the mandible forward.

The jaw-thrust is used for the injured patient because it does not destabilise a possible cervical spine fracture and risk converting a fracture without spinal cord injury to one with spinal cord injury.

This manoeuvre will open 95% of obstructed upper airways. See Figure 7.2.

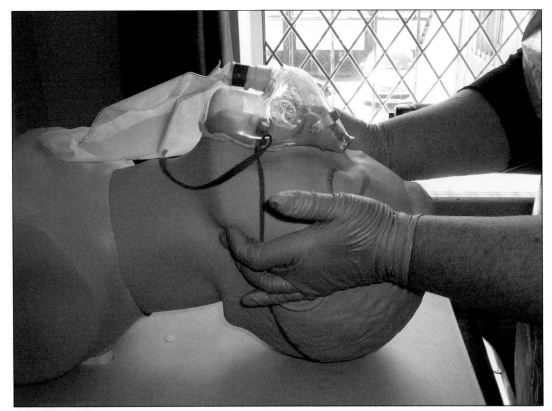

Figure 7.2 Jaw thrust

Suction

Remove blood and secretions from the oropharynx with a rigid suction device (for example, a Yankauer sucker). A patient with facial injuries may have a cribiform plate fracture – in these circumstances suction catheters should not be inserted through the nose, as they could enter the skull and injure the brain.

If attempts to clear the airway do not result in the restoration of spontaneous breathing, this may be because the airway is still not patent or because the airway is patent but there is no breathing. The only way to distinguish these two situations is to put either a pocket mask or facemask over the face and give breaths (either mouth-to-pocket-mask or self-inflating bag to either mask). If the chest rises, this is not an airway problem but a breathing problem. If the chest cannot be made to rise, this is an airway problem.

Clearing the airway may result in improvement in level of consciousness and the patient being able to maintain his own airway.

If the patient cannot maintain their own airway continue with the jaw-thrust or chin-lift or try using an oropharyngeal airway.

Oropharyngeal airway

The oropharyngeal airway (Guedel type) is inserted into the mouth over the tongue. It stops the tongue falling back and provides a clear passage for airflow.

The preferred method is to insert the airway concavity upwards until the tip reaches the soft palate and then rotate it 180 degrees, slipping it into place over the tongue.

Make sure that the oropharyngeal airway does not push the tongue backwards as this will block rather than open the patient's airway.

A patient with a gag reflex may not tolerate the oral airway. See Figure 7.3.

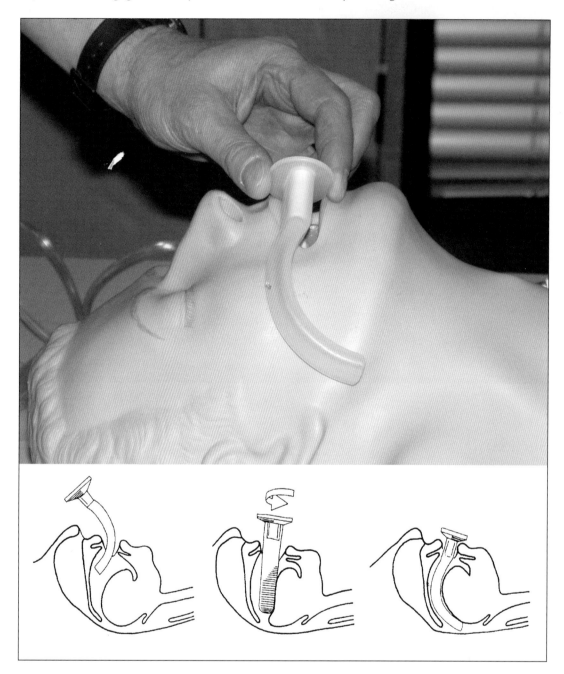

Figure 7.3 Oropharyngeal airway

Nasopharyngeal airway

A nasopharyngeal airway is better tolerated than the oropharyngeal airway by the more responsive patient. It is contraindicated if there is a suspected fractured base of skull. Be aware of the potential for this to cause bleeding, which may soil the lungs of a patient with obtunded laryngeal or pharyngeal reflexes (the unconscious or hypotensive patient). It should only be used if there is an airway problem, an oropharyngeal airway is not tolerated and an anaesthetist is unavailable.

BE VERY RELUCTANT TO USE.

Nasal airways (Figure 7.4) do not have a large part to play in contemporary UK anaesthetic practice because of their potential to cause bleeding. Their use is limited to intensive care units where they might be placed by physiotherapists or anaesthetists to facilitate suctioning of chest secretions.

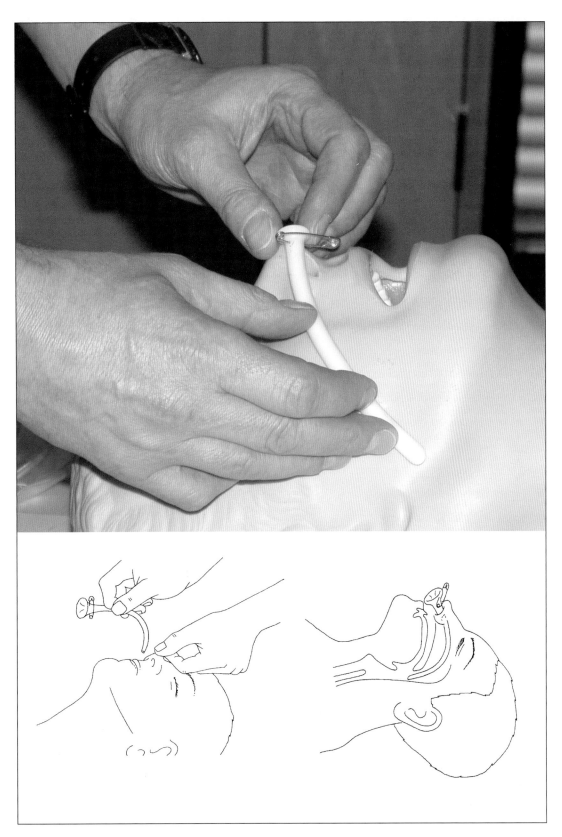

Figure 7.4 Nasopharyngeal airway

Lubricate the airway and insert it through either nostril, straight backwards – not upwards – so that its tip enters the hypopharynx.

A safety pin should be applied across the proximal end before insertion to prevent the tube disappearing into the airway.

Gentle insertion, good lubrication and using an airway that passes easily into the nose will decrease the incidence of bleeding.

The oropharyngeal and nasopharyngeal devices maintain the airway but do not protect it from aspiration.

Advanced airway techniques

Definitive airway is a gold standard for opening, maintaining and protecting the airway. It means that there is a cuffed tube in the trachea attached to oxygen and secured in place. Advanced airway techniques provide a definitive airway.

Advanced airway techniques may be required:

- in cases of apnoea
- when the above techniques fail
- to maintain an airway over the longer term
- to protect an airway
- to allow accurate control of oxygenation and ventilation
- when there is the potential for airway obstruction
- to control carbon dioxide levels in the unconscious patient, as a way of minimising the rise in intracranial pressure.

Advanced airway techniques are:

- endotracheal intubation
- surgical cricothyroidotomy
- surgical tracheostomy.

The circumstances and urgency determine the type of advanced airway technique to be used.

Note: The pregnant woman is at increased risk of gastric regurgitation because she has a mechanical obstruction to gastric emptying and reduced lower oesophogeal barrier as a result of hormonal effects on the smooth muscle. Trauma patients are at increased risk of regurgitation because of reduced gastric emptying. Consequently, the pregnant woman (with or without trauma) without adequate pharyngeal and laryngeal reflexes (unconscious or hypotensive) is at increased risk of pulmonary aspiration. The chemical pneumonitis suffered when a pregnant woman aspirates is more severe than in a nonpregnant woman, as the gastric aspirate is more acidic in pregnancy. Consider early definitive airway.

Endotracheal intubation

In a patient with airway or respiratory compromise, the primary aim is to oxygenate the patient and this can initially be successfully achieved by positioning, use of oropharyngeal airways and use of facemask and self-inflating bag.

If this cannot be achieved, intubation is needed. It should only be carried out without drugs where there is an urgent need for intubation, i.e. in the case of complete airway obstruction or a respiratory arrest, where the airway cannot be otherwise maintained.

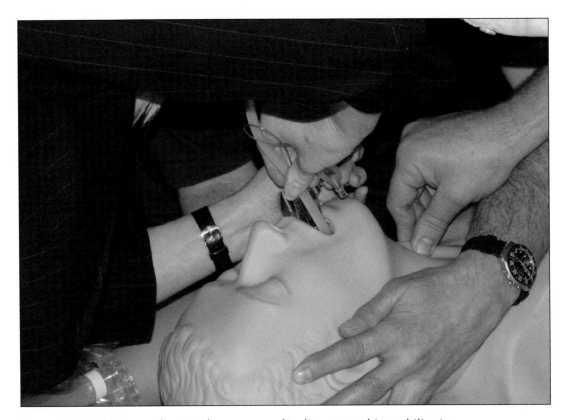

Figure 7.5 Intubation with cricoid pressure and in-line manual immobilisation

It should be emphasised that heavily pregnant women are difficult to ventilate with a bag and mask and to intubate, because of weight gain during pregnancy and the potential for large breasts falling back into the working space. Consequently, for a surgeon or obstetrician, a surgical airway may sometimes be the preferred option.

Oral endotracheal intubation is most commonly used. This uses a laryngoscope to visualise the vocal cords. A cuffed endotracheal tube is placed through the vocal cords into the trachea (Figure 7.5). This skill will be practised in the skill station.

Tracheal intubation without using drugs is not possible unless the patient is very deeply unconscious or has sustained a cardiac arrest. If the patient is unconscious, intracranial pathology is implied and intubation without anaesthetic and muscle relaxation drugs will cause increases in blood pressure and intracranial pressure, which will exacerbate the intracranial condition. Intubation is therefore always a threat to patient wellbeing unless drugs are used.

Anaesthetic involvement in intubation

Drugs should only be used to intubate by those with adequate anaesthetic training

Where anaesthetic skills and drugs are available, endotracheal intubation is the preferred method of securing a definitive airway. This technique comprises:

- rapid sequence induction of anaesthesia ('crash induction')
  - ☐ preoxygenation
  - ☐ application of cricoid pressure
  - ☐ rapid unconsciousness using drugs
  - ☐ no 'bagging'
  - ☐ rapid placement of endotracheal tube in trachea
  - ☐ inflation of cuff before removal of cricoid pressure
- maintenance of cervical spine immobilisation when indicated.

Meticulous care must be taken to keep the cervical spine immobilised if injury to the cervical spine is suspected.

Intermittent oxygenation during difficult intubation

Inability to intubate will not kill. Inability to oxygenate will.

If you can oxygenate by bag and mask, this will keep the patient alive.

Avoid prolonged efforts to intubate without intermittently oxygenating and ventilating. Practise taking a deep breath when starting an attempt at intubation. If you have to take a further breath before successfully intubating the patient, abort the attempt and reoxygenate using the bag and mask technique.

Correct placement of the endotracheal tube

To check correct placement of the endotracheal tube:

- see the endotracheal tube pass between the vocal cords
- listen on both sides in the mid-axillary line for equal breath sounds
- listen over the stomach for gurgling sounds during assisted ventilation for evidence of oesophageal intubation
- monitor end-tidal carbon dioxide levels
- if in doubt about the position of the endotracheal tube, take it out and oxygenate the patient by another method, bag and mask or surgical airway.

See Figure 7.6.

Other methods for maintaining the airway (not definitive airway as still unprotected):

Laryngeal mask airway (LMA) and Combitubes are used to make an airway patent and to maintain it. They do not have a place in the conventional management of the trauma or obstetric patient, at high risk of aspiration, as they do not protect the airway. They would be used only in a dire emergency where the airway could not be opened or maintained by other methods. Manually ventilating via a laryngeal mask can cause further problems in that the stomach can become inflated, further predisposing to regurgitation.

Needle cricothyroidotomy can be used to oxygenate in an emergency but it is not a definitive airway. A cannula-over-needle device is inserted through the cricothyroid membrane and attached to a flow of oxygen from an insufflation device or through oxygen tubing connected to wall oxygen at 15 litres/minute with either a Y-connector, three-way tap or side hole in the tubing at the cannula end of the tubing.

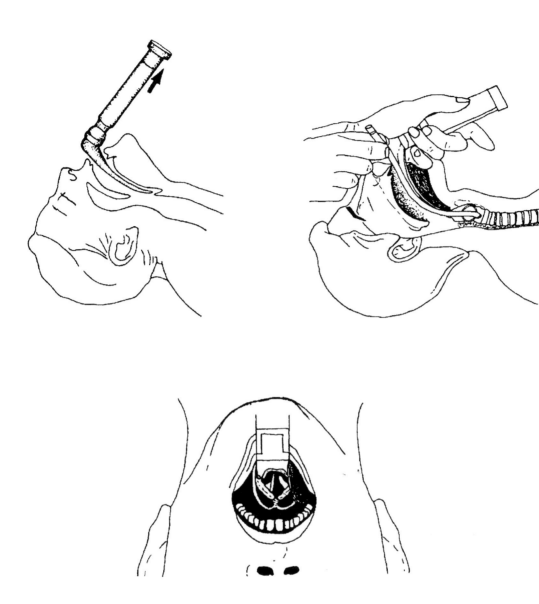

Figure 7.6 Endotracheal intubation

Intermittent insufflation can be carried out by occlusion of the open lumens or side hole, 1 second held on then 4 seconds off. During the 4 seconds off, some exhalation occurs but, if there is complete or near complete airway obstruction proximal to the needle device, intrathoracic pressure can rise (with consequent barotrauma such as tension pneumothorax or pulmonary rupture). This technique does not allow adequate ventilation so CO_2 levels rise. It can only be used for 30–40 minutes. It may buy time for skilled personnel capable of providing a definitive airway to arrive. It is further limited in patients with high intrathoracic pressures (such as the heavily pregnant patient) or chest injuries.

Cannula-over-needle cricothyroiotomy kits, which are superior to the intravenous cannula that was used in the past, are now available. 'Difficult intubation' trolleys would routinely carry one; familiarise yourself with the one in your own unit. This skill will be practised in the skill station. In addition curved hollow needles designed to provide an emergency airway can be directly connected to a high-pressure oxygen source (e.g. Manujet). These techniques allow oxygenation until a definitive airway is secured.

Fibreoptic intubation is an alternative if a suitably skilled anaesthetist is available.

Surgical airway

A surgical airway should not be undertaken lightly and is used when:

- a hypoxic patient needing a definitive airway for resuscitation is too awake to tolerate endotracheal intubation without the use of anaesthetic drugs and there is no anaesthetist available to intubate in this way in the time span in which the definitive airway is required

- trauma to the face and neck makes endotracheal intubation impossible

- a patient with face and neck burns requires airway protection to pre-empt delayed obstruction but expert anaesthetic help is unavailable to carry out endotracheal intubation

- the anaesthetist cannot intubate or ventilate, e.g. at caesarean section.

Surgical cricothyroidotomy

Surgical cricothyroidotomy places a tube into the trachea via the cricothyroid membrane (see Figures 7.7 and 7.8). A small tracheostomy tube (5–7 mm) is suitable. During the procedure, appropriate cervical spine protection must be maintained when indicated. There are also commercially available surgical cricothyroidotomy sets. A cricothyroidotomy can be replaced by a formal tracheostomy (if needed) at a later time.

Emergency tracheostomy

A formal surgical tracheostomy takes longer and is more difficult than a surgical cricothyroidotomy. Commercial sets are available for rapid percutaneous tracheostomy using a Seldinger (guidewire) technique.

Management of ventilation

Once the airway is patent and maintained there may be a separate requirement to assist breathing (ventilation). Spontaneous ventilation (self-ventilation) means the same as breathing. Assisted (artificial) ventilation means the patient is receiving help with breathing. The aim is to improve gaseous exchange in the lungs and to breathe for the patient if spontaneous ventilation has stopped or is inadequate. The indication for assisted ventilation is when ventilation is inadequate as in:

- chest injury

- respiratory depression due to drugs (such as opiates)

- head injury which might be causing respiratory depression and which requires end tidal carbon dioxide levels to be closely controlled to prevent cerebral vasodilatation and a consequent rise in intracranial pressure.

Assisted ventilation can be achieved by the following techniques:

- mouth-to-mouth (or nose) – unlikely in hospital

- mouth to pocket-mask

- self-inflating bag to pocket mask or facemask

- self-inflating bag to endotracheal tube or tracheostomy tube

- automatic ventilation via endotracheal tube or tracheostomy tube.

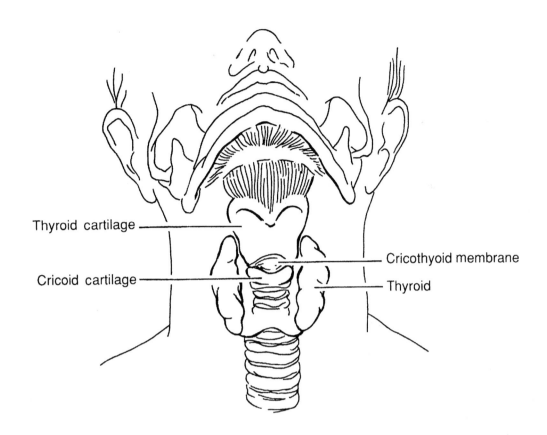

Thyroid cartilage ——————

Cricoid cartilage ——————

—————— Cricothyoid membrane

—————— Thyroid

Figure 7.7 Anatomical landmarks for surgical airway

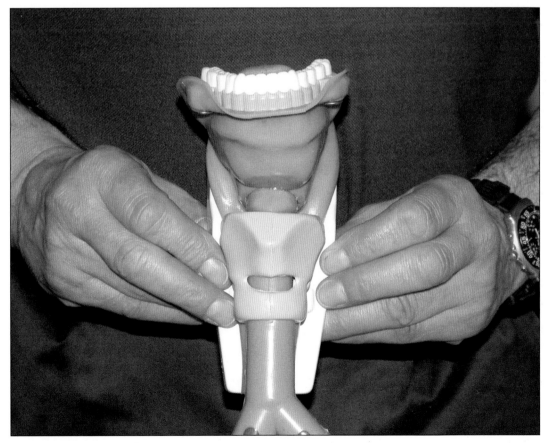

Figure 7.8 Anatomy of airway

Summary

■ Talk, look, listen, feel.

■ Primary aim is to provide adequate oxygenation.

■ Try simple manoeuvres, i.e. chin lift, jaw thrust, suction.

■ Try simple adjuncts, namely the oropharyngeal airway.

■ Tracheal intubation, endotracheal or surgical airway is gold standard because this makes the airway patent, maintains patency and protects the airway.

■ Beware of cervical spine injury during airway management.

Appendix 7A

Practical procedures

Reproduced with permission from the Advanced Life Support Group.

Oropharyngeal airway

Equipment

■ A series of oropharyngeal (Guedel) airways.

■ Tongue depressor.

■ Laryngoscope.

Procedure

The correct size of airway is selected by comparing it with the vertical distance from the angle of the mandible to the centre of the incisors. The airway is inserted in adults and older children as follows:

■ Open the patient's mouth and check for debris. Debris may be inadvertently pushed into the larynx as the airway is inserted.

■ Insert the airway into the mouth either:
    (i)   'upside down' (concave uppermost) as far as the junction between the hard and soft palates and rotate through 180 degrees or
    (ii)   use a tongue depressor or the tip of a laryngoscope blade to aid insertion of the airway 'the right way up' under direct vision.

■ Insert so that the flange lies in front of the upper and lower incisors or gums in the edentulous patient (Figure 7A.1).

■ Check the patency of the airway and ventilation by 'looking, listening, and feeling'.

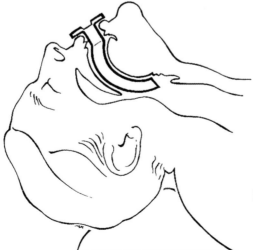

Figure 7A.1 Oropharyngeal airway in situ

Complications

■ Trauma resulting in bleeding.

■ Vomiting or laryngospasm if the patient is not deeply unconscious.

Laerdal pocket mask

Equipment

■ Laerdal pocket mask.

■ Airway manikin.

Procedure

■ With the patient supine, apply the mask to the patient's face, using the thumbs and index fingers of both hands.

■ Use the remaining fingers to exert pressure behind the angles of the jaw (as for the jaw thrust), at the same time pressing the mask on to the face to make a tight seal (Figure 7A.2).

■ Blow through the inspiratory valve for 1–2 seconds, at the same time looking to ensure that the chest rises and then falls.

■ If oxygen is available, add via the nipple at 12–15 litres/minute.

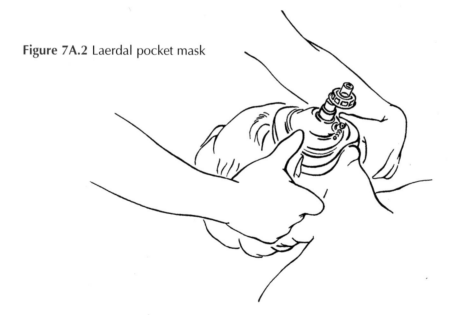

Figure 7A.2 Laerdal pocket mask

Insertion of the laryngeal mask airway

Equipment

■ Lubricant.

■ Syringe to inflate cuff.

■ Adhesive tape to secure laryngeal mask airway.

■ Suction.

■ Ventilating device.

Procedure

■ Whenever possible, ventilate the patient with 100% oxygen using a bag–valve–mask device before inserting the laryngeal mask airway. During this time, check that all the equipment is present and working, particularly the integrity of the cuff.

■ Deflate the cuff and lightly lubricate the back and sides of the mask.

■ Tilt the patient's head (if safe to do so), open the mouth fully and insert the tip of the mask along the hard palate with the open side facing, but not touching the tongue (Figure 7A.3a).

■ Insert the mask further, along the posterior pharyngeal wall, with your index finger initially providing support for the tube (Figure A.3b). Eventually, resistance is felt as the tip of the laryngeal mask airway lies at the upper end of the oesophagus (Figure 7A.3c).

■ Fully inflate the cuff using the air filled syringe attached to the valve at the end of the pilot tube using the volume of air shown in the earlier box (Figure 7A.3d).

■ Secure the laryngeal mask airway with adhesive tape and check its position during ventilation as for a tracheal tube.

■ If insertion is not accomplished in less than 30 seconds, re-establish ventilation using a bag–valve–mask.

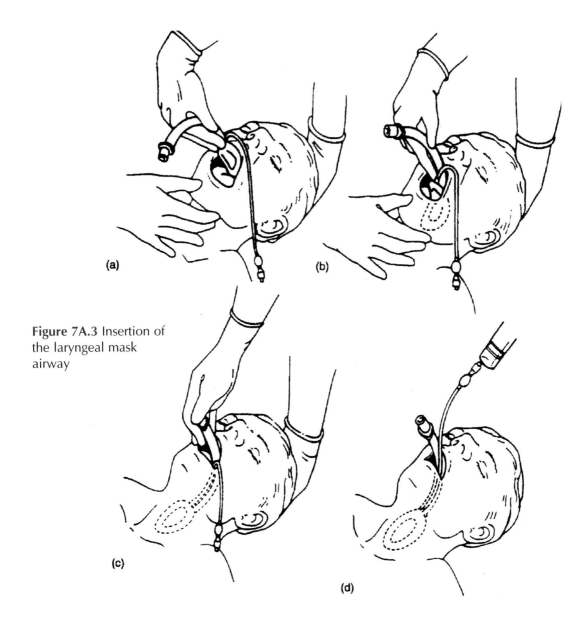

(a)

(b)

Figure 7A.3 Insertion of the laryngeal mask airway

(c)

(d)

Complications

Incorrect placement is usually due to the tip of the cuff folding over during insertion. The laryngeal mask airway should be withdrawn and reinserted.

Inability to ventilate the patient can be because the epiglottis has been displaced over the larynx. Withdraw the laryngeal mask airway and reinsert it, ensuring that it closely follows the hard palate. This may be facilitated by the operator or an assistant lifting the jaw upwards. Occasionally, rotation of the laryngeal mask airway may prevent its insertion. Check that the line along the tube is aligned with the patient's nasal septum; if not, reinsert.

Coughing or laryngeal spasm is usually due to attempts to insert the laryngeal mask airway into a patient whose laryngeal reflexes are still present.

Intubation via the laryngeal mask airway

Insert an introducer through the laryngeal mask airway into the trachea, remove the laryngeal mask airway and then pass the tracheal tube over the introducer into the trachea. Alternatively, a small diameter cuffed tracheal tube (6 mm) may be passed directly through a size-4 laryngeal mask airway into the trachea. A laryngeal mask airway is currently being designed to allow intubation through it with a larger diameter tracheal tube.

The surgical airway

It is important to realise that these techniques are temporary measures, while preparing for a definitive airway.

Needle cricothyroidotomy

Equipment

- Venflons 12–14 gauge.
- Jet insufflation equipment.
- Oxygen tubing with either a three-way tap or a hole cut in the side.
- 20 ml syringe.
- Manikin or sheep's larynx.

Procedure

- Place the patient supine with the head slightly extended.
- Identify the cricothyroid membrane as the recess between the thyroid cartilage (Adam's apple) and cricoid cartilage (approximately 2 cm below the V-shaped notch of the thyroid cartilage) (Figure 7A.4).
- Puncture this membrane vertically using a large-bore (12–14 gauge) intravenous cannula attached to a syringe.
- Aspiration of air confirms that the tip of the cannula lies within the tracheal lumen.
- Angle the cannula at 45 degrees caudally and advance over the needle into the trachea (Figure 7A.5).
- Attach the cannula to an oxygen supply at 12–15 litres/minute either via a 'Y' connector or a hole cut in the side of the oxygen tubing. Oxygen is delivered to the patient by occluding the open limb of the connector or side hole for 1 second and then releasing for 4 seconds.

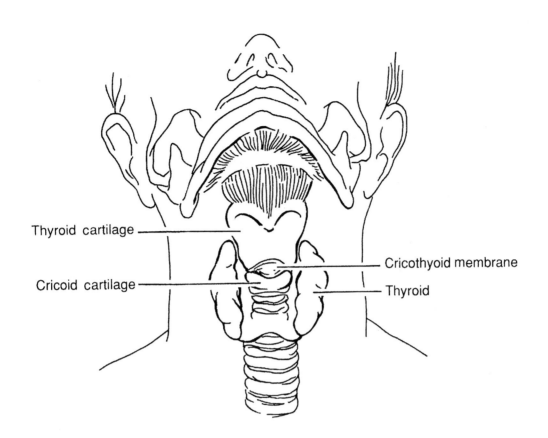

Figure 7A.4 Cricothyroidotomy: relevant anatomy

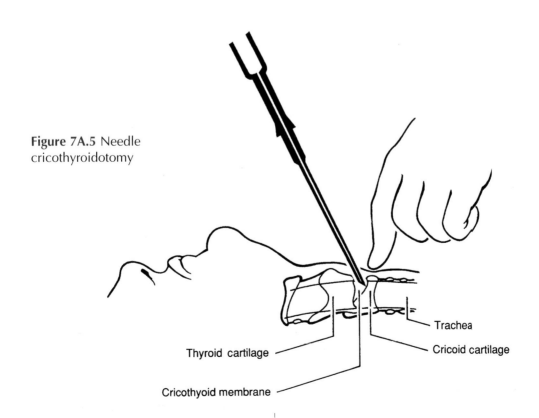

Figure 7A.5 Needle cricothyroidotomy

■ Expiration occurs passively through the larynx. Watch the chest for movement and auscultate for breath sounds, although the latter are difficult to hear.

■ If satisfactory, secure the cannula in place to prevent it being dislodged.

An alternative method of delivering oxygen is to use jet ventilation. This involves connecting the cannula to a high-pressure oxygen source (4 bar, 400 kPa, 60 psi) via luerlock connectors or by using a Sanders injector. The same ventilatory cycle is used.

Complications

■ Asphyxia.

■ Pulmonary barotrauma.

■ Bleeding.

■ Oesophageal perforation.

■ Kinking of the cannula.

■ Subcutaneous and mediastinal emphysema.

■ Aspiration.

■ Occasionally, this method of oxygenation will disimpact a foreign body from the larynx, allowing more acceptable methods of ventilation to be used.

There are two important facts to remember about transtracheal insufflation of oxygen:

■ It is not possible to deliver oxygen via a needle cricothyroidotomy using a self-inflating bag and valve. This is because these devices do not generate sufficient pressure to drive adequate volumes of gas through a narrow cannula. In comparison, the wall oxygen supply will provide a pressure of 400 kPa (4000 cm H_2O), which overcomes the resistance of the cannula.

■ Expiration cannot occur through the cannula or through a separate cannula inserted through the cricothyroid membrane. The pressure generated during expiration is generally less than 3 kPa (30 cm H_2O), which is clearly much less than the pressure required to drive gas in initially. Expiration must occur through the upper airway, even when partially obstructed. If the obstruction is complete, then the oxygen flow must be reduced to 2–4 litres/minute to avoid the risk of barotrauma, in particular the creation of a tension pneumothorax.

Surgical cricothyroidotomy

Equipment

■ Antiseptic solution.

■ Swab.

■ Syringe, needle, and local anaesthetic.

■ Scalpel.

■ Two arterial clips.

■ Endotracheal tube or size-5 tracheotomy tubes.

■ Tape.

■ Gloves.

■ Manikin or sheep's larynx.

Procedure

- Place the patient supine if possible, with the head extended.
- Identify the cricothyroid membrane as described earlier (Figure A.4).
- Stabilise the thyroid cartilage using the thumb, index and middle fingers of the left hand.
- If the patient is conscious, consider infiltrating with local anaesthetic containing epinephrine (adrenaline) (lignocaine 1% with epinephrine 1/200 000).
- Make a longitudinal incision down to the membrane, pressing the lateral edges of the skin outwards to reduce bleeding.
- Incise the membrane transversely and dilate the channel with the scalpel handle to accept a small (4–7 mm) cuffed tracheostomy tube. If one of these is not immediately available, a similarly sized tracheal tube can be used.
- Ensure that the tube enters the tracheal lumen, rather than just running anteriorly in the soft tissues.
- Inflate the cuff and commence ventilation.
- Check the adequacy of ventilation as described earlier and, if satisfactory, the tube can be secured.
- Suction the upper airway via the tube to remove any inhaled blood or vomit.

An alternative technique in these circumstances is the 'Mini-Trach' (Portex). This was originally designed to facilitate the removal of secretions from the chest. The 'kit' contains everything required to create an emergency surgical airway.

- Use a guarded scalpel to puncture the cricothyroid membrane percutaneously to the correct depth.
- Pass the rigid, curved introducer through the puncture site into the trachea.
- Pass the 4-mm PVC flanged tracheal cannula (with a standard 15-mm connector attached) over the introducer into the trachea.
- Remove the introducer and secure the cannula via the flanges with tapes. Ventilate the patient using the devices already described.

Complications

- Similar to needle cricothyroidotomy, except that bleeding is more profuse due to the larger incision
- Vocal cord damage may result in hoarseness.
- Cricoid cartilage damage may cause laryngeal stenosis.

Algorithm 8.1 **Newborn resuscitation**

(Reproduced with permission from the Advanced Life Support Group)

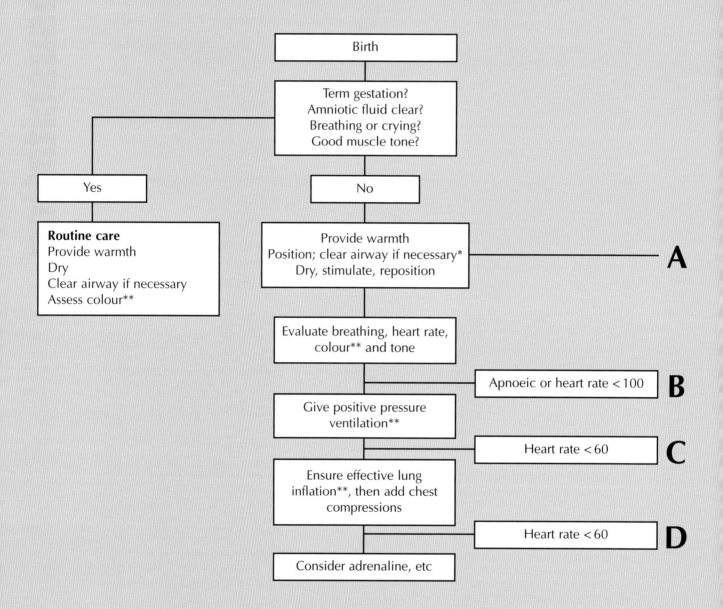

* Tracheal intubation may be considered at several steps
** Consider supplemental oxygen at any stage if cyanosis persists

Chapter 8

Resuscitation of the baby at birth

Reproduced with permission from the Advanced Life Support Group.

Objectives

On successfully completing this topic you will understand:

■ the important physiological differences in the newborn baby

■ the equipment used for resuscitation at birth

■ how to assess the baby at birth

■ how to resuscitate the baby at birth

■ additional measures for special situations.

Introduction

The resuscitation of babies at birth is different from the resuscitation of all other age groups, and knowledge of the relevant physiology and pathophysiology is essential. However, the majority of babies will establish normal respiration and circulation at delivery without help. Ideally, someone trained in newborn resuscitation should be present at all deliveries. All those who attend deliveries should attend courses such as the Newborn Life Support Course, organised by the Resuscitation Council (UK) or the Neonatal Resuscitation Programme, organised by the American Academy of Pediatrics. However, some babies are born in unexpected places, such as accident and emergency departments. For these situations, it is important that clinicians have an understanding of the differences in resuscitating a baby at birth.

Normal physiology

At birth, the baby must change, within a matter of moments, from an organism with fluid-filled lungs whose respiratory function is carried out by the placenta to a separate being whose air-filled lungs can successfully take over this function. Preparation for this begins during labour, when the fluid-producing cells within the lung cease secretion and begin reabsorption of that fluid. Delivery by caesarean section before the onset of labour may slow the clearance of pulmonary fluid from the lungs.

During vaginal delivery some lung fluid, perhaps 35 ml in a term baby, is expelled by passage through the birth canal. In a healthy baby, the first spontaneous breaths may generate a negative pressure of between –40 cm H_2O and –100 cm H_2O (–3.9 and –9.8 kPa), which aerates the lungs for the first time. This pressure difference is 10–15 times greater than that needed for later breathing but appears to be necessary to overcome the viscosity of the fluid filling the airways, the surface tension of the fluid-filled lungs and the elastic recoil and resistance of the chest wall, lungs and airways. These powerful chest movements cause fluid to be displaced from the airways into the lymphatics and circulation.

After delivery, a healthy term baby usually takes its first breath within 60–90 seconds of clamping or obstructing the umbilical cord. Separation of the placenta or clamping of the cord leads to the onset of hypoxia with hypercarbia, which is initially a major stimulant to start respiration. Physical stimuli such as cold air or physical discomfort may also provoke respiratory efforts.

In a 3-kg baby, up to 100 ml of fluid is cleared from the airways following the initial breaths, a process aided by full inflation and prolonged high pressure on expiration, i.e. crying. The effect of the first few breaths is to produce the baby's functional residual capacity. Neonatal circulatory adaptation commences with the detachment of the placenta, but lung inflation and alveolar distension release mediators, which affect the pulmonary vasculature as well as increase oxygenation.

Pathophysiology

Our knowledge of the pathophysiology of fetal asphyxia is based on pioneering animal work in the early 1960s. The results of these experiments, which followed the physiology of newborn animals during acute, total, prolonged asphyxia and subsequent resuscitation are summarised in Figure 8.1.

When the placental oxygen supply is interrupted, the fetus attempts to breathe. Should these attempts fail to inflate the lung with air – as they will inevitably fail to do *in utero* – the baby will lose consciousness. If hypoxia continues, the respiratory centre becomes unable, through lack of sufficient oxygen, to continue initiating breathing and the breathing stops, usually within 2–3 minutes.

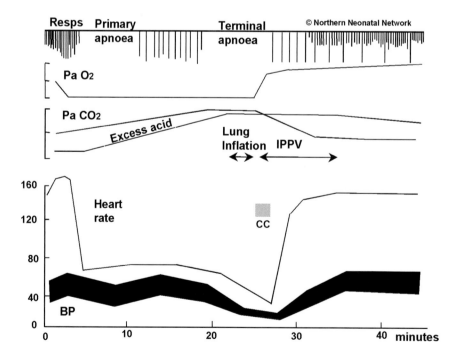

Figure 8.1 Response of babies born in terminal apnoea. In this case lung inflation is not sufficient because the circulation is already falling. However, lung inflation delivers air to the lungs and then a brief period of chest compressions (CC) delivers oxygenated blood to the heart which then responds (reproduced with permission from the Northern Neonatal Network)

Fetal bradycardia ensues but blood pressure is maintained, primarily by peripheral vaso-constriction and diversion of blood away from non-vital organs, and also by an increased stroke volume. After a latent period of apnoea (primary), primitive spinal centres, no longer suppressed by neural signals from the respiratory centre, will initiate primitive gasping breaths. These deep spontaneous gasps are easily distinguishable from normal breaths as they only occur 6–12 times/minute and involve all accessory muscles in a maximal inspiratory effort. After a while, if hypoxia continues, even this activity ceases (terminal apnoea). The time taken for such activity to cease is longer in the newly born baby than in later life, taking up to 20 minutes.

The circulation is almost always maintained until all respiratory activity ceases. This resilience is a feature of all newborn mammals at term, largely due to the reserves of glycogen in the heart. Resuscitation is therefore relatively easy if undertaken before all respiratory activity has stopped. Once the lungs are inflated, oxygenated blood will be carried to the heart and then to the brain provided the circulation is still functional. Recovery will then be rapid. Most infants who have not progressed to terminal apnoea will resuscitate themselves if their airway is patent. Once gasping ceases, however, the circulation starts to fail and these infants are likely to need more extensive resuscitation (Figure 8.1).

Equipment

For many newborn babies, especially those born outside the delivery room, the need for resuscitation cannot be predicted. It is therefore useful to plan for such an eventuality.

Equipment that may be required to resuscitate a newborn baby is listed in Box 8.1.

Box 8.1: Equipment that may be required to resuscitate a newborn baby

- A flat surface
- Radiant heat source and dry towels (or suitable plastic bags for preterm infants)
- Suction with catheters at least 12 Fr
- Face masks
- Bag–valve–mask or T piece with pressure-limiting device
- Source of air and/or oxygen
- Oropharyngeal (Guedel) airways
- Laryngoscopes with straight blades, 0 and 1
- Nasogastric tubes
- Cord clamp
- Scissors
- Tracheal tubes sizes 2.5–4.0 mm
- Umbilical catheterisation equipment
- Adhesive tape
- Disposable gloves

The list will vary between departments; however, most babies can be resuscitated with a flat surface, warmth, knowledge and a way to deliver air or oxygen at a controlled pressure.

Practical aspects of neonatal resuscitation

Most babies, even those born apnoeic, will resuscitate themselves given a clear airway. However, the basic approach to resuscitation is **A**irway, **B**reathing and **C**irculation, with the following initial actions:

■ get help

■ start the clock

■ dry, wrap and keep baby warm

■ assess baby.

Call for help

Ask for help if you expect or encounter any difficulty.

Start clock

Start the clock, if available, or note the time.

Keep the baby warm

Dry the baby off immediately and then wrap in a dry towel. A cold baby has increased oxygen consumption and cold babies are more likely to become hypoglycaemic and acidotic. They also have an increased mortality. If this is not addressed at the beginning of resuscitation it is often forgotten. Most of the heat loss is evaporative heat loss caused by the baby being wet and in a draught – hence the need to dry the baby and then to wrap the baby in a dry towel. Babies also have a large surface area to weight ratio; thus, heat can be lost very quickly. Ideally, delivery should take place in a warm room, and an overhead heater should be switched on. However, drying effectively and wrapping the baby in a warm dry towel is the most important factor in avoiding hypothermia. A naked wet baby can still become hypothermic despite a warm room and a radiant heater, especially if there is a draught (see **Preterm babies**).

Assessment of the newborn baby

The APGAR score was proposed as a tool for evaluating a baby's condition at birth as a means of judging the quality of obstetric anaesthesia. Although the score, calculated at 1 and 5 minutes, may be of some use retrospectively, it is almost always recorded subjectively. It is not used to guide resuscitation.

Acute assessment is made by assessing:

Airway

Breathing (rate and quality)

Circulation:

    Heart rate (fast, slow, absent)

    Colour (pink, blue, pale)

    Tone (unconscious, apnoeic babies are floppy).

Unlike resuscitation at other ages, it is important to assess the situation fully so one can judge the success of interventions. This is especially true of heart rate.

Respiration

Most babies will establish spontaneous regular breathing within 3 minutes of birth that is sufficient to maintain the heart rate above 100 beats/minute and to improve the skin colour. If apnoea or gasping persists after drying, intervention is required.

Heart rate

Listening with a stethoscope at the cardiac apex is the best method to assess the heart rate. Palpating peripheral pulses is not practical and cannot be recommended. Palpation of the umbilical pulse can only be relied upon if it is more than 100 beats/minute. A rate less than this should be checked by auscultation if possible. An initial assessment of heart rate is vital because an increase in the heart rate will be the first sign of success during resuscitation. This initial assessment will categorise the baby into one of the three following groups:

1. Regular breathing, fast heart rate (more than 100 beats/minute) pink, good tone.

    These are healthy babies and they should be kept warm and given to their mothers. The baby will remain warm through skin-to-skin contact with the mother under a cover and may be put to the breast at this stage.

2. Irregular or inadequate breathing, slow heart rate (less than 100 beats/min), blue, normal or reduced tone.

    If gentle stimulation (such as drying) does not induce effective breathing, the airway should be opened and cleared. If the baby responds then no further resuscitation is needed. If there is no response, progress to lung inflation.

3. Not breathing, slow or absent heart rate (less than 100 beats/minute), blue or pale, floppy.

Whether an apnoeic baby is in primary or secondary apnoea (Figure 8.1) the initial management is the same. Open the airway and then inflate the lungs. Reassessment of any heart rate response then directs further resuscitation. Reassess the heart rate and respiration at regular intervals throughout. Apnoea, low or absent heart rate, pallor and floppiness together suggest terminal apnoea.

Resuscitation

After assessment, resuscitation follows:

■ airway

■ breathing

■ circulation

■ use of drugs in a few selected cases.

Airway

The baby should be positioned with the head in the neutral position (Figure 8.2).

The newborn baby's head has a large occiput, which is often exaggerated further by moulding. This tends to cause the neck to flex with consequent obstruction of the airway when the baby is supine on a flat surface. However, overextension may collapse the newborn baby's pharyngeal airway, also leading to obstruction. A towel folded to a thickness of about 2–3 cm and placed under the shoulders may help to maintain the airway in a neutral position.

If the baby is very floppy then jaw thrust may be needed to bring the tongue forward and open the airway (Figure 8.3). Visible secretions may be removed by gentle suction with a paediatric Yankauer or 12–14 Fr suction catheter, although these rarely cause airway obstruction. Blind deep pharyngeal suction should be avoided as it may cause vagally induced bradycardia and laryngospasm. Suction, if it is used, should not exceed –100 mmHg (9.8 kPa). The presence of thick meconium (see below) in a non-vigorous baby is the only indication for considering immediate suction.

Meconium aspiration

Meconium-stained liquor is relatively common and occurs in up to 10% of births. Happily, meconium aspiration is a rare event. Meconium aspiration usually happens in term infants and

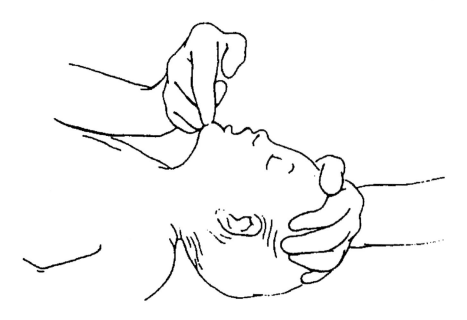

Figure 8.2 Chin lift in infants

before delivery. A large randomised trial has shown no advantage to suctioning meconium from the mouth and nose while the head is on the perineum. This practice is, therefore, no longer recommended. Another randomised trial has shown that, if the baby is vigorous, then intubation followed by immediate suctioning of the trachea offers no advantage either and no specific action (other than drying and wrapping the baby) is needed. However, if the baby is not vigorous (that is, has absent or inadequate respirations, a heart rate of less than 100 beats/minute or hypotonia) then our current state of knowledge suggests that you should inspect the oropharynx with a laryngoscope and aspirate any particulate meconium seen using a wide-bore catheter.

If intubation is possible and the baby is still unresponsive, aspirate the trachea, preferably using the tracheal tube as a suction catheter. However, if intubation cannot be achieved immediately, clear the oropharynx and start mask inflation. If, while attempting to clear the airway, the heart rate falls to less than 60 beats/minute then stop airway clearance, give aeration breaths and start ventilating the baby.

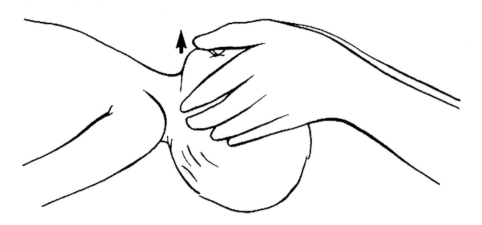

Figure 8.3 Jaw thrust

Breathing (aeration breaths and ventilation)

There is currently insufficient evidence to specify the concentration of oxygen to be used when starting resuscitation at birth. Most experts still use oxygen-enriched air but the absence of oxygen should not delay the delivery of breaths in an apnoeic baby. The priority must be to aerate the lungs. Therefore, the first five breaths should be 'aeration' or 'inflation' breaths in order to replace lung fluid in the alveoli with air/oxygen. These breaths should have a sustained inflation time of 2–3-seconds and are most easily delivered using a continuous gas supply, a pressure-limiting device a T-piece and a mask. Use a transparent, circular mask big enough to cover the nose and mouth of the baby (Figure 8.4). If no such system is available then a 500-ml self-inflating bag with a blow-off valve set at 30–40 cm H_2O can be used. This is especially useful if compressed air or oxygen is not available.

The chest may not move during delivery of the first one to three breaths as fluid is displaced by air with little change in chest volume. Adequate ventilation is usually indicated by either a rapidly increasing heart rate or a heart rate that is maintained at more than 100 beats/minute. Therefore, reassess the heart rate after delivery of the first five breaths. It is safe to assume the lungs have been aerated successfully if the heart rate responds. If the heart rate has not responded, then check for chest movement rather than auscultation. In fluid-filled lungs, breath sounds may be heard even when the lung is not aerated.

Once the lung is aerated and the heart rate has increased or if the chest has been seen to move in response to passive inflation then ventilation should be continued at a rate of 30–40 ventilations/minute.

Continue ventilatory support until regular breathing is established.

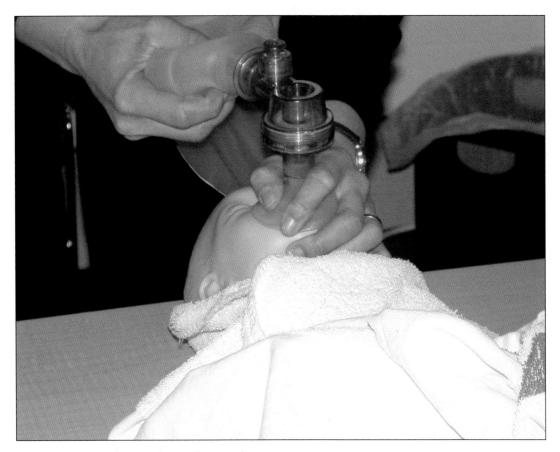

Figure 8.4 Bag value mask ventilation of neonate

Circulation

If the heart rate remains slow (less than 60 beats/minute) even after the lungs have been aerated, chest compressions must be started. However, the most common reason for the heart rate to remain low is that lung inflation has not been successful – chest compressions are rarely needed. Cardiac compromise is always the result of respiratory failure and can only be effectively treated if effective ventilation is occurring.

The most efficient way of delivering chest compressions in the neonate is to encircle the chest with both hands, so that the fingers lie behind the baby and the thumbs are apposed on the sternum just below the inter-nipple line (Figure 8.5). Compress the chest briskly, by one third of its depth. Current advice is to perform three compressions for each ventilation breath (3:1 ratio).

The purpose of chest compression is to move oxygenated blood or drugs to the coronary arteries in order to initiate cardiac recovery. Thus, there is no point in starting chest compression before effective lung inflation has been established. Similarly, compressions are ineffective unless interposed by ventilation breaths of good quality. Therefore, the emphasis must be upon good-quality breaths, followed by effective compressions. Simultaneous delivery of compressions and breaths should be avoided, as the former will reduce the effectiveness of the breaths. Once the heart rate is above 60 beats/minute and rising, chest compression can be discontinued.

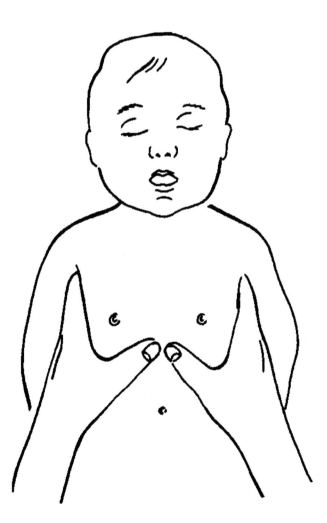

Figure 8.5 Hand encircling

Drugs

If after adequate lung inflation and chest compressions the heart rate has not responded, drug therapy should be considered. However, the most common reason for failure of the heart rate to respond is failure to achieve lung inflation, and there is no point in giving drugs unless the airway is open and the lungs have been inflated. Airway and breathing must be reassessed as adequate before proceeding to drug therapy. Venous access will be required via an umbilical venous line, because ideally drugs should be given centrally. The outcome is poor if drugs are required for resuscitation.

Adrenaline (epinephrine)

The alpha-adrenergic effect of adrenaline (epinephrine) increases coronary artery perfusion during resuscitation, enhancing oxygen delivery to the heart. In the presence of profound unresponsive bradycardia or circulatory standstill, 10 micrograms/kg (0.1 ml/kg 1:10 000) adrenaline (epinephrine) may be given intravenously. Further doses of 10–30 micrograms/kg (0.1–0.3 ml 1:10 000) may be tried at 3–5-minute intervals if there is no response. The tracheal route cannot be recommended, as there are insufficient data. However, if it is used tracheally animal evidence suggests that doses of 30 microgram/kg will be ineffective.

Bicarbonate

Any baby who is in terminal apnoea will have a significant metabolic acidosis. Acidosis depresses cardiac function. Bicarbonate 1–2 mmol/kg (2 ml/kg of 4.2% solution) may be used to raise the pH and enhance the effects of oxygen and epinephrine.

Bicarbonate use remains controversial and it should only be used in the absence of discernible cardiac output despite all resuscitative efforts or in profound and unresponsive bradycardia.

Dextrose

Hypoglycaemia is a potential problem for all stressed or asphyxiated babies. It is treated using a slow bolus of 5 ml/kg of 10% dextrose intravenously, and then providing a secure intravenous dextrose infusion at a rate of 100 ml/kg/day of 10% dextrose. Urinary dipsticks (BM Stix) are not reliable in neonates when reading less than 5 mmol/l.

Fluid

Very occasionally, hypovolaemia may be present because of known or suspected blood loss (fetomaternal haemorrhage, antepartum haemorrhage, placenta or vasa praevia, cord haemorrhage) or it may be secondary to loss of vascular tone following asphyxia. Volume expansion, initially with 10 ml/kg, may be appropriate. Physiological saline can be used; alternatively Gelofusine has been used safely and if blood loss is acute and severe, non-crossmatched O-negative blood should be given immediately. Albumin is no longer recommended. However, most newborn or neonatal resuscitations do not require fluid unless there has been known blood loss or septicaemic shock.

Naloxone

Strictly speaking this is not a drug of resuscitation – it should only be used once it is clear that a baby who has been effectively resuscitated – is pink, with a heart rate of over 100 beats/minute – but is not breathing spontaneously or adequately because of the possible effects of maternal opiates. If respiratory depressant effects are suspected the baby should be given naloxone intramuscularly (200 micrograms in a full-term baby). Smaller doses of 10 micrograms/kg will also reverse the sedation but the effect will only last a short time (perhaps 20 minutes intravenously or a few hours intramuscularly). Intravenous naloxone has a half life shorter than opiates, and there is no evidence to support intra-tracheal administration.

Atropine and calcium gluconate

Atropine and calcium gluconate have no place in newborn resuscitation. Atropine may, rarely, be useful in the neonatal unit, when vagal stimulation has produced resistant bradycardia or asystole (see bradycardia protocol).

Response to resuscitation

The first indication of success will be an increase in heart rate. Recovery of respiratory drive may be delayed. Babies in terminal apnoea will tend to gasp first as they recover before starting normal respirations (Figure 8.3). Those who were in primary apnoea are likely to start with normal breaths, which may commence at any stage of resuscitation.

Tracheal intubation

Most babies can be resuscitated using mask inflation. Swedish data suggest that if this is applied adequately, only 1/500 babies appear to need intubation. However, tracheal intubation remains the gold standard in airway management. It is especially useful in prolonged resuscitations, preterm babies and meconium aspiration. It should be considered if mask ventilation has failed, although the most common reason for failure with mask inflation is poor positioning of the head or failure to use jaw thrust with consequent failure to open the airway.

The technique of intubation is the same as for infants. A normal full-term newborn usually needs a 3.5 mm tracheal tube but 4.0, 3.0 and 2.5 mm tubes should also be available.

Tracheal tube placement must be assessed visually during intubation and in most cases will be confirmed by a rapid response in heart rate on ventilating via the tracheal tube. If in doubt exhaled CO_2 detection will correctly identify most correctly sited tubes in the presence of any cardiac output.

Special cases

Preterm babies

Preterm babies are more likely to get cold (higher surface area to mass ratio, little insulating fat) and more likely to become hypoglycaemic (fewer glycogen stores). There are now several trials that support the practice of placing small preterm babies in plastic bags (with the face exposed) under radiant heat without drying, in order to prevent evaporative heat loss. This technique might also be useful when dealing with the unexpected preterm birth outside a delivery unit but it must be remembered that it does nothing to prevent conductive or radiant heat losses. Large, food-grade microwaveable roasting bags are suitable (see Box 8.2).

The more preterm a baby the less likely it is to be able to establish adequate respirations. Preterm babies (less than 32 weeks) are likely to be deficient in surfactant especially after unexpected or precipitate delivery. The surfactant, secreted by pneumocytes in the alveolar epithelium, reduces alveolar surface tension and prevents alveolar collapse on expiration. Small amounts of surfactant can be demonstrated from about 20 weeks of gestation but a surge in production occurs at 30–34 weeks. Surfactant is released at birth due to aeration and distension of the alveoli. The half-life of the surfactant is approximately 12 hours. Production is reduced by hypothermia (less than 35 degrees C), hypoxia and acidosis (pH less than 7.25). In babies born before 32 weeks, one must anticipate a lack of surfactant. The effort of respiration will be increased, although the musculature will be less developed. They may require help to establish prompt aeration and ventilation, and may subsequently require exogenous surfactant therapy.

Box 8.2: Guidelines for use of plastic bags for preterm babies (less than 29 weeks) at birth

1. Preterm babies born below 29 completed weeks of gestation may be placed in plastic bags, under radiant heat, to maintain their temperature during resuscitation. They should remain in the bag until they are on the neonatal intensive care unit and the humidity within their incubator is at the desired level. This prevents evaporative heat loss but it does not prevent conductive or radiant heat loss. It should not replace all efforts to maintain a high ambient temperature around babies born outside delivery suites.

2. At birth, the baby should not be dried but should be slipped straight into the prepared plastic bag and placed under the radiant heater. This prevents evaporative heat loss. There is no need to wrap in a towel so long as this is done immediately after birth.

3. Suitable plastic bags are food-grade bags designed for microwaving and roasting. They should be large. The bag is prepared with a V cut in the closed end.

4. The bag should be slipped from the head up to the legs, covering in full, and let the head be completely accessible from the V-cut. This is most easily performed if the hand is placed through the V, the head placed in the hand and the bag drawn back down over the baby.

5. The head will stick out of the V-cut and will be dried as usual and resuscitation commenced as per standard guidelines. A hat should be placed on the head to further reduce heat loss.

6. The standard resuscitation would be carried out without any limitations of access, but if the umbilicus is required for any access then a small hole can be made above the area and the desired intervention done.

7. Chest compression can be performed without removing the bag.

8. After the baby is transferred to a neonatal unit, the temperature should be recorded after securing ventilation. The bag is only removed when the incubator humidity is satisfactory, and further care provided as per nursing protocols.

The lungs of preterm babies are more fragile than those of term babies and thus are much more susceptible to damage from over-distension. Therefore, it is appropriate to start with a lower inflation pressure of 2.0–2.5 kPa (20–25 cm H_2O) but do not be afraid to increase this to 30 cm H_2O if there is no heart rate response.

Vigorous passive chest movement in preterm babies (especially below 30 weeks) should be avoided, as it is usually indicates excessive lung inflation with the possibility of causing extensive lung damage (volume trauma).

Actions to be taken in the event of a poor initial response to resuscitation are shown in Box 8.3.

Box 8.3: Actions in the event of poor initial response to resuscitation

1. Check airway and breathing.

2. Check for a technical fault:

    (a) Is mask ventilation effective? Observe chest movement.

    (b) Is the tracheal tube in the trachea? Auscultate both axillae, listen at the mouth for a large leak, and observe movement. Use an exhaled CO_2 detector.

    (c) Is the tracheal tube in the right bronchus? Auscultate both axillae and observe movement.

    (d) Is the tracheal tube blocked? If there is doubt about the position or patency of the tracheal tube replace it. Use an exhaled CO_2 detector.

    (e) Is a longer inflation time required?

    (f) Is the oxygen connected? This is least likely to be a cause.

3. Does the baby have a pneumothorax? This occurs spontaneously in up to 1% of newborns, but those needing action in the delivery unit are exceptionally rare. Auscultate the chest for asymmetry of breath sounds. A cold light source can be used to transilluminate the chest – a pneumothorax may show as a hyper-illuminating area. If a tension pneumothorax is thought to be present clinically, a 21-gauge butterfly needle should be inserted through the second intercostal space in the mid-clavicular line. Alternatively, a 22-gauge cannula connected to a three-way tap may be used. Remember that you may well cause a pneumothorax during this procedure.

4. Does the baby remain cyanosed despite breathing with a good heart rate? There may be a congenital heart malformation, which may be duct-dependent, or a persistent pulmonary hypertension.

5. If, after resuscitation, the baby is pink and has a good heart rate but is not breathing effectively, it may be suffering the effects of maternal opiates. Naloxone 200 micro-grams intramuscularly may be considered. Given intramuscularly this should outlast the opiate effect.

6. Is there severe anaemia or hypovolaemia? In case of large blood loss, 20 ml/kg O-negative blood or a volume expander should be given.

Birth outside the delivery room

Whenever a baby is born unexpectedly, the greatest difficulty lies often in keeping it warm. Skin-to-skin contact of the baby with the mother or another adult will keep most babies warm if the two are then covered against draughts. Drying and wrapping, turning up the heating and closing windows and doors are all important in maintaining temperature. Special care must be taken to clamp and cut the cord to prevent blood loss.

Hospitals with accident and emergency departments should have guidelines for resuscitation at birth, summoning help and post-resuscitation transfer of babies born within the department.

Babies born unexpectedly, outside hospital, will be at greater risk of being preterm and of getting cold. However, the principles of resuscitation are identical to the hospital setting. Transport will need to be discussed according to local guidelines.

Discontinuation of resuscitation

The outcome for a baby with no cardiac output after more than 10 minutes of adequate resuscitation is likely to be very poor. Stopping resuscitation early, or not starting resuscitation at all, may be appropriate in situations of extreme prematurity (less than 23 weeks), birth weight of less than 400 g or in the presence of lethal abnormalities such as anencephaly or confirmed trisomy 13 or 18.

Resuscitation is nearly always indicated in conditions with a high survival rate and acceptable morbidity. Such decisions should be taken by a senior member of the team, ideally a consultant in consultation with the parents and other team members. This means that help must have been called for.

Communication with the parents

It is important that the team caring for the newborn baby informs the parents of the progress whenever possible. This is likely to be most difficult in unexpected deliveries so prior planning to cover the eventuality may be helpful. Decisions at the end of life must involve the parents whenever possible. All communication should be documented after the event.

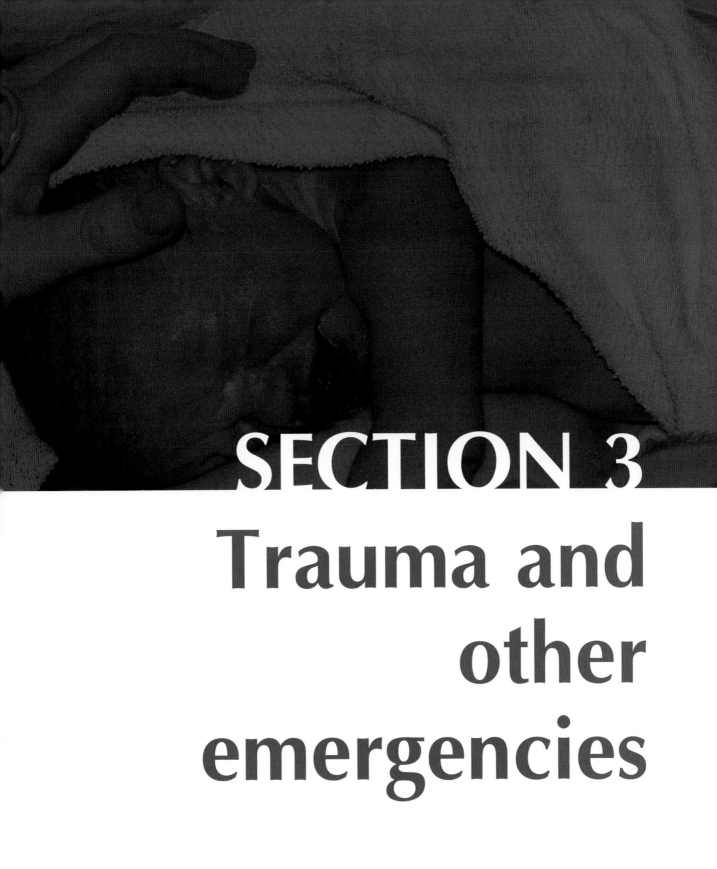

SECTION 3
Trauma and other emergencies

Introduction to trauma

Major trauma is a life-threatening emergency. It is addressed on the first day of the MOET course, alongside cardiorespiratory arrest. Having a correct approach and understanding of major trauma provides the ability to deal with any life-threatening emergency. Trauma is an example of multi-system life-threatening illness.

There are marked differences in the epidemiology of trauma in different countries. In the UK, road traffic accidents are the most common cause of trauma deaths. Trauma in pregnancy is most commonly due to road traffic accidents (equal frequency throughout pregnancy), domestic violence (more common before 18 weeks), falls (between 20 and 30 weeks) and burns. In the UK, there are an estimated 10 000 deaths from trauma each year – approximately 30 deaths each day.

Major trauma is common in young women who are of childbearing years. The Confidential Enquiry into Maternal Deaths 2000–2002 reported suicide as a major cause of maternal mortality and, of the trauma deaths, 65% died violently. It reported 11 cases of murder, eight deaths from road traffic accidents and, of the 391 deaths assessed, 51 of these women had suffered from domestic violence. The obstetrician is most likely to be called to any case of trauma in the pregnant woman.

A survey of trauma deaths showed 33% to be preventable. Preventable deaths occurred from hypoxia and hypovolaemia. Forty percent of deaths occur at the scene of the accident; 30% die in hospital; 30% survive but, of these, only 18% make a full functional recovery; 9% have moderate disability (usually orthopaedic, such as knee ligaments) and 3% have severe disability (usually neurological, spinal-cord injury, head injury). Trauma occurs in up to 7% of pregnancies. Abruption occurs in up to 70% of major injuries and in 5% of minor injuries in pregnancy. Uterine rupture occurs in less than 1% of major injuries but with maternal death in 10% of those. However, uterine rupture occurred in two of the eight deaths described in the 2000–2002 Confidential Enquiries. Fetal loss occurs in up to 40% major and 2% minor injuries. Fetal loss occurs in 35% traumatic abruptions and is invariable in traumatic rupture. The seat belt 'above and below the bump, not over it' advice is repeated in the 2000–2002 CEMD report.

Analysis of trauma data shows a trimodal death distribution:

1. Instantaneous

Within seconds to minutes of the injury. Deaths are due to head injury, spinal-cord injury and exsanguination.

2. Early

These extend from the first few minutes to a few hours. Examples include airway and respiratory compromise, continuing haemorrhage and subdural and extradural haematoma. It is in this phase, often referred to as 'the golden hour' of trauma management, that properly trained individuals can save many lives.

3. Late

These occur from a few hours to days or even weeks after injury. The majority are due to sepsis with associated multi-organ dysfunction. This course is primarily aimed at preventing potential deaths in the 'early' phase. However, the 'late' outcome (death due to multi-organ

85

dysfunction) can also be significantly influenced by vigorous and correct initial management; for example, restoration of tissue perfusion – oxygenation, antibiotics and, vitally, by recognising the need for early surgical intervention, followed by intensive medical and nursing care. The course also aims to reduce and prevent disability.

The pathophysiological response to trauma is altered in pregnancy and thereby the clinician's assessment of trauma may be adversely affected. The obstetrician, obstetric anaesthetist and midwife have a role in understanding anatomical and physiological changes and adapting trauma care to the pregnant woman and the fetus. They have a particular role in the protection of the fetus, the institution of fetal monitoring, identifying the need to empty the uterus, the timing of delivery and the consideration of fetomaternal haemorrhage. The use of ultrasound should be encouraged.

In the management of the nonpregnant trauma patient, hypotensive resuscitation is generally supported as means of reducing bleeding before definitive haemostasis can be achieved (by surgery or embolisation), although the permissible depth and length of hypotensive resuscitation is currently unknown. There is however no place for hypotensive resuscitation in pregnancy as it causes shut down of perfusion to the fetoplacental unit.

Clear chronological records of assessment of injuries, treatment and reassessment findings should be made and signed, timed and dated.

Communication with the patient, with relatives and with the multidisciplinary team is essential for success.

Algorithm 9.1 Thoracic emergencies

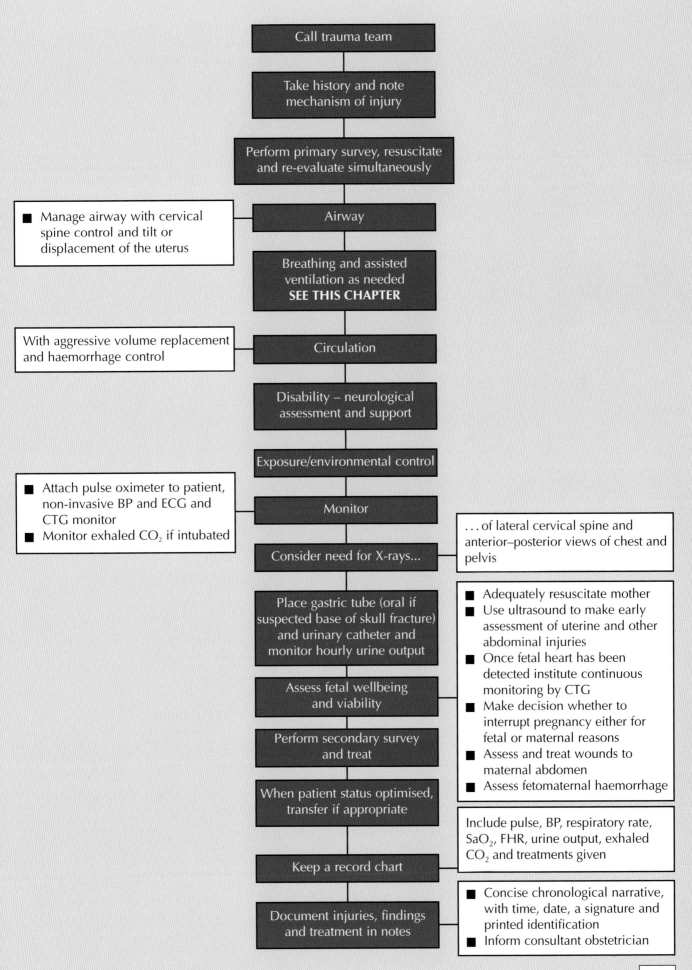

Call trauma team

Take history and note mechanism of injury

Perform primary survey, resuscitate and re-evaluate simultaneously

Airway
- Manage airway with cervical spine control and tilt or displacement of the uterus

Breathing and assisted ventilation as needed **SEE THIS CHAPTER**

Circulation
- With aggressive volume replacement and haemorrhage control

Disability – neurological assessment and support

Exposure/environmental control

Monitor
- Attach pulse oximeter to patient, non-invasive BP and ECG and CTG monitor
- Monitor exhaled CO_2 if intubated

Consider need for X-rays...
...of lateral cervical spine and anterior–posterior views of chest and pelvis

Place gastric tube (oral if suspected base of skull fracture) and urinary catheter and monitor hourly urine output

Assess fetal wellbeing and viability
- Adequately resuscitate mother
- Use ultrasound to make early assessment of uterine and other abdominal injuries
- Once fetal heart has been detected institute continuous monitoring by CTG
- Make decision whether to interrupt pregnancy either for fetal or maternal reasons
- Assess and treat wounds to maternal abdomen
- Assess fetomaternal haemorrhage

Perform secondary survey and treat

When patient status optimised, transfer if appropriate

Include pulse, BP, respiratory rate, SaO_2, FHR, urine output, exhaled CO_2 and treatments given

Keep a record chart

Document injuries, findings and treatment in notes
- Concise chronological narrative, with time, date, a signature and printed identification
- Inform consultant obstetrician

Chapter 9

Thoracic emergencies

Introduction and incidence

The 2002–2002 report of the Confidential Enquiries into Maternal Deaths in the UK described five cases of dissecting aortic aneurysm with rupture into the pericardium causing cardiac tamponade, and five deaths from coronary artery aneurysm. Chest injuries are common in patients with major trauma and they are responsible for around one-quarter of trauma deaths. Many of these deaths can be prevented by the prompt recognition of life-threatening conditions and the early initiation of simple methods of treatment. Very few patients will require surgery. Most are treated by the simple methods taught on this course of needle thoracocentesis and chest drain placement. Prompt and effective resuscitation of the mother, including the avoidance of aortocaval compression is the most effective way of ensuring good fetoplacental perfusion.

Types of injury

Chest injuries are usually classified as penetrating, blunt or both.

It must be appreciated that, while there may be external signs of thoracic injury, intra-abdominal organs including the gravid uterus may also have been damaged, particularly in the later stages of pregnancy. The reverse is also true, in that obvious abdominal trauma may extend into the chest. In general, penetrating injuries will require surgical exploration.

Initial assessment and management

An accurate incident history is vital. For example, the driver of a car in collision with a tree would be at risk of a traumatic brain injury, cervical-spine trauma, traumatic aortic rupture, lung and myocardial contusion and abdominal trauma, in addition to many other bony and soft-tissue injuries.

The principles of management are:

■ Primary survey and resuscitation: life-threatening injuries discovered during the primary survey should be dealt with immediately.

■ Assessment of fetal wellbeing and viability.

■ Secondary survey: careful head-to-toe examination should identify any other injuries sustained.

■ Definitive care.

Life-threatening injuries to identify and treat

Mnemonic for life-threatening injuries

A   Airway obstruction

T   Tension pneumothorax

O   Open pneumothorax

M   Massive haemothorax

F   Flail chest

C   Cardiac tamponade

Airway obstruction

See Section 2 Chapter 6.

Tension pneumothorax

The classical signs of tracheal deviation, hyper-resonant percussion note, reduced air entry and venous hypertension may be very late or absent. The diagnosis should be considered in any trauma patient with respiratory distress and shock.

If there is any doubt, needle thoracocentesis to decompress and subsequent intercostal drain placement should be performed without delay and are very safe when done correctly.

Open pneumothorax (sucking chest wound)

A large chest-wall defect will suck air through it with each inspiration and cause a progressive decline in pulmonary function.

Principles of management: the defect should be covered in such a way as to prevent air being sucked in but allow accumulated air to escape. An Asherman seal will be effective for small wounds or a dressing taped securely on three sides for larger wounds.

An intercostal drain should be placed remote to the site of injury.

Massive haemothorax

Large haemothoraces are usually caused by damage to a systemic or pulmonary vessel. Clinical signs include evidence of hypovolaemia, decreased air entry and dullness to percussion.

The drainage of a large collection without wide-bore intravenous access can lead to circulatory collapse when the tamponade effect is acutely lost, so intravenous access should be secured prior to drainage. After the placement of an intercostal drain, operative intervention will usually be necessary if the initial loss is greater than 1500 ml or continuing losses exceed 200 ml/hour. However, most haemothoraces are managed conservatively.

Flail chest

When a segment of the chest wall loses continuity with rest of the thoracic cage, that segment moves paradoxically with respiration and the segment is called a flail. The importance is the hypoxia caused by trauma to the underlying lung and this can be severe. The bony injury can be extremely painful and this impairs oxygenation further. The principles of management include high concentration oxygen, insertion of an intercostal drain, careful fluid management and effective analgesia. A period of mechanical ventilation may be required in severe cases.

Cardiac tamponade

This occurs infrequently with blunt or penetrating trauma to the chest and can be difficult to detect. Signs include arterial hypotension, venous hypertension and muffled heart sounds. It should be suspected in a patient with chest trauma and hypotension. Ultrasound can quickly confirm the diagnosis. The treatment is needle pericardiocentesis and should be performed under ultrasound and ECG control.

Secondary survey

After completion of the primary survey and necessary resuscitation and assessment of fetal wellbeing, a full top-to-toe secondary examination should identify any potentially lethal or non-lethal injuries sustained. In addition, a thorough assessment of fetal wellbeing can be performed at this time. X-ray of the chest taken in the primary survey should be reviewed. The chest film should be examined for bony injury and its relevance, air or blood in a pleural cavity, contusion and position of gastric and tracheal tubes and any central venous catheters placed.

Any abnormality should be interpreted according to the mechanism of injury and the likelihood of underlying thoracic injury.

Potentially lethal chest injuries

These may not be obvious during the primary survey. They are usually labelled as two contusions and four disruptions:

■ pulmonary contusion

■ myocardial contusion

■ diaphragmatic disruption

■ tracheobronchial disruption

■ oesophageal disruption

■ aortic disruption.

Pulmonary contusion

Pulmonary contusion is usually as a result of blunt trauma to the chest and presents as hypoxia that may progress to respiratory failure. The key to successful management is to maintain a high index of suspicion, as the young pregnant population may hide the initial signs well. Any signs of respiratory impairment such as tachypneoa, use of accessory muscles, cyanosis etc. should prompt immediate referral to the intensive care unit. Young pregnant patients should have excellent oxygenation when breathing high-flow oxygen. If they have not, then significant contusion should be suspected.

Myocardial contusion

Myocardial contusion should be suspected whenever there is a history of blunt chest injury, although proof of significant contusion is difficult to obtain. Patients may have extrasystoles, abnormal complexes or even haemodynamically significant arrhythmia.

Diaphragmatic disruption

Diaphragmatic disruption is usually associated with blunt abdominal injury and is usually found on the left side. Compression causes a radial tear in the diaphragm, allowing abdominal contents to herniate into the chest. Abdominal structures may have been damaged by the injury itself, by the placement of an intercostal drain or may become ischaemic while in the chest cavity. Oxygenation and ventilation can be severely affected.

The diagnosis should be suspected with blunt trauma to the chest or abdomen and is confirmed by the presence of a gastric tube above the diaphragm on chest X-ray. The diaphragm is usually repaired without delay.

Tracheobronchial disruption

Injuries to the larynx, trachea or bronchi need urgent attention from a senior anaesthetist. Laryngeal and tracheal injuries are rare and present with airway obstruction, subcutaneous emphysema and hoarseness. In addition, they suggest the presence of other injuries to thorax or abdominal structures. Bronchial injuries are often fatal. They may present as a pneumothorax with a continuing air leak after drain placement. Surviving patients usually require surgical repair.

Oesophageal disruption

This is usually the result of a penetrating injury, although can be caused by blunt trauma to the upper abdomen. The diagnosis is suggested by:

1. History
    - pain out of proportion to other injuries
    - left-sided pneumothorax
    - particulate matter from the drain.
2. Mediastinal air.

Surgical repair is the treatment of choice if the diagnosis is made early but the mediastinitis can be fatal.

Traumatic aortic disruption

The mechanism of injury here is usually a decelerating injury such as a car crash or a fall and those that survive to hospital have a laceration in the region of the ligamentum arteriosum and a contained haematoma. The diagnosis is made using a high index of suspicion from the history and the chest X-ray appearance of a widened mediastinum. This leads to further investigation such as CT, angiography or transoesophageal echocardiography. The treatment is surgical repair.

Summary

- Chest trauma in pregnancy provides a combination of injury to major thoracic structures and the disadvantage of a large gravid uterus that can easily impair venous return and compromise respiration.

- Most injuries can be identified by careful assessment and managed with simple measures including the avoidance of aortocaval compression.

- Knowledge of the pathophysiology of these injuries allows the obstetrician to take part in the decision-making process and prioritise maternal and fetal treatment appropriately.

Appendix 9A

Practical procedures

Reproduced with permission from the Advanced Life Support Group.

Needle thoracocentesis

Equipment

■ Alcohol swab.

■ Intravenous cannula (16 gauge minimum).

■ 20-ml syringe.

Procedure

■ Identify the second intercostal space in the midclavicular line on the side of the pneumothorax (the opposite side to the direction of tracheal deviation).

■ Swab the chest wall with surgical preparation or an alcohol swab.

■ Attach the syringe to the cannula.

■ Insert the cannula into the chest wall, just over the rib, aspirating all the time.

■ If air is aspirated, remove the needle, leaving the plastic cannula in place.

■ Tape the cannula in place and proceed to chest drain insertion (see later) as soon as possible.

Complications

■ Local haematoma.

■ Lung laceration.

If needle thoracocentesis is attempted, and the patient does not have a tension pneumothorax, the chance of causing a pneumothorax is 10–20%. Patients must have a chest X-ray, and will require chest drainage if ventilated.

Chest drain insertion

Equipment

■ Skin preparation and surgical drapes.

■ Local anaesthetic.

■ Scalpel.

■ Scissors.

■ Large clamps (2).

■ Chest drain tube without trochar.

■ Suture.

■ Underwater seal.

■ 10-ml syringe with orange, blue and green needles.

Procedure

■ Identify relevant landmarks (usually the fifth intercostal space anterior to the midaxillary line) on the side with the pneumothorax (Figure 9A.1).

■ Swab the chest wall with surgical preparation or an alcohol swab.

■ Use local anaesthetic if necessary.

■ Make a 2–3 cm transverse skin incision along the line of the intercostal space, towards the superior edge of the sixth rib (thereby avoiding the neurovascular bundle).

■ Bluntly dissect through the subcutaneous tissues just over the top of the rib and puncture the parietal pleura with the tip of the clamp.

■ Put a gloved finger into the incision and clear the path into the pleura.

■ Advance the chest drain tube into the pleural space without the trochar.

■ Ensure that the tube is in the pleural space by listening for air movement and by looking for fogging of the tube during expiration.

■ Connect the chest drain tube to an underwater seal.

■ Suture the drain in place, and secure with tape.

■ Obtain a chest X-ray.

Complications

■ Damage to intercostal nerve, artery or vein.

■ Introduction of infection.

■ Tube kinking, dislodging or blocking.

■ Subcutaneous emphysema.

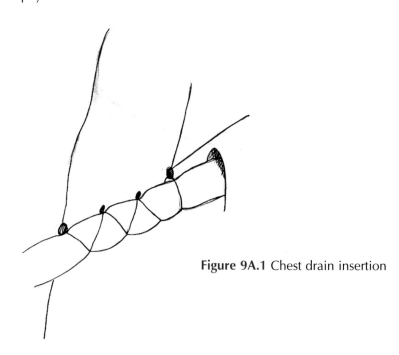

Figure 9A.1 Chest drain insertion

■ Persistent pneumothorax due to faulty tube insertion, leaking around chest drain, leaking underwater seal, bronchopleural fistula.

■ Failure of lung to expand due to blocked bronchus.

■ Anaphylactic or allergic reaction to skin preparation.

Trauma and other emergencies

Algorithm 10.1 **Shock**

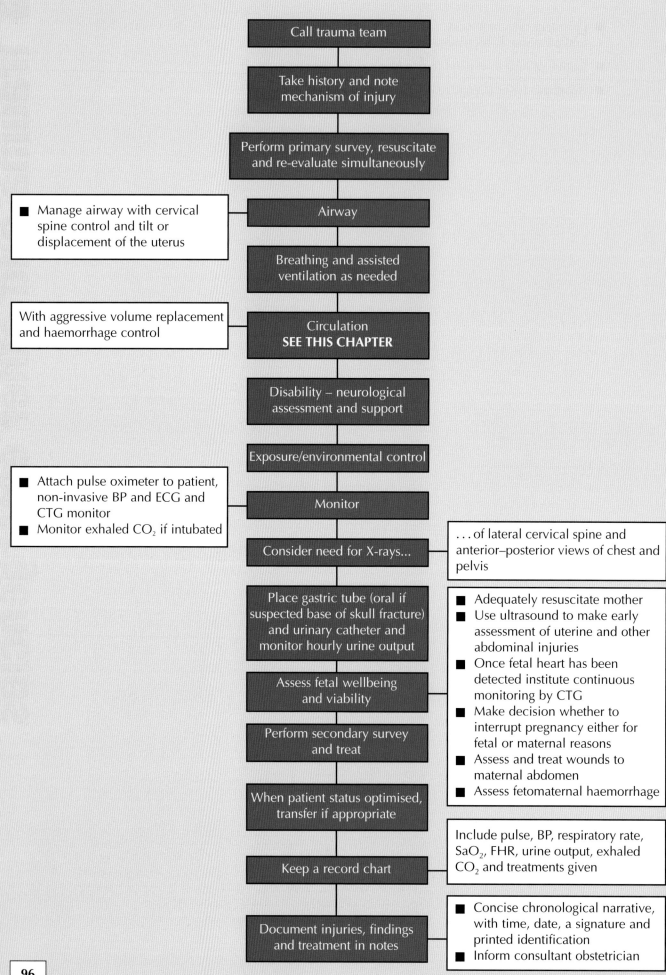

Call trauma team

Take history and note mechanism of injury

Perform primary survey, resuscitate and re-evaluate simultaneously

Airway
- Manage airway with cervical spine control and tilt or displacement of the uterus

Breathing and assisted ventilation as needed

Circulation
SEE THIS CHAPTER
- With aggressive volume replacement and haemorrhage control

Disability – neurological assessment and support

Exposure/environmental control

Monitor
- Attach pulse oximeter to patient, non-invasive BP and ECG and CTG monitor
- Monitor exhaled CO_2 if intubated

Consider need for X-rays...
...of lateral cervical spine and anterior–posterior views of chest and pelvis

Place gastric tube (oral if suspected base of skull fracture) and urinary catheter and monitor hourly urine output

Assess fetal wellbeing and viability
- Adequately resuscitate mother
- Use ultrasound to make early assessment of uterine and other abdominal injuries
- Once fetal heart has been detected institute continuous monitoring by CTG
- Make decision whether to interrupt pregnancy either for fetal or maternal reasons
- Assess and treat wounds to maternal abdomen
- Assess fetomaternal haemorrhage

Perform secondary survey and treat

When patient status optimised, transfer if appropriate

Keep a record chart
Include pulse, BP, respiratory rate, SaO_2, FHR, urine output, exhaled CO_2 and treatments given

Document injuries, findings and treatment in notes
- Concise chronological narrative, with time, date, a signature and printed identification
- Inform consultant obstetrician

Chapter 10

Shock

Objectives

On successfully completing this topic you will be able to:

■ define shock

■ relate the physiological changes to the cardiovascular system in pregnancy and how they affect the presentation of hypovolaemia

■ recognise shock

■ discuss the principles of treatment of hypovolaemic shock

■ identify other shock syndromes and understand their management.

Definition

Shock is inadequate tissue perfusion. Inadequate tissue perfusion means imminent cell death. In obstetric emergencies and in trauma, hypovolaemia is by far the most common cause of shock.

The treatment of shock is directed towards restoring cellular and organ perfusion with adequately oxygenated blood. To maintain organ perfusion an adequate cardiac output is required.

$$\text{cardiac output (CO)} = \text{stroke volume (SV)} \times \text{heart rate (HR)}$$

Stroke volume is determined by the venous return to the heart otherwise known as preload, and will be reduced if there is a low circulating volume of blood, or if the vascular system is operating at a low pressure due to vasodilatation.

Physiological changes to the cardiovascular system in pregnancy

During pregnancy, the plasma volume and red-cell volume increase to make a total increase in circulating blood volume. The pregnant woman may lose 1200–1500 ml of blood before showing any signs of hypovolaemia (35% of her circulating blood volume). The compensatory mechanism that allows this involves the shutting down of blood flow to the fetoplacental unit. Blood loss in the mother therefore may first be reflected by fetal distress. The fetal heart rate should be monitored to assess this.

In the heavily pregnant woman, the uterus may lie on the vena cava and reduce the venous return to the heart. Vena caval and aortic compression may reduce cardiac output by up to 30%. This is known as supine hypotension syndrome. Hypotension for any reason is exacerbated by vena caval obstruction. To prevent this the heavily pregnant woman must always be tilted or have the uterus manually displaced to the left to reduce the pressure on the inferior vena cava (see Figure 4.1).

> # To prompt uterine tilt early in the process of resuscitation, remember:
> # "Hello. How are you Mrs Tilt?"

Recognition of hypovolaemia

The most common cause of hypotension in trauma is hypovolaemia but hypotension is a very late sign, developing only when significant blood loss has occurred. Successful outcome depends on the early recognition of shock, restoration of volume and control of haemorrhage.

Signs of hypovolaemia are:

■ increase in heart rate

■ cold, pale, sweaty, cyanosed skin with delayed capillary refill

■ alteration of mental state

■ fall in urine output

■ narrowed pulse pressure

■ hypotension (late sign).

Increase in heart rate

Increase in heart rate is an early compensation for hypovolaemia or vasodilatation, both of which can cause hypotension and shock. A maternal heart rate of greater than 100 beats/minute should be considered sinister until proved otherwise. Most, but not all, women will demonstrate a tachycardia if bleeding significantly but paradoxical bradycardia has also been observed.

Skin, capillary refill, mental state and urine output

The skin, brain and kidneys can be thought of as 'end organs' which reflect adequacy of perfusion to all tissues.

Capillary refill (capillary return time, CRT)

This is a quantification of skin perfusion. It can be assessed by compressing a fingernail for 5 seconds. The test is normal if colour returns within two seconds of releasing compression (i.e. a CRT of less than 2 seconds – the time taken to say the words 'capillary refill'). Capillary refill can be prolonged but may be insignificant if the patient is cold.

Mental state

If the woman is conscious and talking sensibly, she is not only breathing through an open airway, she is perfusing her cerebral cortex with sufficient oxygenated blood (50% of the normal cardiac output). Increasing hypovolaemia and subsequent cerebral hypoxia cause alterations in the level of consciousness. These alterations begin with anxiety and, if untreated, may proceed through confusion and aggression to eventual unresponsiveness and death.

Narrowed pulse pressure

This is caused by an increase in diastolic blood pressure, which reflects a vasoconstriction occurring as a compensation for hypovolaemia.

Classification of circulating volume lost

Haemorrhage is the acute loss of circulating blood. In the nonpregnant adult, 7% of body weight is circulating blood, approximately 5 litres in a 70-kg adult or 70 ml/kg of body weight. In term pregnant women, the circulating volume increases by about 40% (100 ml/kg of body weight).

The classification in Table 10.1 applies to the nonpregnant woman. It is useful in identifying the signs of hypovolaemia and relating them to the level of loss.

Think of a tennis match!

Table 10.1. Classification of circulating volume lost in nonpregnant patient

Class	Loss of circulating volume (%)	Amount in a 70-kg adult (ml)	Symptoms and treatment
I	0–15	<750	This is fully compensated by the diversion of blood from the splanchnic pool. There are no abnormal symptoms and signs other than minimal tachycardia. In otherwise healthy patients this blood loss does not require blood replacement.
II	15–30	750–1500	Requires peripheral vasoconstriction to maintain systolic blood pressure. Symptoms are tachycardia, tachypnoea and the pulse pressure is narrowed because of raised diastolic blood pressure; Crystalloid fluid replacement will be required.
III	30–40	1500–2000	There is tachycardia, tachypnoea, changes in mental status and a measurable fall in systolic blood pressure because peripheral vasoconstriction fails to compensate for the increasing loss. Note it is only at this stage of loss that there is a fall in systolic pressure. Patients with this blood loss may require crystalloid, colloid and blood transfusion.
IV	>40	>2000	Immediately life-threatening. Symptoms are tachycardia, fall in blood pressure, narrowing of pulse pressure, negligible urine output, altered mental status. Loss of more than 50% circulating volume results in loss of consciousness. These patients require transfusion and immediate surgical intervention.

Pitfalls in the recognition of shock

◼ In pregnancy, as described above.

◼ Some pregnant women do not mount a tachycardia or can even produce a bradycardia which is very misleading and makes the recognition of serious haemorrhage very difficult. It is not clear why this should occur.

◼ People with pacemakers have a fixed upper-heart rate.

◼ Athletes may have a very slow baseline heart rate.

◼ People on beta-blockers are relatively unable to mount a tachycardia.

◼ Haemoglobin level may be a useful measure of acute blood loss. In the very acute phases of loss the haemaglobin measurement will not change. However, the rapid movement of fluid from the extracellular space into the intravascular compartment in compensation for the loss, or the provision of intravenous fluids to restore circulating volume will result in a fall in haematocrit. It is always worth tracking the haematocrit if there is any suspicion of haemorrhage as this may be the only indicator in a slow steady bleed. If it has fallen quickly with early signs of hypovolaemia this is suggestive of very severe loss.

Principles of treatment of hypovolaemic shock

Primary survey and resuscitation according to the ABC principle.

Clear the Airway (protect the cervical spine when appropriate) and deliver oxygen at 10–15 litres/minute via tight-fitting facemask with reservoir bag. Correct any life-threatening Breathing difficulties.

Circulation: diagnosis of hypovolaemic shock must be promptly followed by restoration of adequate circulating volume and stopping the bleeding.

Consider haemorrhage to be of two types:

◼ compressible

◼ non-compressible.

Compressible haemorrhage is controllable by direct pressure, limb elevation, packing, or by reduction and immobilisation of fractures or, in obstetric situations, compression of the uterus.

Non-compressible haemorrhage may be found in a body cavity (chest, abdomen, pelvis or retroperitoneum). Splinting, in the case of a pelvic fracture, or surgery may be needed to control bleeding. Call the appropriate surgeon.

Blood loss in trauma may be in five sites ('blood on the floor and four more'):

1.   external ('on the floor')
2.   chest
3.   abdomen
4.   pelvis and retroperitoneum
5.   around long-bone fractures (especially the femur).

Note: The presence of significant amounts of blood in the chest will be identified during Breathing in the primary survey. Identification of other sites of bleeding is an essential element of Circulation.

Be highly suspicious in all cases of blunt abdominal injuries.

Some idea of blood volumes lost from different injuries can be seen from Table 10.2.

Table 10.2. Blood volumes lost from different injuries

Injury	Blood volume lost (litres)
Closed femoral fracture	1.5
Fractured pelvis	3.0
Fractured ribs (each)	0.15
One blood-filled hemithorax	2.0
A closed tibial fracture	0.5
An open wound the size of an adult hand	0.5
A clot the size of an adult fist	0.5

Replacement of lost volume

Intravenous access is best achieved by inserting as large a cannula as possible into each ante cubital fossa. Short, wide-bore cannulae deliver the best flow. If peripheral cannulation cannot be achieved consider:

- intravenous cutdown (Figure 10.1)
- femoral vein cannulation (avoid if possible in the pregnant woman)
- central venous access, if appropriate personnel.

Always warm fluids.

Crystalloids are physiological solutions that remain only temporarily in the circulation (about 30 minutes) before passing into the intercellular space. They are useful for the immediate replacement of lost volume. Initially, 2 litres of crystalloid (Hartmann's solution or Ringer lactate) should be infused through wide-bore cannulae.

Crystalloids do, however, distribute outside the intravascular compartment and are therefore less effective in maintaining intravascular volume. An overload may cause pulmonary and cerebral oedema (care in pre-eclampsia/eclampsia). Colloids remain longer in the intravascular compart-

Table 10.3. Response to resuscitation by intravenous fluids

Response type	Intervention needed
I	Signs improve and remain improved. No further fluid challenge is required.
II	An initial but unsustained improvement then regression to abnormal levels of these vital signs. This means that either the fluid has been redistributed from the intravascular compartment to the extravascular compartment or blood loss continues.
	Give a further intravenous challenge of two units of colloid and ensure blood is available. If the vital signs return to acceptable levels, the response was due to redistribution of fluid. If vital signs remain abnormal then this is a Type III response.
III	Continue intravenous colloid or warmed blood at flow rates sufficient to sustain resuscitation. This patient needs urgent surgery within the hour.
IV	No response to rapid intravenous infusion of crystalloid, colloid and/or blood. This patient needs immediate surgery (to 'turn off the tap') if she is to survive.

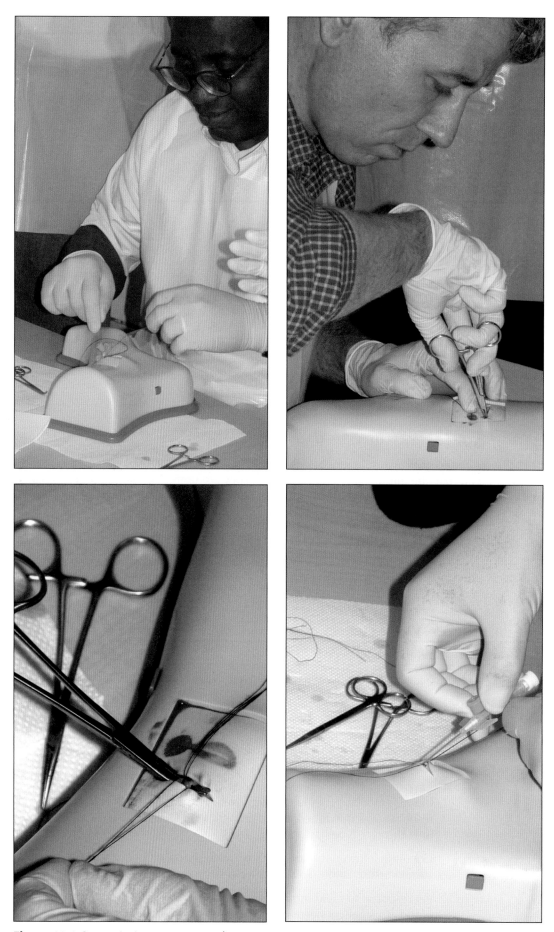

Figure 10.1 Stages in intravenous cutdown

ment. However, the use of colloids has some rare additional risks, such as anaphylaxis. The crystalloid versus colloid debate is complex but it is generally agreed that an initial infusion of crystalloid is appropriate for emergency situations requiring volume resuscitation.

Treatment regimen

The response to resuscitation by intravenous fluids and the need for further intravenous fluids and/or surgery can be considered under four headings (Table 10.3).

Management problems

Cooling

Transfusion of large amounts of fluid can cause hypothermia. Take measures to prevent this. (see Chapter 17).

Continuing haemorrhage

Consider all potential sources of blood loss. Concealed haemorrhage is life threatening and must be strongly considered in all hypovolaemic patients who respond poorly or do not respond to treatment: response types III and IV. Urgent surgery is required. Consider the possibility of coagulopathy when large volumes of fluids have been infused. Remember that stored blood contains fewer clotting factors than fresh blood. Clotting factors may be required (see Chapter 17).

Fluid overload

Fluid overload is unlikely to occur in severely injured, previously fit, young adults. Fluid replacement should be titrated against haemodynamic effects, especially when estimates of loss can be calculated from the mechanism of injury and the haemorrhage is compressible.

Acid-base imbalance

Metabolic acidosis may develop with severe or long-standing shock as a result of inadequate tissue perfusion and subsequent anaerobic metabolism. The way to treat is to adequately resuscitate.

Other types of shock

Hypovolaemic shock is the most common in obstetrics and in trauma. The differential diagnosis should also include septic, cardiogenic, neurogenic and anaphylactic shock. Clues can be gained from the history, careful primary and secondary survey, selected additional tests and the response to treatment.

Septic shock

Septic shock is a recognised complication of delivery, where the source of infection will be the genital tract, but could occur with any source of infection, for example a urinary tract or chest infection.

The mechanism of shock is one of vasodilatation caused by bacterial toxins.

If there has been no haemorrhage (or if haemorrhage has been adequately corrected) the patient, although hypotensive, will have a tachycardia and, initially, warm pink skin and a wide pulse pressure (a full bounding pulse).

10

Trauma and other emergencies

The very sick septic patient will be tachycardic, cyanosed and peripherally shut down.

Septic patients have a metabolic acidosis, detectable on sampling of arterial or venous blood. See Chapter 19 for the management of sepsis in pregnancy. In trauma, sepsis is most likely to occur in patients with penetrating abdominal injuries and in whom the peritoneal cavity has been contaminated by intestinal contents.

Cardiogenic shock

Myocardial dysfunction may occur following cardiac tamponade, myocardial contusion, air embolus, pulmonary embolus, tension pneumothorax or myocardial infarction.

Ideally, all patients with blunt thoracic injury should have constant ECG monitoring.

Measuring cardiac enzymes will not alter the acute management of myocardial infarction and are poor indicators of myocardial contusion.

Treatment may include vasopressors and inotropes. Intensive care help will be required.

Neurogenic shock

See Chapter 13.

Anaphylactic shock

See Chapter 34.

Summary

■ Hypovolaemia is the cause of shock in most obstetric and trauma patients.

■ A high index of suspicion is essential during assessment.

■ Management requires replacement of lost volume and immediate control of haemorrhage either by direct compression, splintage or, where necessary, by urgent surgery.

Algorithm 11.1 Abdominal emergencies in pregnancy

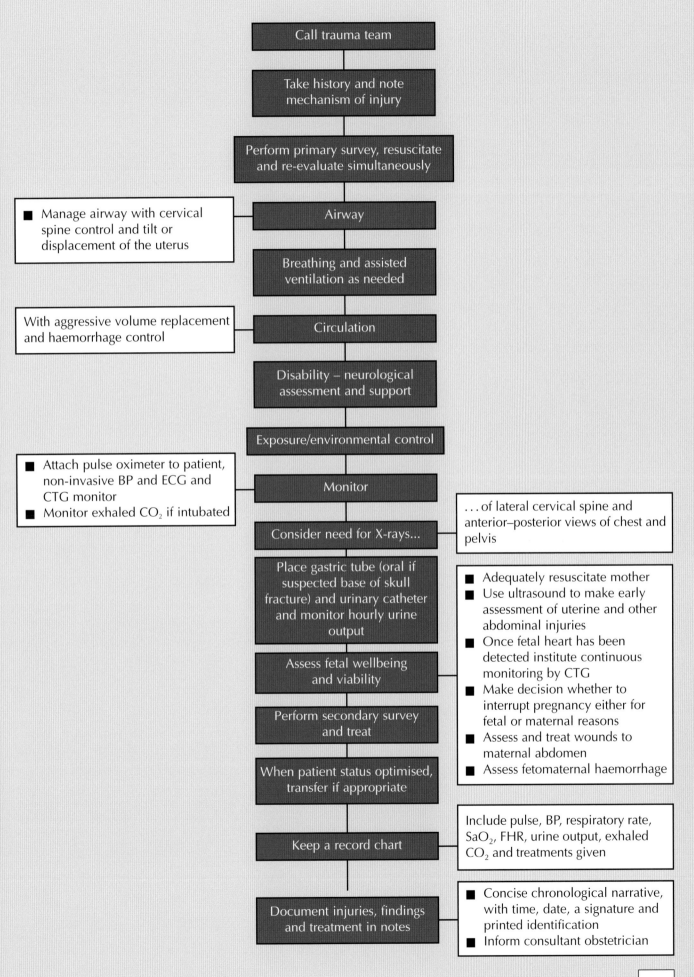

Call trauma team

Take history and note mechanism of injury

Perform primary survey, resuscitate and re-evaluate simultaneously

Airway
- Manage airway with cervical spine control and tilt or displacement of the uterus

Breathing and assisted ventilation as needed

Circulation
- With aggressive volume replacement and haemorrhage control

Disability – neurological assessment and support

Exposure/environmental control

Monitor
- Attach pulse oximeter to patient, non-invasive BP and ECG and CTG monitor
- Monitor exhaled CO_2 if intubated

Consider need for X-rays...
...of lateral cervical spine and anterior–posterior views of chest and pelvis

Place gastric tube (oral if suspected base of skull fracture) and urinary catheter and monitor hourly urine output

Assess fetal wellbeing and viability
- Adequately resuscitate mother
- Use ultrasound to make early assessment of uterine and other abdominal injuries
- Once fetal heart has been detected institute continuous monitoring by CTG
- Make decision whether to interrupt pregnancy either for fetal or maternal reasons
- Assess and treat wounds to maternal abdomen
- Assess fetomaternal haemorrhage

Perform secondary survey and treat

When patient status optimised, transfer if appropriate

Keep a record chart
Include pulse, BP, respiratory rate, SaO_2, FHR, urine output, exhaled CO_2 and treatments given

Document injuries, findings and treatment in notes
- Concise chronological narrative, with time, date, a signature and printed identification
- Inform consultant obstetrician

Chapter 11

Abdominal emergencies in pregnancy

Objectives

On successfully completing this topic you will:

- be able to assess the patient who has sustained abdominal trauma and recognise the possibility of injury

- be able to assess the pregnant woman with abdominal pain and diagnose potentially life-threatening conditions

- be aware of the changes in anatomy and physiology that occur in pregnancy and be aware of how they may alter the response to trauma and affect presentation of acute abdominal conditions

- be aware of the diagnostic procedures available for the investigation of abdominal trauma

- be familiar with the investigation and treatment of abdominal pain in pregnancy

- be aware of the role of ultrasound in pregnancy-related trauma especially the role of focused assessment by sonography for trauma (FAST)

- be aware of the role of diagnostic peritoneal lavage and its indications.

Background and incidence

Abdominal injuries in pregnancy are on the increase, both from accidental and non-accidental causes. Apparently fairly trivial trauma to the uterus may be responsible for significant placental abruption fatal to the fetus. Abdominal pain in pregnancy is common and missed or delayed diagnoses of intra-abdominal pathology occur not infrequently.

Abdominal injuries are a recurring cause of preventable deaths associated with major trauma in the pregnant and nonpregnant woman alike. The prompt and accurate assessment of the presence of intra-abdominal injury and its likely source can be challenging and the existence of a gravid uterus makes the decision harder. These factors apply also to the assessment of acute abdominal pain in pregnancy.

Obstetricians should become involved early in the trauma process when pregnancy is obvious or suspected. They need to be familiar with the patterns of abdominal injury in the pregnant and nonpregnant patient and their degree of priority. They need to be aware of the effects of pregnancy on the response to blood loss both of mother and fetus. The mother, especially in later pregnancy, tolerates blood loss well; the fetus tolerates maternal blood loss very badly and is a good 'monitor' of maternal hypovolaemia by demonstrating fetal distress on monitoring.

Pregnancy also may make the assessment of the abdomen more challenging. The peritoneum is less sensitive, the omentum is less able to contain local inflammation and areas of maximum tenderness may be shifted due to organ displacement secondary to the enlarging uterus, such as in appendicitis.

The 2000–2004 CEMD report makes recommendations for the use of seat belts in pregnancy: 'Above and below the bump – not over it'. Three-point seat belts should be worn throughout pregnancy, with the lap strap placed as low as possible beneath the 'bump', lying across the thighs, with the diagonal shoulder strap above the bump, lying between the breasts. The seat belt should be adjusted to fit as snugly as comfortably possible and, if necessary, the seat should be adjusted to enable the seat belt to be worn properly.

Between 2000 and 2002, eight women died from road traffic accidents while still pregnant and one died after delivery. Three of the women who died were not wearing seat belts. Three of these were still pregnant and one died after delivery. The women who were not wearing seat belts and whose life might have been saved were 'young girls or others with marked features of social exclusion'.

Introduction

You must be able to identify those patients who require immediate or emergency intervention either obstetric or surgical. A high index of suspicion is required and early consultation with other specialties. Unrecognised or underestimated abdominal injury is unfortunately still not an uncommon cause of preventable death. Up to 50% of young patients with significant intra-abdominal haemorrhage will have minimal or no signs on initial assessment. Deceleration injuries give a strong clue to the likelihood of blunt trauma, with the resulting risk of damage to viscera and damage to the uterus.

Abdominal pain, especially of acute onset in the woman with a viable fetus, is a medical emergency and both mother and fetus need urgent assessment.

Anatomy and physiology

The uterus is initially protected from injury in the first trimester by the bony pelvis and by the fact that the uterine wall is thick. Subsequently, it is the uterus that provides some protection to the abdominal contents and becomes increasingly vulnerable. As pregnancy progresses, the uterus becomes thinner. The uterus is elastic but the placenta is not, leading to the risk of the placenta shearing off the uterine wall in the case of trauma (placental abruption). In addition to abruption, there is the potential for solid and hollow visceral injury. Uterine rupture and amniotic fluid embolisation may occur. Incorrectly placed seat belts on the pregnant abdomen predispose to rupture. These conditions may not immediately occur to members of the trauma team without obstetric prompting.

In the context of haemorrhage, the physiological changes associated with pregnancy generally increase maternal tolerance to blood loss. By the third trimester, the plasma volume has expanded by 50%. While maternal tolerance to blood loss is increased, the fetus is particularly sensitive to comparatively small reductions in maternal circulating blood volume. The placental bed blood flow reduces well before the mother shows any of the classical signs of blood loss. This is in response to maternal catecholamines as well as hypovolaemia. Therefore, even modest blood loss requires careful investigation and monitoring. Significant abdominal trauma in pregnancy is associated with a high likelihood of fetal death, either early or delayed.

Fluid replacement should be aggressive to maintain blood volume and hypotensive resuscitation (maintaining a blood pressure to keep the mother conscious), such as is used for ectopic pregnancies on their way to theatre, is inappropriate.

Types of injury are blunt or penetrating. The vast majority of injuries in the UK are of blunt origin. Many are associated with motor vehicle accidents, although the incidence of violent injuries is increasing, particularly domestic violence.

Primary survey and resuscitation

A good history provides vital clues to the likelihood of abdominal injury and takes very little time. It should include 'MIST:

■ Mechanism of injury

■ Injuries already identified

■ Symptoms and signs

■ Treatment already received.

Details should also include the mechanism of restraint, if any, and details of the pregnancy. Women often carry their own obstetric notes. An 'AMPLE' history may also be useful:

■ Allergies

■ Medication

■ Previous medical history

■ Last meal

■ Events and environments related to the injury.

The principles of management are that life-threatening problems to airway and breathing should be dealt with immediately. It is, however, essential to tilt the woman as soon as possible to avoid aortocaval compression with resulting functional hypovolaemia.

Abdominal problems may cause a '**C**' problem.

It may be obvious from a brief examination during the primary survey that continuing haemorrhage is from an abdominal source and further investigation may not be necessary. Resuscitation should continue on the way to theatre for laparotomy.

Far more frequently, intra-abdominal bleeding may only be suspected and further investigations are required, and the gravid uterus makes such investigation more difficult.

The fetal heart should be checked early in suspected abdominal injury, as the occurrence of placental abruption is fairly common after significant blunt trauma to the abdomen. In the hurly-burly of the emergency room it may be difficult to hear the fetal heart with the Pinard stethoscope and a Doppler or ultrasound machine should be obtained if possible. This may be necessary to confirm the presence of a fetal heart but will also, depending on the skill of the operator, allow a FAST examination to be carried out. The mother, if conscious, is certain to be concerned about fetal wellbeing.

In addition to basic measures, such as blood grouping and crossmatching, a Kleihauer test should be carried out, even if the woman is rhesus positive, to give information about the extent of fetomaternal transfusion. The patient should be tilted, oxygen administered and intravenous fluid commenced.

A fuller examination of the abdomen, including vaginal and rectal examination, should be performed as soon as is practical. The presence of uterine contractions should be noted, as should the presence of amniotic fluid in the vagina, cervical effacement and dilatation and the relationship of the fetal presenting part to the ischial spines. Only a very gentle examination of the pelvis should be attempted if a fracture is suspected. This should be one experienced person gently pressing inwards on the pelvic bones. Under no circumstances should there be an attempt to demonstrate the 'open book fracture'. In the emergency situation the pelvis should be immobilised, e.g. with a pelvic binder or failing that a sheet will do. Stabilisation of the pelvis by external fixation may be part of resuscitation, i.e. to 'turn off the tap'.

Bleeding into the uterine muscle or into the uterine cavity is an irritant and contractions may be the first sign of a developing abruption. Distension, tenderness, guarding, rigidity suggest injury, although a seemingly normal examination does not exclude a potentially serious injury. A gastric tube and a urinary catheter should be put in place, and X-rays of the chest and pelvis should be taken and reviewed.

Aids to diagnosis

The most common investigations to detect intra-abdominal injury are diagnostic peritoneal lavage, FAST and abdominal CT scanning with intravenous contrast. While the way in which these are used varies in different institutions, the following principles generally apply.

Diagnostic peritoneal lavage

The placement of a catheter in the peritoneal cavity requires skill and a gentle touch. However, pregnancy is not a contraindication, provided that an approach above the umbilicus is used. While highly sensitive for intra-abdominal bleeding, false positives do occur and the invasive nature of the procedure has led to a decline in its use. In most institutions, it has been replaced by other investigations.

Ultrasound

A brief ultrasound examination of the left and right upper quadrant, the pelvis and the pericardium (FAST) by an experienced operator has become the initial investigation of choice in many trauma units. Good results have been achieved in pregnant trauma patients. Precise information can be obtained concerning the nature and extent of intra-abdominal bleeding and the examination is non-invasive and is easily repeatable. It may, however, fail to identify small amounts of intraperitoneal fluid, bowel or pancreatic injuries and a negative examination should be viewed with caution after a major trauma. It has the advantage that it visualises the fetal heart to obtain an accurate fetal heart rate, but is not good at diagnosing an early or evolving abruption.

Computed tomography

CT scanning provides a highly sensitive and specific examination in suspected abdominal injury. The principle disadvantage is the risk associated with transfer to a remote department away from resuscitation and operative facilities. Radiation risks have been considerably reduced in recent years. CT should only be used for stable patients where further elucidation of the precise injuries are required. In the patient with a viable pregnancy, abdominal delivery followed by a trauma laparotomy is likely to be the safer option for baby and mother.

Assessment of fetal wellbeing and viability

Data on outcome after maternal abdominal trauma suggest maternal outcomes similar to those for nonpregnant patients but there is a high likelihood of fetal loss. It cannot be over-emphasised that the best way of achieving a good fetal outcome is by thorough evaluation and resuscitation of the mother, thereby ensuring good placental perfusion and oxygenation. Once maternal stability has been achieved and life-threatening injuries have been dealt with, delivery may be expedited if fetal wellbeing is in question. A resuscitative laparotomy may be indicated for both fetal and maternal reasons. Hypotensive resuscitation is not appropriate for the pregnant woman with a live, viable fetus. The correct treatment is to turn off the tap.

Secondary survey

A complete examination of the abdomen should be carried out regardless of whether serious injury is suspected. Even limited musculoskeletal trauma may affect the progress of the pregnancy and interrupting the pregnancy may make management easier. Regular obstetric evaluation will be required.

Solid and hollow visceral injury

Injuries to the liver and spleen are less common with the protection of the gravid uterus in late pregnancy but they still occur. If a patient's cardiovascular system is stable, experienced centres may elect to treat selected patients conservatively. This is particularly the case in women where the fetus is not viable. There should be a very low threshold for caesarean section. Hollow visceral injuries can be very difficult to detect and a high index of suspicion is required to pick them up. A careful maternal and fetal examination and ultrasound examination should reveal significant uterine injuries. Injuries to the genitourinary tract, the pancreas and retroperitoneum can be difficult to detect and specialised radiological investigations may be required.

It should be remembered that the peritoneum is less sensitive in pregnancy.

Pelvic trauma

There is very little literature concerning serious pelvic injuries in the later stages of pregnancy. However, uncontrolled haemorrhage from pelvic fractures continues to be a cause of potentially avoidable death after major trauma in the nonpregnant population and the management principles are common to both groups.

Pelvic fractures may cause fracture to the fetal head, especially if the head is engaged. The precise mechanism of injury provides considerable information as to the type of pelvic injury sustained. An anteroposterior X-ray of the pelvis is a mandatory investigation in any major trauma. Serious injuries are usually obvious, although the pelvis may only be confirmed as the source of bleeding once abdominal, thoracic and external sources have been excluded.

Venous and arterial haemorrhage should be initially treated with manual attempts to return the pelvis to its anatomical position. Both these manoeuvres and the application of an external fixator (required to maintain anatomical reduction) may be difficult in the later stages of pregnancy. Often, delivery by caesarean section will be required to salvage the baby and achieve control of pelvic haemorrhage. It may be necessary to empty the uterus by caesarean section even if the baby is dead to gain access and control haemorrhage. A high index of suspicion of the pelvis as a potential source of life-threatening bleeding should be maintained until control by other means has been established.

Acute abdominal conditions presenting in pregnancy

Abdominal pain is common in pregnancy. Heartburn, indigestion, upper abdominal discomfort, nausea, vomiting, constipation and diarrhoea frequently occur. However, sudden onset of these symptoms accompanied by pain should ring alarm bells.

History

The acute onset of abdominal pain suggests rupturing or tearing including ruptured ectopic, ruptured uterus, ruptured aneurysm (splenic, renal, epigastric or aortic), rupture of an abscess or perforation of an ulcer. Acute abruption also presents with severe abdominal pain and should be the presumptive diagnosis until ruled out.

11

Trauma and other emergencies

Pain which increases over a comparatively short time is more characteristic of acute degeneration of a fibroid, acute cholecystitis, acute pancreatitis, strangulated hernia, ureteric colic, strangulation or infarction of the bowel.

Site of the pain

Right upper-quadrant pain is fairly common in pregnancy and may be caused by a variety of conditions including, most seriously, rupture of the capsule of the liver (rarely diagnosed preoperatively) and associated with pre-eclampsia, hepatitis, cholecystitis and pyelonephritis.

Left upper-quadrant pain is unusual but should always be taken seriously and splenic rupture and splenic artery rupture both need to be excluded. Both of these conditions occur more frequently in pregnancy.

Back pain is common in pregnancy.

Pain from pancreatitis is felt in the back and may be partially relieved by leaning forward. Pain from cholecystitis is commonly referred to the area of the lower ribs posteriorly or between the shoulder blades; hyperaesthesia may be present over the lower ribs to the right (Boas's sign).

Pain from renal pathology is usually felt in the loin.

Low abdominal pain is often difficult to diagnose and is often never satisfactorily explained.

Management of the commoner surgical conditions in pregnancy

Appendicitis

Appendicitis is more common in the first two trimesters but perforation is more common in the third. It has long been recognised that there is a higher morbidity for mother and baby in pregnancy and therefore a relatively high negative laparotomy is acceptable.

Laparoscopy may be helpful in early pregnancy and laparoscopic appendicectomy may be feasible. Later in pregnancy the position of the appendix shifts upwards and laterally and a muscle splitting incision should be made over the site of maximum tenderness.

Cholecystitis

Cholecystitis should be treated in the same way in the pregnant woman as in the nonpregnant. The trend is away from conservative management towards surgical treatment.

Pancreatitis

Acute pancreatitis carries 10% mortality in pregnancy but it is fortunately uncommon.

Colonic pseudo-obstruction (Ogilvie's syndrome)

Colonic pseudo-obstruction, so called Ogilvie's syndrome, can be a complication of caesarean section, as well as other abdominal operations.

There is increasing abdominal distension, which may be dramatic. Bowel sounds may sound obstructive. Abdominal X-rays will show distension of the caecum with or without ascending and transverse colon dilatation. The critical diameter of the caecum is suggested to be 9 cm. Dilatation greater than this diameter markedly increases the risk of spontaneous perforation.

Water-soluble contrast enemas can aid diagnosis and colonoscopy may be used to decompress the bowel if simple measures to manage ileus are not successful.

Intestinal obstruction in pregnancy is increasing due to the increasing incidence of surgical interventions in young women leading to adhesions.

Sigmoid volvulus

Volvulus is increased in pregnancy.

The symptoms of intestinal obstruction, absolute constipation, vomiting and colicky abdominal pains are the same in the pregnant and the nonpregnant woman. Fetal assessment should be carried out to determine if the baby should be delivered at the time of laparotomy.

Fatal abdominal problems in pregnancy

The 1997–1999 CEMD report listed three fatalities from intestinal obstruction, one of which was said to demonstrate the difficulty in diagnosing acute abdominal pain in pregnancy, and two of which demonstrated substandard care. There were two deaths from pancreatitis, one from a splenic artery aneurysm, one from intra-abdominal bleeding, one from liver failure and one from liver rupture.

These cases point out the need to carry out a structured laparotomy when operating for malignancy and hypovolaemic shock, if a patient has hypovolaemic shock that cannot be explained by blood loss, on the floor, in the chest or due to fractures in the pelvis or long bones (blood on the floor and four places more: chest, abdomen, pelvis and long bones).

The laparotomy should be a structured 'trauma' laparotomy with an experienced general surgeon to hand. These deaths are classified as indirect deaths.

The 2000–2002 CEMD report again records seven deaths which were as follows: three deaths from intestinal obstruction and/or perforation of the bowel; there was one death each from peritonitis, pancreatitis, a pancreatic cyst and ruptured oesophagus.

A number of avoidable factors were identified.

■ There was failure to recognise the significance of a falling blood pressure and a rising pulse and despite these observations a patient was sent home post-caesarean section without medical review.

■ There was failure to make a provisional diagnosis despite an admission of a patient with abdominal pain who required intravenous fluids.

■ Symptoms were ascribed to a mental disorder despite abnormal biochemical results being available.

■ A patient with known bowel disease was not being seen by senior members of staff despite being given repeated doses of pethidine analgesia and a steroid injection.

■ There was delay in carrying out surgery in an isolated unit.

■ Extreme obesity caused a delay in diagnosis and difficulty achieving intravenous access.

■ There was failure of a senior anaesthetist to attend a known high-risk case despite concerns being passed on with regard to expected anaesthetic difficulties.

■ There was lack of a tertiary centre to take a patient with major pulmonary problems although many hours were spent on the telephone trying to find a bed.

The above factors emphasise the importance of women at high risk being confined in units with adequate facilities and quick access to specialist help and also to the significance of changes in pulse and blood pressure in a previously healthy pregnant woman.

Summary

■ Acute abdominal problems in pregnancy are increasing due to an increase in trauma and the increased exposure of young women to surgical procedures.

■ These deaths are classified as indirect deaths.

■ It must always be remembered how well young, fit, pregnant women compensate for blood loss.

■ Obstetricians should call on advice from other specialties early in the case of non-obstetric disease. Few people have experience of dealing with major trauma in pregnancy but if the woman is pregnant the obstetrician will be involved early and their input required.

Algorithm 12.1 The unconscious patient

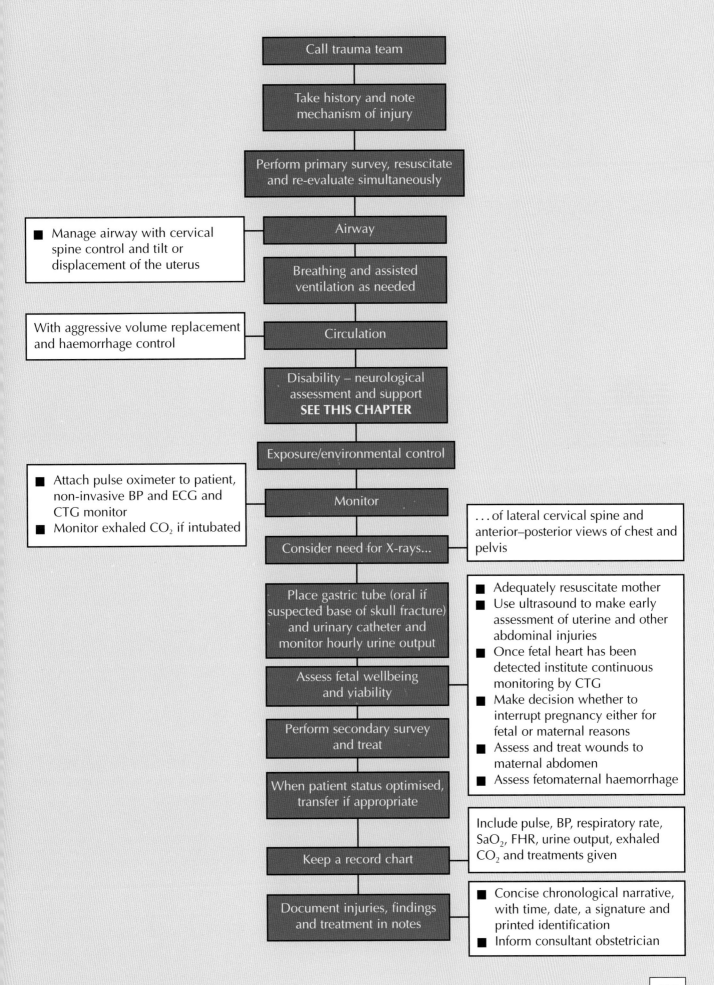

Call trauma team

Take history and note mechanism of injury

Perform primary survey, resuscitate and re-evaluate simultaneously

Airway
- Manage airway with cervical spine control and tilt or displacement of the uterus

Breathing and assisted ventilation as needed

Circulation
- With aggressive volume replacement and haemorrhage control

Disability – neurological assessment and support **SEE THIS CHAPTER**

Exposure/environmental control

Monitor
- Attach pulse oximeter to patient, non-invasive BP and ECG and CTG monitor
- Monitor exhaled CO_2 if intubated

Consider need for X-rays...
...of lateral cervical spine and anterior–posterior views of chest and pelvis

Place gastric tube (oral if suspected base of skull fracture) and urinary catheter and monitor hourly urine output

Assess fetal wellbeing and viability
- Adequately resuscitate mother
- Use ultrasound to make early assessment of uterine and other abdominal injuries
- Once fetal heart has been detected institute continuous monitoring by CTG
- Make decision whether to interrupt pregnancy either for fetal or maternal reasons
- Assess and treat wounds to maternal abdomen
- Assess fetomaternal haemorrhage

Perform secondary survey and treat

When patient status optimised, transfer if appropriate

Keep a record chart
Include pulse, BP, respiratory rate, SaO_2, FHR, urine output, exhaled CO_2 and treatments given

Document injuries, findings and treatment in notes
- Concise chronological narrative, with time, date, a signature and printed identification
- Inform consultant obstetrician

Chapter 12

The unconscious patient

Objectives

On successfully completing this topic you will be able to:

■ describe the principles of treatment of the unconscious patient

■ understand the concept of secondary brain injury and how to prevent it

■ identify types of lesion amenable to surgery (extradural and subdural haematoma).

Incidence

The 2000–2002 Confidential Enquiries described 17 deaths due to subarachnoid haemorrhage, four to intracerebral haemorrhage and 13 deaths from epilepsy. The 1997–99 report had reported 11 deaths due to subarachnoid haemorrhage, five due to intracerebral haemorrhage, five due to cerebral thrombosis and nine due to epilepsy. The management of the unconscious patient as a result of whatever cause should therefore be a basic skill of every obstetrician and midwife. The obstetric team should be aware of the potential causes of a decreased level of consciousness and treat the underlying cause as appropriate.

Causes of decreased level of consciousness:

A B Failure of airway or breathing: hypoxia/hypercarbia

C Failure of circulation: hypotension or cardiac arrest

D Failure of central nervous system:

☐ eclampsia or epileptic

☐ intracranial haemorrhage, trauma, thrombosis, tumour or infection

☐ drugs, alcohol or poisoning.

Principles of treatment

Primary and secondary brain injury

Primary brain injury is the neurological damage produced by the initial event such as a brain haemorrhage. Secondary (further) brain injury is the neurological damage caused by lack of oxygen delivery to the brain. This may be caused by:

■ A B Failure of ventilation caused by airway obstruction or inadequate breathing resulting in poor oxygenation. In addition, both airway obstruction and inadequate breathing may lead to a rise in arterial carbon dioxide levels. This has direct consequences on intracranial pressure (see below).

- C Failure of circulation due to hypotension

- D intracerebral damage may cause an excessive rise in intracranial pressure leading to reduced cerebral perfusion pressure (CPP).

Cerebral perfusion

Cerebral perfusion refers to the supply of oxygenated blood to the brain. The blood supply to the brain is more complex than other organs because the brain is enclosed inside a rigid box. The volume of this box is fixed so one component can only increase in volume at the expense of another, or at the expense of an increase in intracranial pressure (ICP). The main components inside the box are:

- brain substance or space occupying lesions

- cerebral spinal fluid

- cerebral blood vessels and the blood contained within these vessels

- extracellular fluid.

Cerebral perfusion pressure (CPP) depends on the mean arterial pressure (MAP) pushing blood into the brain and the resistance to this blood flow from the intracranial pressure due to box contents.

$$CPP = MAP - ICP$$

- Any factors affecting mean arterial pressure or intracranial pressure will affect cerebral perfusion pressure.

- Adequate blood pressure (MAP) must be maintained to maintain CPP.

- Rises in volume of box contents may need to be controlled if the normal mechanism of cerebral autoregulation of intracranial pressure has failed:

  ☐ Brain substance or space occupying lesions can increase in volume as a result of tumour or blood clot. These may need surgery.

  ☐ Cerebral spinal fluid can increase in volume if there is an obstruction to free drainage of the fluid, e.g. by blood clots leading to hydrocephalus. Cerebral spinal fluid can be drained by temporary or permanent surgical shunts.

  ☐ Cerebral blood content can increase in volume if the arterial carbon dioxide levels are allowed to rise resulting in cerebral vasodilatation. Carbon dioxide levels can be reduced by maintaining a clear airway and controlling ventilation to a normal level of $PaCO_2$.

  ☐ Extracellular fluid levels can increase as a result of response to injury, such as around tumours or following cell damage caused by a major head injury. This is difficult to treat but careful fluid management avoiding excess intravenous fluids will be part of the care.

  ☐ Raised intracranial pressure may also be due to obstruction of venous drainage from the head. This may be due to pressure on the neck veins, head down position or excess intrathoracic pressure.

Normal MAP = 70–90 mmHg

Normal ICP = 10 mmHg

If CPP is less than 50 mmHg, cerebral hypoxia may follow

(There are limits beyond which the MAP itself will contribute to a rise in intracranial pressure: systolic BP > 160 mmHg)

Priorities in management to prevent secondary brain injury

1. **Primary survey and resuscitation.**

2. **Secondary survey.**

3. **Assessment of fetal wellbeing and viability.**

It follows that preventing a rise in intracranial pressure or a fall in cerebral perfusion is vital in the overall management of head injury.

1. Primary survey and resuscitation

A Airway

Clear the airway. A patient with a reduced level of consciousness is more likely to have a compromised airway as the tongue falls back into the posterior pharynx. Further, she is at risk of aspiration as she has obtunded laryngeal reflexes.

B Breathing

Adequate ventilation ensures that the brain receives blood containing enough oxygen, thereby preventing further brain injury. Adequate ventilation prevents the accumulation of carbon dioxide. Ventilation may be impaired by a reduced level of consciousness.

Raised intrathoracic pressure (as happens in tension pneumothorax) will compromise venous drainage from the head and raise ICP.

C Circulation

An adequate blood pressure is required to maintain cerebral perfusion pressure. Use fluids and vasopressors appropriately. Hypotension resulting from other injuries must be swiftly recognised and managed to prevent secondary brain injury. It is equally important to remember that excessive fluids are rarely needed in an isolated head injury and may contribute to worsening cerebral oedema.

Never assume that the brain injury is the cause of hypotension. Scalp lacerations may bleed profusely but hypotension secondary to an isolated brain injury is uncommon and usually fatal. Always presume that hypotension is due to hypovolaemia outside the brain, not brain injury, and look for a source of blood loss elsewhere.

Cushing's response (progressive hypertension, bradycardia and slowing of respiratory rate) is an acute response to rapidly rising intracranial pressure and is a pre-morbid sign. This needs urgent attention, which may include establishing controlled ventilation, use of mannitol and/or urgent surgery.

D Disability

A decrease in level of consciousness is the marker of brain injury. Generally, the more deeply unconscious a patient becomes, the more serious is the injury.

AVPU: a rapid assessment of conscious level is made in the primary survey. Is the patient **A**lert, responding to **V**oice, only responding to **P**ain or **U**nresponsive?

Pupillary responses may help to identify the degree of intracranial compromise and the possibility of a unilateral space-occupying lesion.

Additional measures:

■ avoid head-down position, head up if possible

■ avoid ties around the neck, e.g. for an endotracheal tube

■ control fluid therapy carefully

■ avoid rises in intrathoracic pressure

■ rapid access to surgery may be required to evacuate blood clot

■ high-dose steroids may reduce swelling associated with brain tumours.

2. Assessment of fetal wellbeing and viability

When the mother is adequately resuscitated, the further wellbeing of the fetus must be considered. Timing of delivery should be considered in the patient about to undergo neurosurgical treatment or a prolonged period of intensive care, or who is unlikely to recover consciousness. Delivery of the term fetus may be appropriate if a prolonged period of intensive care is anticipated. Physiological complications that develop in the long-term intensive care patient (coagulopathy, sepsis, etc.) may complicate a continuing pregnancy.

3. Secondary survey

The neurological examination assesses:

■ pupillary function

■ lateralising signs, e.g. limb weakness

■ level of consciousness by the Glasgow Coma Scale.

The mini-neurological examination serves to determine the severity of the brain injury and the likelihood of a surgically treatable lesion. When applied repeatedly, it can be used to determine objectively any neurological deterioration. It is supplemented by CT scanning.

Pupillary function

Evaluate the pupils for their equality and response to bright light. A difference in diameter of the pupils of more than 1 mm is abnormal but a local injury to the eye may be responsible for this abnormality. Normal reaction to a bright light is brisk constriction of the pupil; a more sluggish response may indicate brain injury. Pressure on the third cranial nerve (oculomotor) will result in a dilated pupil on the same side ('ipsilateral') as the injury.

Lateralising signs, such as limb weakness

Observe spontaneous limb movements for equality. If movement is negligible then assess the response to a painful stimulus. Any delay in onset of movement or lateralisation of movement following a painful stimulus is significant. Obvious limb weakness localised to one side suggests an intracranial injury causing brain compression on the opposite side. Damage to the motor or sensory cortex (or tracts leading from them) will result in a motor or sensory deficit on the opposite side to the injury.

Level of consciousness

Glasgow Coma Scale provides a quantitative assessment of the level of consciousness. It is the sum of scores awarded (Table 12.1) for three types of response:

Table 12.1. Glasgow Coma Scale scoring

Response	Points
Eye opening	
Spontaneous, that is, open with normal blinking	4
Eye opening to speech on request	3
Eye opening only to pain stimulus	2
No eye opening despite stimulation	1
Verbal response	
Orientated, spontaneous speech	5
Confused conversation but answers questions	4
Inappropriate words, that is, garbled speech but with recognisable words	3
Incomprehensible sounds or grunts	2
No verbal response	1
Motor response	
Obeys commands and moves limbs to command	6
Localizes, for example, moves upper limb to pain stimulus on head	5
Withdraws from painful stimulus on limb	4
Abnormal flexion or decorticate posture	3
Extensor response, decerebrate posture	2
No movement to any stimulus	1

■ Eye opening (E)
The scoring of eye opening is not possible if the eyes are so swollen as to be permanently shut. This fact must be documented.

■ Verbal response (V)
The scoring of verbal response is not possible if the patient cannot speak because of endotracheal intubation. This fact must be documented.

■ Motor response (M)
The best response obtained for either of the upper extremities is recorded even though worse responses may be present in other extremities.

The Glasgow Coma Scale is scored differently in children.

Subsequent reassessment can be used to detect any deterioration. For example, if the Glasgow Coma Scale has decreased by two points or more, deterioration has occurred. A decrease of three points or more is a bad prognostic indicator and demands immediate treatment.

Severity of head injuries is classified as follows:

Score 8 or less = Severe

Score 9 to 12 = Moderate

Score 13 to 15 = Minor

Changes in vital signs

Dramatic changes in the Glasgow Coma Scale are often preceded by more subtle changes in vital signs indicating deterioration. Rising intracranial pressure due to brain swelling or expanding haematomas inside the head can cause pressure on the respiratory and cardiovascular centres in the brain stem. This produces respiratory or cardiovascular abnormalities such as changes in heart rate and blood pressure, change in breathing pattern and rate.

Types of head injury

Primary brain injury may be diffuse or focal.

Diffuse primary brain injury

Blunt injury to the brain may cause diffuse brain injury, particularly when rapid head motion (acceleration or deceleration) leads to widespread damage within the brain substance. Such injuries form a spectrum extending from mild concussion to severe injury known as diffuse axonal injury.

Concussion is a brain injury accompanied by a brief loss of consciousness and, in its mildest form, may cause only temporary confusion or amnesia. With mild forms of concussion, most patients will be slightly confused and may be able to describe how the injury occurred. They are likely to complain of mild headache, dizziness or nausea. The mini-neurological examination will not show lateralising signs. With more severe concussion there is a longer period of unconsciousness, longer amnesia (for time both before and after the injury) and there may be focal signs. The duration of amnesia needs to be recorded.

Diffuse axonal injury is so severe as to cause a characteristically long coma in 44% of cases. The overall mortality rate is over 30%, rising to 50% in its most severe form. The treatment of such injury involves prolonged controlled ventilation in an intensive care unit.

Focal primary brain injury

Contusions are caused by blunt injury producing acceleration and deceleration forces on the brain tissue, resulting in tearing of the small blood vessels inside the brain. Contusions can occur immediately beneath the area of impact, when they are known as coup injuries, or at a point distant from the area of impact in the direction of the applied force, when they are known as contrecoup injuries. If the contusion occurs near the sensory or motor areas of the brain, these patients will present with a neurological deficit. Precise diagnosis requires appropriate imaging (CT scanning).

Haematomata within the skull may arise either from meningeal vessels or from vessels within the brain substance. They are defined anatomically; such a classification is useful as it has implications in terms of remediable surgery, urgency and prognosis.

Intracerebral haematomata

Extradural haemorrhage

Extradural haemorrhage is caused by a tear in a dural artery, most commonly the middle meningeal artery. This can be torn by a linear fracture crossing the temporal or parietal bone and injuring the artery lying in a groove on the deep aspect of the bone.

Isolated extradural haemorrhage is unusual, accounting for only 0.5% of all head injuries and less than 1.0% of injuries causing coma. The importance of early recognition of this injury lies in the fact that, when treated appropriately, the prognosis is good because of the lack of underlying serious injury to brain tissue. If unrecognised, the rapidly expanding haematoma causes intracranial pressure to rise, reducing cerebral perfusion and leading to cerebral hypoxia, coma and death.

The typical symptoms and signs of extradural haemorrhage are:

■ loss of consciousness followed by a lucid interval (which may not be a complete return to full consciousness)

■ secondary depression of consciousness

■ dilated pupil on the side of injury

■ weakness of the arm and leg on the contralateral side to the injury.

Subdural haemorrhage

Subdural heamorrhage is more common than extradural haemorrhage and is found in 30% of all severe head injuries. The mortality rate is up to 60% because, in addition to the compression caused by the subdural blood clot, there is often major injury to the underlying brain tissue. The haematoma can arise from tears in the bridging veins between the cortex and the dura or from laceration of the brain substance and the cortical arteries.

The typical symptoms and signs of subdural haemorrhage are:

■ varying levels of consciousness, depending on the underlying brain damage and rate of haematoma formation

■ dilated pupil on the side of the injury

■ weakness of the arm and leg on the contralateral side to the injury.

Initial treatment:

■ prevent secondary brain injury

■ urgent evacuation of the haematoma where surgically amenable.

Delay in the treatment of extradural haemorrhage beyond 2 hours and delay in the treatment of subdural haemorrhage beyond four hours worsens the prognosis.

Subarachnoid haemorrhage

Where haemorrhaging has occurred into the subarachnoid space, the irritant effect of the bloody cerebrospinal fluid causes headache, photophobia and neck stiffness. On its own, this is not serious but prognosis is poor if it is associated with a more severe head injury.

Intracerebral laceration

Through-and-through injuries, side-to-side injuries and injuries in the lower region of the brain stem all have a poor outcome.

All foreign bodies found protruding from the skull must be left in place. These should only be removed at a neurosurgical unit. Skull X-rays will show the angle and depth of penetration. Care must be taken during transfer to ensure that there is no further penetration.

Open brain injury in a conscious patient carries a good prognosis if surgery is not delayed. Scalp haemorrhage should be stopped, entrance and exit wounds covered with sterile dressings and the patient transferred to a neurosurgical unit.

Other injuries

Scalp wounds

The scalp is arranged in layers. It is highly vascular and a laceration will often result in profuse haemorrhage. The bleeding point should be located and the haemorrhage arrested. This may include the use of haemostatic surgical clips and ligatures, particularly where the laceration is deep. Direct pressure may not be sufficient. The wound should be inspected carefully for signs of skull fracture and irrigated to remove debris and dirt.

Gentle palpation of the scalp wound wearing a sterile glove may enable you to diagnose the presence of a skull fracture. If an open or depressed fracture is detected, close the wound with sutures, apply a dressing, give antibiotics and transfer the patient to a neurosurgical unit. Do not remove any bone fragments at this stage.

Skull fractures

Although skull fractures are common, many major brain injuries will occur without the skull being fractured and many skull fractures are not associated with severe brain injury. Where the mini-neurological examination identifies the presence of a severe brain injury, time taken to search for a skull fracture should never delay definitive management. The significance of a skull fracture is that it identifies a patient with a higher probability of having or developing an intracranial haematoma. All patients with skull fractures should be admitted for observation.

- Linear skull fractures

  These are particularly important when the fracture crosses the line of intracranial vessels indicating an increased risk of intracranial haemorrhage.

- Depressed skull fractures

  All depressed skull fractures should be transferred for neurosurgical unit assessment. They may be associated with underlying brain injury and require operative elevation to reduce the risk of infection.

- Open skull fractures

  By definition, there is direct communication between the outside of the head and brain tissue because the dura covering the surface of the brain is torn. This can be diagnosed if brain tissue is visible on examination of the scalp wound or if cerebrospinal fluid is seen to be leaking from the wound. These fractures all require operative intervention and the risk of infection is high. Give prophylactic antibiotics.

- Basal skull fractures

  The base of the skull does not run horizontally backwards but diagonally. Basal skull fractures will produce signs along this diagonal line. They can be diagnosed clinically in the presence of cerebrospinal fluid leaking from the ear (otorrhoea) or the nose (rhinorrhoea). When cerebrospinal fluid is mixed with blood it may be difficult to detect. Bruising in the mastoid region (Battle's sign) also indicates basal skull fracture but the bruising usually takes 12–36 hours to develop. Blood seen behind the tympanic membrane (haemotympanum) may also indicate a basal skull fracture. Fractures through the cribriform plate are frequently associated with bilateral periorbital haematomas. Subconjunctival haematoma may occur from direct orbital roof fracture, in which case there is no posterior limit to the haematoma.

  All these signs may take several hours to develop and may not be present in a patient seen immediately after injury. Basal skull fractures are very difficult to diagnose from plain X-ray films.

Summary

■ Remember the **A B C D E** routine.

■ Prevent secondary injury by: preventing hypoxia, hypercarbia and hypovolaemia.

■ Establish a working diagnosis.

■ Constantly repeat the mini-neurological examination.

■ Consider the best management of the fetus.

12

Trauma and other emergencies

Algorithm 13.1 Spine and spinal cord injuries

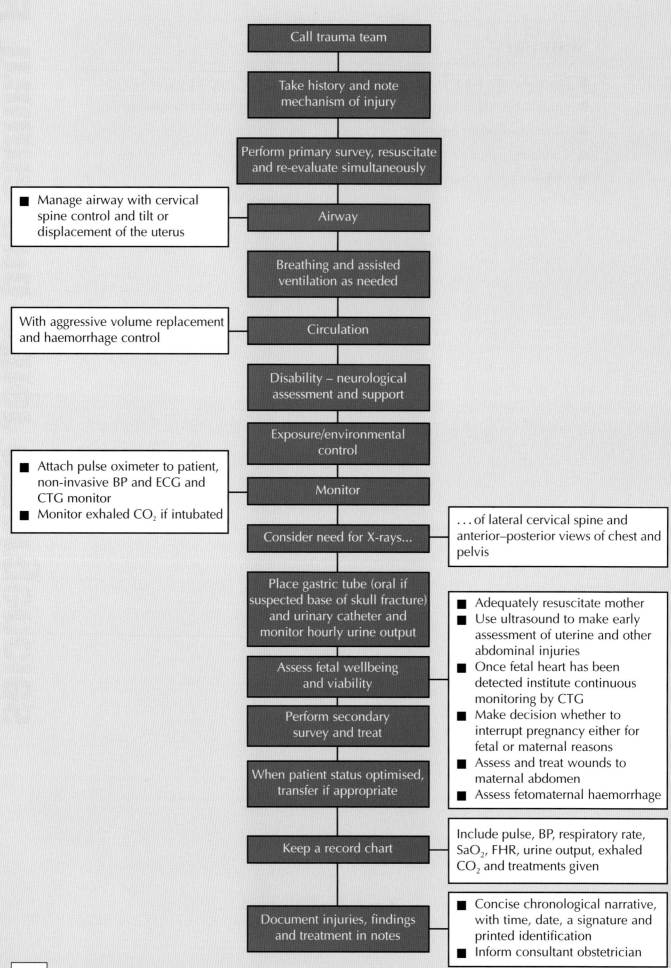

Call trauma team

Take history and note mechanism of injury

Perform primary survey, resuscitate and re-evaluate simultaneously

- Manage airway with cervical spine control and tilt or displacement of the uterus

Airway

Breathing and assisted ventilation as needed

With aggressive volume replacement and haemorrhage control

Circulation

Disability – neurological assessment and support

Exposure/environmental control

- Attach pulse oximeter to patient, non-invasive BP and ECG and CTG monitor
- Monitor exhaled CO_2 if intubated

Monitor

Consider need for X-rays...

...of lateral cervical spine and anterior–posterior views of chest and pelvis

Place gastric tube (oral if suspected base of skull fracture) and urinary catheter and monitor hourly urine output

Assess fetal wellbeing and viability

- Adequately resuscitate mother
- Use ultrasound to make early assessment of uterine and other abdominal injuries
- Once fetal heart has been detected institute continuous monitoring by CTG
- Make decision whether to interrupt pregnancy either for fetal or maternal reasons
- Assess and treat wounds to maternal abdomen
- Assess fetomaternal haemorrhage

Perform secondary survey and treat

When patient status optimised, transfer if appropriate

Keep a record chart

Include pulse, BP, respiratory rate, SaO_2, FHR, urine output, exhaled CO_2 and treatments given

Document injuries, findings and treatment in notes

- Concise chronological narrative, with time, date, a signature and printed identification
- Inform consultant obstetrician

Chapter 13

Spine and spinal cord injuries

Objectives

On successfully completing this topic you will be able to:

■ recognise circumstances in which spinal trauma is likely to occur

■ understand the importance and techniques of spinal immobilisation

■ identify and evaluate spinal trauma.

Introduction

In the context of this chapter, spinal injuries refer to injuries to the bony spinal column, the spinal cord or both. There can be an injury to the bony spine without injury to the spinal cord, but there is significant risk of cord injury in these circumstances.

Failure to immobilise a patient with a spinal injury can cause neurological damage or exacerbate it. Failure to immobilise a patient with an injury to the bony spine (without cord injury at that stage) can cause injury to the spinal cord. Evaluation of the spine and exclusion of spinal injuries can be safely deferred as long as the person's spine is protected.

A spinal injury should always be suspected:

■ in falls from a height

■ in vehicle collisions, even at low speed

■ when pedestrians have been hit by a vehicle

■ where persons have been thrown

■ in sports field injuries, e.g. rugby

■ in a person with multiple injuries

■ in a person with injury above the clavicle (including the unconscious patient – 15% of unconscious patients have some form of neck injury)

■ in the conscious patient complaining of neck pain and sensory and/or motor symptoms.

Persons who are awake, sober, neurologically normal and have no neck pain are extremely unlikely to have a cervical spine fracture. However, neurosurgical or orthopaedic opinion should always be taken if an injury is suspected or detected.

The cervical spine is more vulnerable to injury than the thoracic or lumbar spine.

Approximately 10% of patients with a cervical spine fracture have a second associated non-contiguous fracture of the vertebral column. Hence if a cervical spine fracture is diagnosed, other spinal fractures should be suspected.

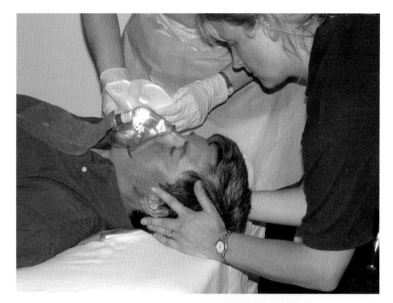

Manual immobilisation

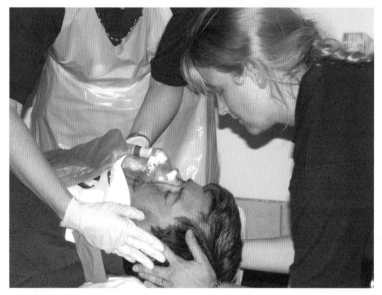

Immobilisation and collar application

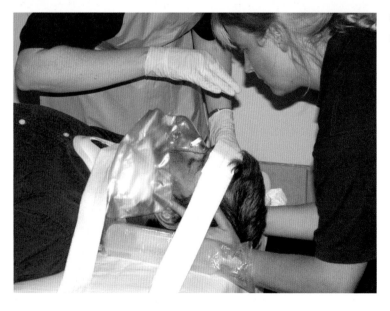

Collar, blocks (sandbags) and straps (tapes)

Figure 13.1 Immobilisation techniques

Immobilisation techniques

If injury to the spine is suspected, the whole spine should be immobilised until examination, X-ray and supplementary radiological investigations have excluded spinal injury. Injury can only be excluded by an orthopaedic or neurosurgeon or a suitably skilled A&E doctor.

Immobilisation should be carried out by maintaining the spine in the neutral position.

Immobilisation of the spine is done by:

- manual in-line immobilisation of the head or
- semi-rigid cervical collar plus blocks on a backboard (which may be a head board or full spine board and straps) (Figures 13.1 & 13.2).

Collars are correctly sized by using manufacturer's instructions.

Spine board

The thoracic and lumbar spine should be immobilised by a long spine board. Inadequate or even prolonged immobilisation with a spine board has its own complications, with the possibility of worsening any injury and the risk of pressure sores if prolonged immobilisation is undertaken. Hence, the long backboard is usually a transportation device. Early assessment by neurosurgeon or orthopaedic surgeon is undertaken to allow removal from the device. If this is not feasible the injured patient should be log-rolled every 2 hours while maintaining spinal integrity.

To avoid supine hypotension in the heavily pregnant patient, the right hip should be elevated to four to six inches with a towel and the uterus displaced manually. Alternatively the whole patient can be tilted to the left if on a long spine board by putting a wedge under the board (Figure 13.3). If a pelvic fracture is suspected, manual displacement of the uterus is recommended rather than elevation of the hip.

Evaluation of a patient with a suspected spinal injury

Spinal injuries may cause problems that are identified in the primary survey, affecting airway breathing, or circulation or the injury may itself be identified during the secondary survey.

Spinal assessment

A log-roll must be performed (Figure 13.4). This is a coordinated, skilled manoeuvre by trained personnel. At least four persons are required to perform this: one to maintain manual in-line mobilisation of the patient's head and neck, one for the torso with pelvis, one for the hips and legs with the fourth directing the procedure and move the spine board so as to turn the patient from the supine to the lateral position without causing damage to the spinal cord.

Look for bruising, deformity and localised swelling of the vertebral column. Palpate for localised tenderness or gaps between spinous processes. At this point it is appropriate to carry out a per rectum examination.

Neurological assessment

Of the many tracts in the spinal cord the three that can be assessed clinically are:

- corticospinal tract: controls muscle power on the same side of the body and is tested by voluntary movement and involuntary response to painful stimuli

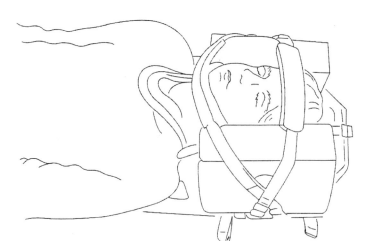

Figure 13.2 Immobilisation of the cervical spine

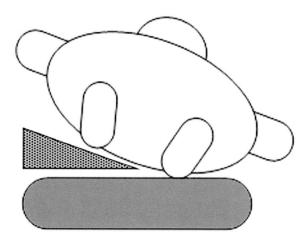

Figure 13.3 Cardiff wedge

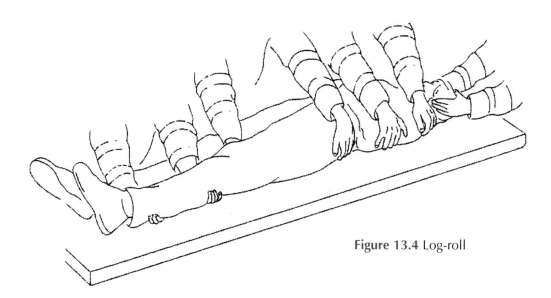

Figure 13.4 Log-roll

- spinothalamic tract: transmits pain and temperature sensation from the opposite side of the body and is tested generally by pinprick
- posterior columns: carry position sense from the same side.

Each can be injured on one or both sides.

If there is no demonstrable sensory or motor function below a certain level bilaterally, this is referred to as a complete spinal injury. If there is remaining motor or sensory function with some loss this is an incomplete injury (better prognosis). Sparing of sensation in the perianal region may be the only sign of residual function. Sacral sparing is demonstrated by presence of sensation perianally and/or voluntary contraction of the anal sphincter.

An injury does not qualify as incomplete on the basis of preserved sacral reflexes, e.g. bulbo-cavernous or anal wink. Priapism is due to unopposed parasympathetic drive and is suggestive of a spinal injury.

The neurological level is the most caudal segment with normal sensory and motor function on both sides.

For completeness, the key dermatomes are given in Figure 13.5.

Each nerve root innervates more than one muscle and most muscles have innervation from more than one nerve root. Certain movements, however, are identified as representing a single nerve root.

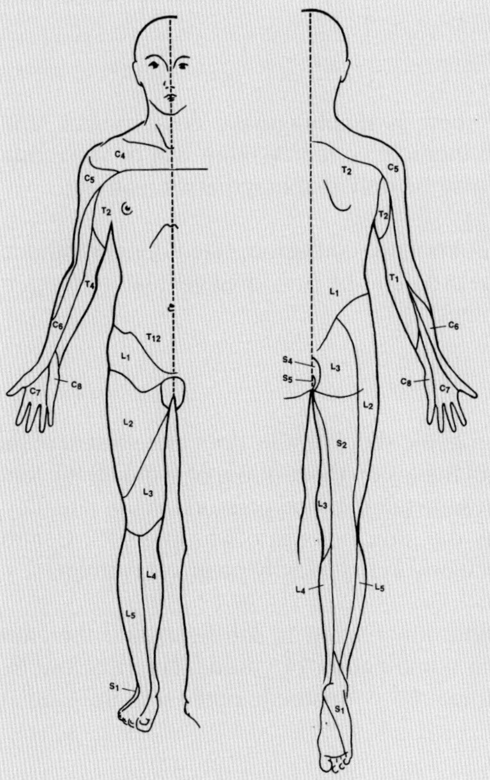

Dermatome	Area
Sensory	
C5	Area over deltoid
C6	Thumb
C7	Middle finger
C8	Little finger
T4	Nipple
T8	Xiphisternum
T10	Umbilicus
T12	Symphysis
L4	Medial aspect shin
L5	Web of first and second toes
S1	Lateral border of foot
S4/5	Perianal
Motor	
C5	Deltoid (shoulder abduction)
C6	Wrist extension
C7	Elbow extension
C8	Flexion of middle finger
T1	Abduction of small finger
L2	Hip flexion
L3	Knee extension
L4	Dorsiflexion
L5	Extension of big toe
S1	Plantar flexion

Figure 13.5 Dermatomes used for sensory and motor testing

A broad distinction can be made between lesions above and lesions below T1 (as determined by sensory and motor testing). Lesions above T1 result in quadriplegia and lesions below T1 result in paraplegia. There is a discrepancy between neurological injury level and level of bony injury because spinal nerves travel up or down the canal from the point of entry through bone to join the spinal cord. The level quoted is the neurological level.

Principles of treatment

The principles of treatment are primary survey and resuscitation, assessment of fetal wellbeing and viability, then secondary survey and protection from further injury.

A spinal injury may present in either the primary survey or the secondary survey.

- Deal with life-threatening conditions according to the **A B C** but avoid any movement of the spinal column.

- Establish adequate immobilisation and maintain it until you are certain there is no spinal injury.

- Make an early referral to a neurosurgeon or orthopaedic surgeon if a spinal injury is suspected or detected.

- Be aware of associations of spinal injury or effects on other systems and injuries.

Effect or associations identified in the primary survey

Airway obstruction

Trauma that has caused damage to the spine is likely to have caused injury above the clavicle. This may take the form of an injury to the airway or a head injury, which puts the patient at risk of airway problems.

Breathing problems

If the injury is above the fourth cervical vertebra there is diaphragmatic compromise. With injuries between the fourth cervical and the twelfth thoracic vertebrae there will be intercostal embarrassment and, depending on the level, there may be only diaphragmatic breathing.

Complicating factors are rib fractures, flail chest, pulmonary contusion, haemopneumothorax and aspiration pneumonitis. Vigorously address these problems by providing ventilatory support, chest drainage and, if the patient can feel pain, analgesia.

Neurogenic shock

Spinal injury may cause a **C**irculation problem. Neurogenic shock results from impairment of the descending sympathetic pathways. Below the level of the lesion there is loss of sympathetic tone to the vessels and therefore vasodilatation, which causes a fall in blood pressure. In this situation, blood pressure is not restored by fluid alone but by the judicious use of vasopressors. Central venous pressure monitoring may be indicated, particularly in the heavily pregnant woman.

Injury above the T4 level causes loss of sympathetic innervation to the heart and therefore bradycardia. With an injury above the T4 level the combination of vasodilatation below the level of the lesion and the bradycardia caused by impaired sympathetic outflow to the cardiac accelerators can cause profound hypotension.

Atropine may be needed to counteract bradycardia. It may be ineffective and an isoprenaline infusion may be required. Advice from intensivists should be taken.

Abdominal injuries

Abdominal injuries may present as a **C** problem. Inability to feel pain due to spinal injury may mask serious intra-abdominal injury. The only symptom pointing to an intra-abdominal problem may be referred shoulder-tip pain. Ileus is usual in a paralysed patient; so a nasogastric tube should be passed.

Locomotor

Musculoskeletal problems may present a life-threatening hypovolaemia but be less readily detected in a patient with spinal cord injury because of the inability to feel pain.

Skin

In a high cord lesion, temperature control function is lost and the patient may become hypothermic or hyperthermic.

Secondary survey

Any injury may be masked by the absence of pain. A vigilant approach to detection is needed. Correct management of upper limb injuries may have a profound effect on the eventual mobility of a quadriplegic.

Bladder

Patients with spinal cord injury and urinary retention need continuous catheter drainage. The recording of urinary output is a good monitor of response to resuscitation.

Recovery and rehabilitation

In a pregnant woman who has sustained severe spinal trauma, the pregnancy may still remain unaffected as long as the vital parameters have been stable. Initial care of the woman with suspected spinal injury determines outcome of the pregnancy.

Summary

- Appropriate immobilisation of the injured patient during primary resuscitation is a vital part of care until further investigation can be carried out

- Spinal injuries may be a cause of ABC problems which should be treated first

- Hypotension due to spinal shock may require vasopressors rather than excess fluids

---

Trauma and other emergencies

Appendix 13A

Practical procedures

Reproduced with permission from the Advanced Life Support Group.

Procedures

■ Manual cervical spine immobilisation.

■ Application of a cervical collar.

■ Application of headblocks and straps.

■ Log-rolling.

Cervical spine immobilisation

All patients with serious trauma (e.g. fall, road traffic accident, assault) must be treated as though they have a cervical spine injury. It is only when adequate investigations have been performed and a neurosurgical or orthopaedic consultation obtained, if necessary, that the decision to remove cervical spine protection should be taken. Manual in-line cervical stabilisation should be continued until a hard collar has been applied, and sandbags and tape or head blocks and straps or sandbags and tape are in position as described below (Figure 13A.1).

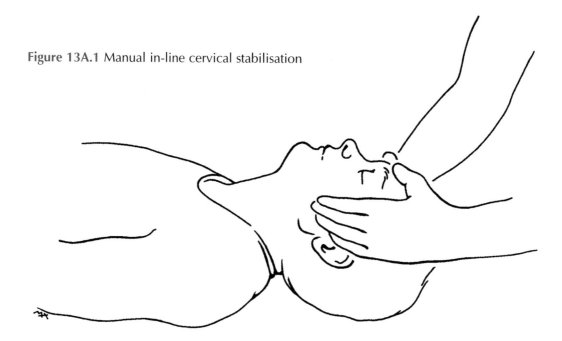

Figure 13A.1 Manual in-line cervical stabilisation

Two techniques are described. It is necessary to apply both to achieve adequate cervical spine control.

Once the collar is in place, the neck is largely obscured. Before placing the collar look for the following signs quickly and without moving the neck:

- distended veins
- tracheal deviation
- wounds
- laryngeal crepitus
- subcutaneous emphysema
- earrings or necklaces (if these are left on they may obscure c-spine x-rays)

Application of a cervical collar

The key to successful, effective, collar application lies in selecting the correct size.

Minimum equipment

- Measuring device.
- Range of hard collars or a multi-sized collar.

Method

- Assess peripheral sensation.
- Ensure that manual in-line cervical stabilisation is maintained throughout by a second person.
- Using the manufacturer's method, select a correctly sized collar.
- Assemble the collar as necessary.
- Taking care not to cause movement, pass the flat part of the collar behind the neck.
- Fold the shaped part of the collar round and place it under the chin.
- Fold the flat part of the collar with its integral joining device (usually Velcro tape) around until it meets the shaped part.
- Reassess the correct fit of the collar.
- If the fit is wrong, slip the flat part of the collar out from behind the neck, taking care not to cause movement. Select the correct size and recommence the procedure.
- If the fit is correct secure the joining device.
- Ensure that manual in-line cervical stabilisation is maintained until head blocks and straps or sandbags and tape are in position.

Application of headblocks and tape

Equipment

- Two headblocks.
- Attachment system.

Method

- Ensure that manual in-line cervical stabilisation is maintained by a second person throughout.
- Place a headblock either side of the head (Figure 13A.2).

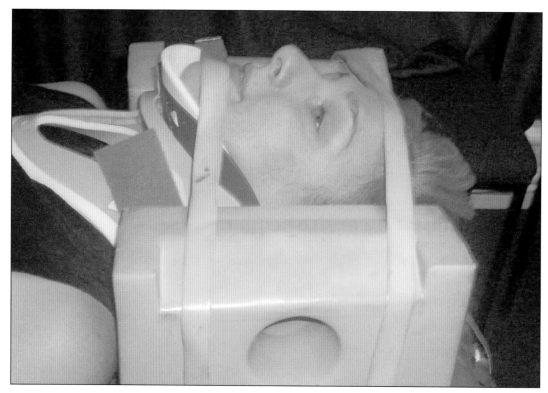

Figure 13A.2 Application of headblocks

■ Apply the forehead strap and attach it securely.

■ Apply lower strap across the chin piece of the hard collar and attach it securely.

■ Apply tape across the chin piece of the hard collar and securely attach it to the long spinal board.

■ Attach body straps to the board.

■ Reassess peripheral sensations.

Exception

A patient who is fitting or combative should not be restrained. In such cases, a hard collar should be applied and no attempt made to immobilise the head with head blocks or sandbags and tape.

Log-rolling

In order to minimise the chances of exacerbating unrecognised spinal cord injury, non-essential movements of the spine must be avoided until adequate examination and investigations have excluded it. If manoeuvres that might cause spinal movement are essential (for example, during examination of the back in the course of the secondary survey) then log-rolling should be performed (Figure 13A.3). The aim of log-rolling is to maintain the alignment of the spine during turning of the patient. The basic requirements are an adequate number of carers and good team command.

Method

■ Gather together enough staff to roll the patient. Four people will be required.

■ Place the staff as shown in Table 13A.1.

■ Ensure each member of staff knows what they are going to do as shown in Table 13A.2.

■ Carry out essential manoeuvres as safely as possible.

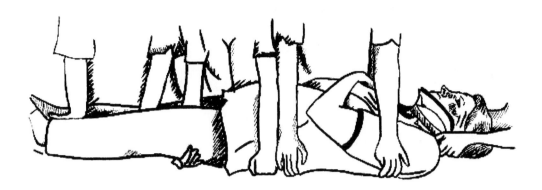

Figure 13A.3 Log-rolling an adult

Table 13A.1. Position of staff in log-rolling an adult

Staff member no.	Position
1	Head
2	Chest and flank
3	Pelvis and thigh
4	Lower legs

Table 13A.2 Tasks of individual members of staff

Staff member position		Task
Head		Hold either side of the head (as for manual in-line cervical stabilisation) and maintain the orientation of the head with the body in all planes during turning. Communicate with the patient and explain the procedure to the patient. **Control the log-roll by telling other staff when to roll and when to lay the patient back onto the trolley.**
Chest	Roll over or back only on the instruction of the person controlling the head and do not remove hands once the patient is supine until told to do so	Reach over the patient and carefully place one hand over the shoulder and one hand over the flank. When told to roll the patient, support the weight of the chest and torso and maintain stability. Watch the movement of the head at all times and roll the chest and torso at the same rate.
Pelvis		Place one hand over the pelvis on the iliac crest and the other under the thigh of the far leg. When told to roll the patient, watch the movement of the head and chest at all times and roll the pelvis at the same rate without adducting the legs.
Legs		Support the weight of the far leg by placing both hands under the lower leg. When told to roll the patient, watch the movement of the chest and pelvis and roll the leg at the same rate without adducting the legs.

Algorithm 14.1 Musculoskeletal trauma

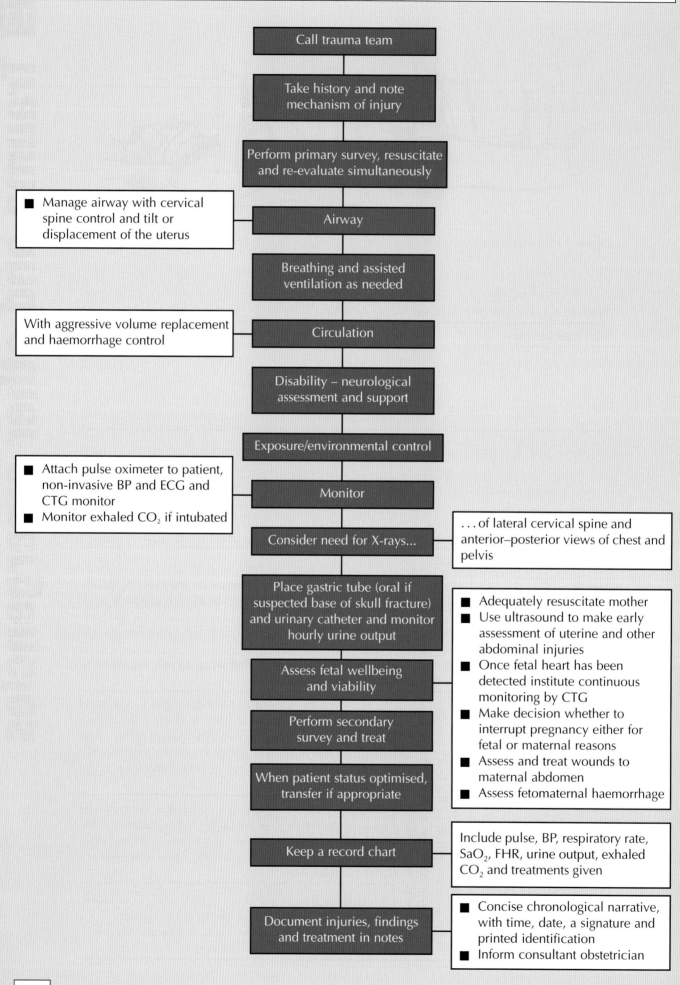

Call trauma team

Take history and note mechanism of injury

Perform primary survey, resuscitate and re-evaluate simultaneously

Airway
- Manage airway with cervical spine control and tilt or displacement of the uterus

Breathing and assisted ventilation as needed

Circulation
- With aggressive volume replacement and haemorrhage control

Disability – neurological assessment and support

Exposure/environmental control

Monitor
- Attach pulse oximeter to patient, non-invasive BP and ECG and CTG monitor
- Monitor exhaled CO_2 if intubated

Consider need for X-rays...
...of lateral cervical spine and anterior–posterior views of chest and pelvis

Place gastric tube (oral if suspected base of skull fracture) and urinary catheter and monitor hourly urine output

Assess fetal wellbeing and viability
- Adequately resuscitate mother
- Use ultrasound to make early assessment of uterine and other abdominal injuries
- Once fetal heart has been detected institute continuous monitoring by CTG
- Make decision whether to interrupt pregnancy either for fetal or maternal reasons
- Assess and treat wounds to maternal abdomen
- Assess fetomaternal haemorrhage

Perform secondary survey and treat

When patient status optimised, transfer if appropriate

Keep a record chart
Include pulse, BP, respiratory rate, SaO_2, FHR, urine output, exhaled CO_2 and treatments given

Document injuries, findings and treatment in notes
- Concise chronological narrative, with time, date, a signature and printed identification
- Inform consultant obstetrician

Chapter 14

Musculoskeletal trauma

Objectives

On successfully completing this topic you will be able to:

■ understand the principles of management of a patient with musculoskeletal trauma

■ identify and treat life-threatening injuries

■ identify and treat limb-threatening injuries.

Principles of management

Primary survey and resuscitation

Within the primary survey, life-threatening injuries are identified and treated. Where musculo-skeletal injuries threaten life it is usually as a Circulation problem. There is a need to recognise hypovolaemia, a rapid inspection to identify sites of major bleeding and measures to stop the bleeding. Beyond the initial resuscitation phase, renal failure can result from traumatic rhabdomyolysis caused by crush injuries and fat embolism is an uncommon but lethal complication of long-bone fractures.

It is important to realise that the patient may have multiple injuries. Knowledge of the mechanism of the injury is important in this; a fall from a height can result in cervical spine and other vertebral fractures and/or fractures of the calcanei and long bones. Some fractures are not easy to detect and are found only after repeated examination.

Assistance from an orthopaedic/emergency physician should be summoned immediately.

Life-threatening injuries

Life-threatening injuries include:

■ major pelvic disruption with haemorrhage

■ major arterial haemorrhage

■ long-bone fractures

■ crush syndrome with hyperkalaemic cardiac arrest and later traumatic rhabdomyolysis.

Major pelvic disruption with haemorrhage

Major pelvic disruption tears the pelvic venous plexus. Where a pelvic injury is suspected, the patient should be resuscitated, immobilised; a sheet can be wrapped around the pelvis as a sling. The input of an orthopaedic surgeon is required urgently to stabilise the pelvis. Caesarean section should be considered if there is an unstable pelvic fracture.

Major arterial haemorrhage

Assess for external bleeding, and suspect if changes in colour, temperature or pulse volume. Treatment comprises resuscitation, compression and immediate orthopaedic input.

Long-bone fractures

Haemorrhage from limb injuries is often compressible. Compression is carried out by:

- pressing on an obvious source of bleeding

- immobilising to reduce bleeding, e.g. splinting or definitive surgery/external fixator.

With open limb wounds the loss may be evident. Loss may be suspected when a limb is swollen and deformed. Equally, loss may only be detected by recognising the signs of hypovolaemia: a closed fracture of the femoral shaft may easily result in the loss of 2 litres into the surrounding tissues. Loss into long bones is one of the four areas for major occult blood loss (chest, abdomen, pelvis and retroperitoneum and long-bone fractures). This requires resuscitation, immobilisation and immediate orthopaedic input.

Crush injuries with hyperkalaemic cardiac arrest and later traumatic rhabdomyolysis

Crush injuries cause damage to muscle cells, releasing potassium and myoglobin into the circulation. High levels of potassium in the blood can cause cardiac arrest. Myoglobin blocks renal tubules, leading to renal failure. To avoid renal failure, intravenous fluids should be given in sufficient volume to produce a minimum of 100 ml urine/hour.

An ECG monitor may give warning of hyperkalaemia (broad bizarre complexes; tented T-wave).

Crush injuries may result in later amputation because of cell damage.

Adjuncts to the primary survey are:

- **fracture immobilisation**, which has the following effects:
  - prevents further blood loss
  - protects circulation
  - prevents further soft tissue damage
  - helps to control pain
  - reduces the risk of fat embolism.

- **X-rays of skeletal injuries**: in the main, these are taken as part of the secondary survey. However, an anterioposterior view of the pelvis is taken during the primary survey in all multiply injured patients and other X-rays may be taken during the primary survey depending on initial clinical findings.

Secondary survey

Limb-threatening injuries

Limb-threatening injuries are identified in the secondary survey and must be treated promptly.

The system of examination of the limbs is **look, feel, circulatory assessment, X-rays**.

Establish the Mechanism of injury, Injuries found, Symptoms and signs and Treatment. The mnemonic is **MIST**.

Examination

There should be a rapid inspection to identify musculoskeletal injuries.

- **Look**

    Examine the limbs for obvious wounds, deformity and the presence of any swelling. Note the colour and compare it with the contralateral limb. Note the perfusion of the limb and describe it in the notes; record capillary return time.

    Describe the wounds (with a sketch if appropriate) and their relationship to any fracture. This will avoid the need for repeated disturbance of the dressings. Note and record any skin loss, especially over fractures.

- **Feel**

    Palpate for tenderness or crepitus, which will reveal the presence of a fracture. Is there loss of sensation to touch? If so, record where; draw a picture.

- **Move**

    Check all the limbs for active movements where possible. The ability to move all major joints suggests that the joint and nerve muscle unit is intact.

- **Circulatory assessment**

    Assess in each limb the temperature, the capillary return time, sensation and the peripheral pulses. Alteration in temperature, pulse discrepancy, pallor and motor dysfunction may suggest an arterial injury.

- **Fracture assessment**

    Is the fracture open or closed? Any fracture with a wound adjacent to it must be assumed to be an open fracture. Note any bone protrusion. Splinting may reduce the risk of a closed fracture becoming an open fracture. Surgical toilet of the bone may be required later.

- **X-rays**

    X-ray of the pelvis and other life-threatening injuries are taken during the primary survey; others are taken during the secondary survey.

Types of limb-threatening injuries

Types of limb-threatening injuries are:

- open fractures and joint injuries

- vascular injuries including traumatic amputations

- compartment syndrome

- nerve injuries secondary to fracture dislocation.

Open fractures and joint injuries

With an open fracture, control haemorrhage by direct pressure, firm compression, bandaging and elevation of the limb. Gross contamination, such as earth and bits of clothing, should be removed and the wound copiously irrigated before applying a dry sterile compression dressing. Severe soft tissue wounds are immobilised to relieve pain and to control haemorrhage.

Wounds are described in the notes to avoid repeated disturbance of the dressing before definitive treatment. Repeated wound inspection increases the risk of infection. The fracture is then treated as for any other fracture.

Dislocations and fracture-dislocations are identified by X-ray. Dislocations are extremely painful when attempts are made to move the joint and this helps early recognition. Such early recognition can allow prompt reduction, especially if there is altered blood supply to the limb, for example in posterior dislocation of the knee occluding the popliteal artery.

All dislocations are reduced at the earliest opportunity. They are often relatively easy to reduce soon after injury. Distal circulation is checked and the joint immobilised after reduction.

Vascular injuries and traumatic amputations

A major vascular injury may be suspected by:

- obvious arterial or venous haemorrhage from the wound
- an expanding haematoma
- absent distal pulses (70%)
- delayed capillary return
- differing skin colour and temperature compared with the contralateral limb
- increasing pain at the site of the injury
- decreasing sensation.

Repeated assessment of the circulation is necessary.

Vascular injury is more likely if the injury is proximal to the knee or elbow. Fractures or fracture-dislocations around the knee or elbow are commonly associated with injury to the femoral and brachial artery, respectively.

Compartment syndrome

Compartment syndrome occurs when the interstitial pressure in a fascial compartment exceeds the capillary pressure, as a result of haemorrhage or oedema within the involved compartment. Initially, venous flow stops and as the pressure increases the arterial supply also stops. The presence of a distal pulse does not exclude a compartment syndrome. Ischaemia of nerves and muscles occurs with rapid and irreversible damage. The distal pulses may be present throughout. The compartments most commonly affected are the anterior tibial compartment and the flexor compartment of the forearm.

Causes include crush injuries, prolonged limb compression, open or closed fractures, ischaemia of the limb and tight plasters or dressings. There are reports of compartment syndrome associated with the Lloyd Davies position, possibly caused by arterial hypoperfusion due to the leg being above the level of the heart, possibly caused by venous obstruction from kinking of the veins at the groin or external pressure from stirrups or compression cuffs, or possibly caused by an increase in compartment pressure due to weight of limb in stirrups or passive plantar flexion of foot.

The main presenting symptom is severe pain in an injured limb that is adequately immobilised. The pain is aggravated by passive stretching of the muscles in the involved compartment. Active movements are absent. The compartments are swollen, tense, tender and the distal sensation may be altered.

Untreated, this will lead to rapid loss of life or limb or permanent disability. Prompt recognition and emergency surgery are needed. If the limb is in plaster or has circumferential dressings, split them completely down to the skin and open them widely. If symptoms do not improve within 15 minutes, any dressings overlying open wounds should be removed and the underlying muscle examined. Its colour should look like raw, red meat; if it does not, suspect compartment syndrome. Such a limb requires urgent fasciotomy.

Nerve injuries secondary to fracture dislocation

Some injuries are often associated with neurological damage; for example, a dislocated hip and sciatic nerve injury or a dislocated elbow and median nerve injury. Altered sensation or motor power, or both suggests nerve involvement. Orthopaedic surgeons must be involved immediately.

14

Trauma and other emergencies

Definitive care

Definitive care continues in the hands of the orthopaedic surgeons.

Summary

■ Manage life-threatening injuries first; they usually present as a Circulation problem.

■ Call orthopaedic surgeons

■ Suspect, detect and treat limb-threatening injuries.

Suggested further reading

Browner BD, Jupiter JB, Levine AM, Trafton PG, editors. *Skeletal Trauma*. Philadelphia, PA: WB Saunders; 1991.

Hansen ST, Swiotkowski MF. *Orthopaedic Trauma Protocols*. New York: Raven Press; 1993.

Algorithm 15.1 Burns

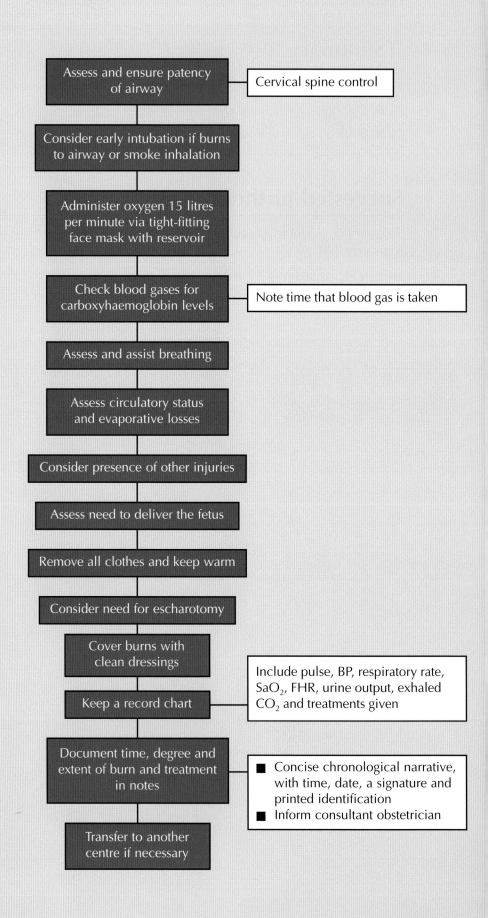

Assess and ensure patency of airway

Cervical spine control

Consider early intubation if burns to airway or smoke inhalation

Administer oxygen 15 litres per minute via tight-fitting face mask with reservoir

Check blood gases for carboxyhaemoglobin levels

Note time that blood gas is taken

Assess and assist breathing

Assess circulatory status and evaporative losses

Consider presence of other injuries

Assess need to deliver the fetus

Remove all clothes and keep warm

Consider need for escharotomy

Cover burns with clean dressings

Keep a record chart

Include pulse, BP, respiratory rate, SaO_2, FHR, urine output, exhaled CO_2 and treatments given

Document time, degree and extent of burn and treatment in notes

- Concise chronological narrative, with time, date, a signature and printed identification
- Inform consultant obstetrician

Transfer to another centre if necessary

Chapter 15

Burns

Objectives

On successfully completing this topic you will be able to:

- understand the impact of a thermal injury on the airway, breathing and circulation
- recognise actual or impending thermal injuries to airway, breathing and circulation
- describe the immediate management of airway breathing and circulation in a patient with burns
- assess the severity of burns
- discuss the management of the fetus in the pregnant patient with burns.

Introduction and incidence

The incidence of pregnancy in women admitted to hospital with burn injuries has been found to be 6.8–7.8%. The burned pregnant woman should be managed jointly by burns team and obstetricians. This may necessitate transfer to a burns centre with appropriate transfer of care to a local obstetrician.

A surface area burn of 25–50% has a mortality rate of 63% for both mother and fetus. Burns may cause immediately life-threatening problems that will be identified and simultaneously treated in the primary survey. The severity of the burn injury depends on the effect of the burn on the ABCs and the area and depth of the burn.

Immediate first aid

The burning process must be stopped: extinguish the flames by laying the affected part on the ground or wrapping the patient in a blanket or equivalent. Gently remove burned clothing. Small burns can be cooled with clean, cold water. Burns should be covered to avoid hypothermia.

Primary survey and resuscitation

There must be early suspicion and aggressive management of the ABCs.

Airway and Breathing injuries should be suspected and particularly if:

- the burn was sustained in an enclosed space
- there is hoarseness, loss of voice, stridor or wheeze
- there is evidence of burns around the lips, mouth and nose

■ there is singeing to the nasal hair or eyebrows

■ there is soot around the mouth or nose or the patient is coughing up carbonaceous sputum

■ there is respiratory distress and alteration in level of consciousness.

Airway burns may result in airway obstruction. Respiratory injuries may result in critically impaired gas exchange. It should be noted that, because of the physiological changes of pregnancy, there is an increased risk of airway complications in pregnancy as compared with the nonpregnant woman, and therefore there must be early control of the airway. Airway injury from burns can be immediate or delayed so the airway must be continually observed and early intubation should be considered particularly if the patient is to be transferred.

Respiratory injury may be caused directly by smoke or by inhalation of the products of combustion. Respiratory damage can occur in the burns patient in the absence of respiratory injury. Inhalation of carbon monoxide is usual if the burn has been sustained in an enclosed area. A carboxyhaemaglobin level of greater than 10% signifies significant inhalation of carbon monoxide. There are, however, usually no physical symptoms at a level of less than 20%. Carbon monoxide levels of 60% result in death. Oxygen delivery relies on haemoglobin binding to oxygen. Carbon monoxide has a greater affinity for haemoglobin than oxygen so displaces oxygen from the haemoglobin molecule thereby causing reduced oxygen delivery to the tissues. The patient must be given 100% oxygen to compete at haemoglobin sites with the carbon monoxide. Note the time of the burn and the time that the arterial sample for carboxyhaemoglobin level is taken. Cyanide can be absorbed by inhalation.

Attend to problems of the airway, breathing and ventilation as identified in the primary survey. Early intubation and ventilation is advisable if there is suspicion of **A** or **B** problem or in the presence of carbon monoxide poisoning.

Circulatory losses should be suspected and particularly in extensive burns.

Assess circulatory status and evaporative losses by heart rate, urine output, blood pressure and 'rule of nines' (Table 15.1). The haematocrit will guide fluid replacement. Place a urinary catheter to monitor output – aim for 50 ml/hour.

Secure IV access and replace fluids with warmed crystalloid solution. The patient requires 2–4 ml/kg/percentage of body surface area burned in the first 24 hours from the time of the burn. Half of this volume is given in the first 8 hours following the burn and half in the next 16 hours.

Vigorous fluid replacement should be given in the presence of myoglobinuria (secondary to rhabdomyolysis). The advice of burns surgeons and intensivists should be taken as to whether forced alkaline diuresis is appropriate.

Table 15.1. The 'rule of nines'

Body surface area	Area burned (%)
Head and neck	9
Each upper limb	9
Front of trunk*	18
Back of trunk	18
Each lower limb	18
Perineum	1

* The gravid abdomen would represent a larger proportion of the total body surface area

Severity of the burn

Severity of the burn depends on:

■ the body surface area burned

■ the depth of the burn.

The rule of nines is used to assess the body surface area burned (Table 15.1).

For children below 30 kg (approximately 12 years), the head represents 18% and the lower limbs 14% each.

The area of the patient's palm represents about 1% of the body surface area.

Depth of the burn

First-degree burns are characterised by erythema and pain without blisters. Partial thickness or second-degree burns are red, mottled, blistered, swollen, may look wet and are very painful.

Full-thickness or third-degree burns are dark and leathery, mottled or translucent. They are painless, usually dry and are hard to the touch.

Assess need to deliver the fetus

Obstetric management has to be individualised. Within hours, the mother becomes hyper-metabolic causing hyperthermia, increased oxygen consumption, tachypnoea, tachycardia and an increase in serum catecholamine levels. Maternal acidosis is a predictive factor. In burns of 50% or greater, urgent delivery should be carried out if second- or third-trimester pregnancy, as fetal survival is not improved by waiting.

If the burn is less than 30% body surface area, the prognosis is good for both mother and fetus (dependent upon gestational age) and depends on the prevention of complications such as hypoxia, hypovolaemia and sepsis.

There are limited data on the management of electrical burns in pregnancy. The amniotic fluid and uterus are good conductors of electricity. There are reports of long-term oligohydramnios and intrauterine growth restriction. However, it is generally felt that there is an 'all or nothing' effect on the fetus: either death results or the prognosis is comparatively good.

Secondary survey and definitive care

Burned tissue may constrict the blood supply to the limbs. The procedure of cutting through burned tissue to restore blood supply (and prevent rhabdomyolysis) is called escharotomy. Call for general/plastic surgical assistance.

Early attention to measures to prevent sepsis is important. Sepsis is the major cause of death due to burns in pregnancy. Prophylactic systemic antibiotics are recommended.

There should be a high index of suspicion for venous thrombosis.

Summary

■ Management of the burned pregnant woman involves the joint working of burns surgeons and obstetricians

■ Assess the actual or potential effect of the burn on the **ABCs**.

■ Simultaneously remedy the actual or potential effect of the burn on the **ABCs** with early recourse to intubation especially in the burned pregnant woman.

■ Assess the severity and depth of surface burns and arrange definitive care.

■ Arrange the timely delivery of the fetus.

■ Conduct secondary survey and definitive care.

Suggested further reading

Chama CM, Na'Aya HU. Severe burn injury in pregnancy. *J Obstet Gynaecol* 2002;22:20–2.

Deitch EA, Rightmire DA, Clothier J, Blass N. Management of burns in pregnant women. *Surg Gynecol Obstet* 1985;161:1–4.

Matthews RN. Obstetric implications of burns in pregnancy. *Br J Obstet Gynaecol* 1982;89:603–9.

Polko LE, McMahon MJ. Burns in pregnancy. *Obstet Gynecol Surv* 1998;53:50–6.

Schmitz JT. Pregnant patients with burns. *Am J Obstet Gynecol* 1971;110:57.

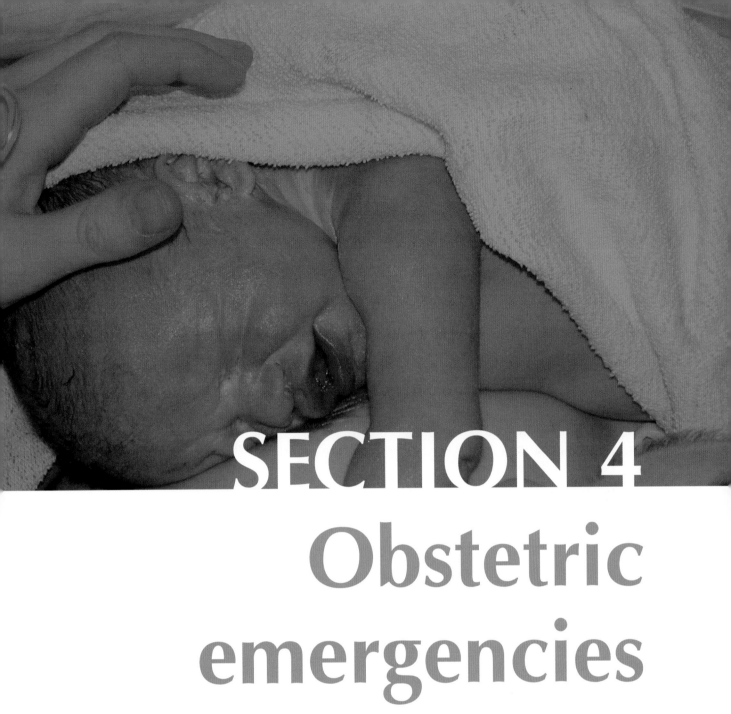

SECTION 4
Obstetric emergencies

Algorithm 16.1 Pre-eclampsia/eclampsia

- Place in semi-prone position
- Call for HELP – duty obstetric and anaesthetic SpRs; senior midwife
- Inform consultants – obstetrician and anaesthetist

Do not leave patient alone

Airway

- Assess
- Maintain patency
- Apply oxygen

- Assess
- Protect airway
- Ventilate as required

Breathing

- Evaluate pulse and BP
- If absent, initiate CPR and call the arrest team
- Secure IV access as soon as safely possible

Circulation

- **Loading dose MgSO$_4$:** 4 g MgSO$_4$ in 20% solution IV over 10–20 minutes. Add 8 ml of 50% MgSO$_4$ solution to 12 ml physiological saline

- **Maintenance dose MgSO$_4$:** 1 g per hour infusion. Add 25 g MgSO$_4$ (50 ml) to 250 ml physiological saline 1 g MgSO$_4$ = 12 ml per hour IV

- **If seizures continue or recur:** MgSO$_4$ 2 g ≤ 70 kg; 4 g ≥ 70 kg IV as per loading dose over 5–10 minutes. If this fails: diazepam 10 ml IV or thiopentone 3–5 mg/kg IV paralyse and intubate

- **Monitor:** Hourly urine output, respiratory rate, O$_2$ saturation & patellar reflexes – every 10 minutes for first 2 hours and then every 30 minutes
  Check serum magnesium if toxicity is suspected on clinical grounds

- **Stop infusion:** Check magnesium levels and review management with consultant if:
  Urine output < 100 ml in 4 hours
  <u>or if</u>   Patellar reflexes are absent
  <u>or if</u>   Respiratory rate < 16/minute
  <u>or if</u>   Oxygen saturation < 90%

- Always get suppression of reflexes before respiratory depression

- **Antidote:** 10% calcium gluconate 10 ml IV over 10 minutes

Control seizures

Control hypertension

- **Treat hypertension** if systolic BP > 170 mmHg or diastolic BP > 110 mmHg or MAP > 125 mmHg Aim to reduce BP to around 130–140/90–100 mmHg **Beware maternal hypotension and FHR abnormalities** – monitor FHR with continuous CTG

- **HYDRALAZINE** 10 mg IV slowly Repeated doses of HYDRALAZINE 5 mg IV 20 minutes apart may be given if necessary
  Close liaison with anaesthetists: may require plasma expansion

- **LABETALOL** 50 mg IV slowly if BP still uncontrolled
  If necessary repeat after 20 minutes or start IV infusion: 200 mg in 200 ml physiological saline at 40 mg/hour, increasing dose at half-hourly intervals as required to a maximum of 160 mg/hour

If not postpartum . . . Deliver

- The continuation of pregnancy is not an option if eclampsia occurs
- **STABILISE THE MOTHER BEFORE DELIVERY**
- **DELIVERY IS A TEAM EFFORT** involving obstetricians, midwives, anaesthetists and paediatricians
- Ergometrine should not be used in severe pre-eclampsia and eclampsia
- Consider prophylaxis against thromboembolism
- Maintain vigilance as the majority of eclamptic seizures occur after delivery

OBSERVATIONS
Pulse oximeter   BP
Respirations
Temperature
ECG
Test urine for protein
Hourly urine output
Fluid balance charts
FHR – monitor continuously

INVESTIGATIONS
FBC & platelets
U&Es
Urate   LFT
Coagulation screen
Group & hold serum
MSSU
24-hour urine collections for:
- total protein & creatinine clearance
- catecholamines

Chapter 16

Pre-eclampsia and eclampsia

Objectives

On successfully completing this topic you will be able to:

- manage severe hypertension in pregnancy
- prevent and treat eclamptic fits
- manage fluid balance in pre-eclampsia/eclampsia
- investigate, recognise and treat the complications of the condition.

Definitions

Pre-eclampsia and eclampsia

Pre-eclampsia is pregnancy-induced hypertension in association with proteinuria or oedema or both. Virtually any organ system may be affected.

The MAGPIE trial defined severe pre-eclampsia as:

- diastolic blood pressure greater than 110 mmHg on two occasions or
- systolic blood pressure greater than 170 mmHg on two occasions and proteinuria greater than 3+ or
- diastolic blood pressure greater than 100 mmHg on two occasions and proteinuria greater than 2+ and at least two signs or symptoms of imminent eclampsia.

Eclampsia was defined as the occurrence of one or more convulsions superimposed on pre-eclampsia.

In the Yorkshire series of severe pre-eclampsia, the criteria for inclusion were either:

severe hypertension: systolic blood pressure over 170 mmHg
or diastolic blood pressure over 110 mmHg
with at least proteinuria of a +
or 1 g on a semiquantitative assessment
(three blood pressure readings in a 15-minute period)

or

moderate hypertension: systolic blood pressure over 140 mmHg
or diastolic blood pressure over 90 mmHg
with at least proteinuria ++
or 3 g on a semi-quantitative assessment

(three blood pressure readings in a 45-minute period)
and any symptoms of:

headache

visual disturbance

epigastric pain

signs of clonus

papilloedema

liver tenderness

platelet count falling to below 100×10^9/l

ALT rising to above 50 iu/l.

Ultimately, as many criteria are subjective, women should be managed according to a careful clinical assessment rather than relying on overly precise criteria.

HELLP syndrome (haemolysis, elevated liver enzymes and low platelets) is an important variant of pre-eclampsia. Strictly, a diagnosis of HELLP syndrome needs confirmation of haemolysis, either by measuring LDH levels, as commonly done in the USA, or by blood film to look for fragmented red cells. ALT levels above 75 iu/l are seen as significant and levels above 150 iu/l are associated with increased morbidity to the mother. The platelet count should be below 100×10^9 to support the diagnosis.

Epidemiology

Eclampsia rates may be falling (Table 16.1). The reduction is mostly in the postpartum group, which suggests that standardised care for pre-eclampsia around the time of delivery, with proven interventions, is associated with a reduction in the rate of eclampsia.

Deaths from pre-eclampsia have reduced from 11.9/million maternities in 1985–1987 to 7.0/million maternities in 2000–2002. This latest CEMD report identified 14 deaths from pre-eclampsia and eclampsia. Nine died from cerebral causes with substandard care in 50% of cases. Particular areas of care highlighted for improvement were the control of hypertension and the management of fluid balance (see below).

There is other serious morbidity with pre-eclampsia. In the Yorkshire series, pulmonary oedema occurred in 2.3% of cases and renal support in 0.55% of cases. Although all women recovered renal function by 3 weeks, 6.9% of cases became oliguric, 4.3% of women had platelets below 50×10^9 and an ALT greater than 70 iu/ml. No specific measure of haemolysis was included, so the incidence of HELLP syndrome cannot be confirmed; 1.2% of women needed coagulation factor replacement and 0.5% of women needed treatment for a retinal detachment. The mortality rate for babies up to the time of discharge was 47.2/1000.

Table 16.1. Incidence of eclampsia

	Cases/10 000 maternities	
	BEST survey (1992) n (%)	Yorkshire series (1999–2003) n (%)
Antenatal	1.9 (38)	2.1 (55)
Intrapartum	0.9 (18)	0.5 (13)
Postnatal	2.2 (44)	1.2 (32)
Total	4.9	3.9

Management of severe pre-eclampsia and eclampsia

The general principles are:

- senior and multidisciplinary involvement
  - ☐ obstetrician
  - ☐ midwife
  - ☐ anaesthetist
  - ☐ haematologist
  - ☐ intensive care team
  - ☐ paediatrician

- working to a standardised pattern of management (guidelines) which should only be deviated from by senior staff (consultants)

- regular review of all parameters with an awareness of complications

- prompt control of hypertension

- meticulous fluid balance to avoid iatrogenic fluid overload

- consideration of seizure prophylaxis.

Confidential Enquiry recommendations

The 2000–2002 CEMD report made the following recommendations with regards to pre-eclampsia and eclampsia:

Service provision
Guidelines and protocols

- Clear, written management protocols for severe pre-eclampsia should guide initial and continuing treatment in hospital.

- Severe, life-threatening hypertension must be treated effectively. Management protocols should recognise the need to avoid very high systolic blood pressures associated with the risk of cerebral haemorrhage. It is recommended that clinical protocols identify a systolic blood pressure above which urgent and effective antihypertensive treatment is required.

- The early involvement of consultant obstetricians in the management of women with suspected or proven pre-eclampsia and eclampsia is essential.

- There should be early engagement of intensive care specialists in the care of women with severe pre-eclampsia.

Individual practitioners

- Pregnant women with a headache of sufficient severity to seek medical advice, or new epigastric pain, should have their blood pressure measured and urine tested for protein, as a minimum.

- Automated blood pressure recording systems can systematically underestimate blood pressure in pre-eclampsia, to a serious degree. Blood pressure values should be compared at the beginning of treatment, with those obtained by conventional sphygmomanometers.

- In women presenting with potentially severe pre-eclampsia (e.g. symptoms, sudden heavy proteinuria, markedly disordered liver function and/or haematological tests) but with unexceptional blood pressure measurements, alarming rises in blood pressure should be anticipated. Consideration should be given to early administration of anti-hypertensive drugs.

■ Magnesium sulphate is the anticonvulsant drug of choice in the treatment of eclampsia.

■ To avoid potentially serious consequences of fluid overload, careful monitoring of fluid input and output, with appropriate fluid restriction, will be required.

Symptoms and signs

Pre-eclampsia is a multi-system disorder and its clinical presentation in terms of symptoms and signs reflects this. Women presenting with multi-system involvement present the more difficult clinical challenge. Awareness of the complications that can occur allows anticipation and prompt management.

The following need to be considered:

■ headache, visual disturbances, vomiting and epigastric pain

■ nondependent (especially facial) or pulmonary oedema

■ right upper-quadrant abdominal tenderness

■ optic vasospasm

■ recently developed hypertension greater than 160/110 mmHg with proteinuria greater than 1 g in 24 hours

■ hyperreflexia with clonus

■ rapidly changing biochemical/haematological picture.

Complications are shown in Table 16.2.

Table 16.2. Complications of pre-eclampsia/eclampsia

	Complication
Maternal	Eclampsia
	Severe hypertension
	Risk of cerebrovascular accident
	Oliguria leading to renal failure
	Liver failure or liver rupture
	Disseminated intravascular coagulation and/or HELLP syndrome
	Placental abruption with haemorrhage
	Pulmonary oedema
	Acute respiratory distress syndrome
	Pulmonary haemorrhage
	Aspiration pneumonia
	Retinal detachment
Fetal	Prematurity
	Intrauterine growth restriction
	Respiratory distress syndrome
	Acute fetal distress (particularly with lowering of blood pressure)
	Intrauterine death

Initial assessment of the woman

Antenatal

One of the main focuses of antenatal care is to detect women at risk of pre-eclampsia and increase the level of care provided. Risk factor identification is important and evidence based guidelines have been produced for community care. The Pre-eclampsia Community Guideline (PRECOG) highlights the value of more detailed assessment of women with either new hypertension or new proteinuria.

Acute management

The initial assessment of a woman with pre-eclampsia involves assessment of maternal and fetal condition. As these are potentially sick women, it is appropriate that senior obstetric and anaesthetic staff should be involved in their assessment and management.

The classification of severity is primarily based on the level of blood pressure and the presence of proteinuria. However, after making an initial diagnosis, other organ involvement becomes important in assessing maternal risk and this includes fetal assessment.

Atypical presentations of pre-eclampsia include women presenting initially with convulsions, abdominal pain or general malaise. In these cases, pre-eclampsia should always be considered and the blood pressure should be measured and the urine analysed. Clinical symptoms can be important features of worsening disease, particularly headache and abdominal pain. Increasing oedema is not in itself a sign that should determine management. Maternal tendon reflexes are difficult to perform in a reproducible way, so are not of value to assess the risk of convulsion although the presence of clonus may be helpful. Tendon reflexes are of help when assessing magnesium toxicity

Taking the blood pressure

It is important to have a standard method of blood pressure assessment but there are concerns about automated methods. Automated methods can systematically underestimate particularly the systolic blood pressure. It has been suggested that mercury sphygmomanometers should be used to establish baseline blood pressure as a reference unless the automated machine has been validated in pregnancy. However, many units no longer have mercury sphygmomanometers so a baseline check with another validated device would be an alternative, although these are limited.

When taking the blood pressure, the woman should be rested and, ideally, sitting at a 45-degree angle. The blood pressure cuff should be of the appropriate size. This is particularly important in overweight women and a large cuff should be available. The cuff should be at the level of the heart. There are fluctuations in blood pressure in normal circumstances so multiple readings are needed to confirm the diagnosis. Roundings of blood pressure are avoided by automated measurement. There is now a consensus that Korotkoff phase 5 is the preferable measurement of diastolic blood pressure.

In the initial assessment phase, the blood pressure should be checked each 15 minutes until the woman is stabilised and then half hourly. If intravenous antihypertensive drugs are being administered, the blood pressure may need to be assessed every 5 minutes while the effect of treatment is being titrated against the response.

Measuring proteinuria

Proteinuria is associated with the classic pathological finding of glomeruloendotheliosis. It is not a sign of renal damage but a pathophysiological change that will usually recover after delivery. The usual screening test is visual dipstick assessment but significant false negative as well as false positive rates are reported. A two-plus dipstick measurement can be taken as evidence of proteinuria but ideally a more accurate test, such as 24-hour urine, is required to confirm this. In circumstances where immediate delivery is required this will not be possible. Newer techniques such as protein/creatinine ratios have not been fully evaluated but may be a valid alternative. A level of 30 mg/nmol urinary protein/creatinine appears to be equivalent to 0.3 g/mmol/24 hours.

Basic investigations

Blood should be sent for:

Serum electrolytes	(Na, K, urea, creatinine, urate)
Liver function tests	(albumin, ALT or AST, bilirubin)
Full blood count	(haemoglobin, white cell count, platelets)
Clotting	(PT, KCCT + fibrinogen, FDPs)
Group-and-save serum	

Urine should be tested for protein and sent for culture.

All tests should be checked daily or more frequently if abnormal.

Coagulation

If the platelet count is above $100 \times 10^9/l$ and liver function tests are normal, the likelihood that the clotting results will be abnormal is very low. Some units choose not to perform clotting tests without a platelet count but in the acute presentation it may be appropriate if the woman is unwell with clinical signs of concern to establish the baseline clotting studies at the outset. However, there is no direct correlation between platelet count and liver damage and assessment of liver enzyme levels (usually by AST or ALT) is required. An AST level of above 75 iu/l is seen as significant and a level above 150 iu/l is associated with increased morbidity to the mother.

A diagnosis of HELLP syndrome should not be made on liver function tests alone but needs confirmation of haemolysis, either by LDH levels as commonly measured in the USA or by blood film. If HELLP syndrome is suspected, a blood film should be carried out to look for fragmented red cells.

Renal function

Renal function is a marker of placental dysfunction and increased renal excretion in normal pregnancy lowers serum levels of uric acid. Although, in pre-eclampsia, a rise in uric acid correlates with poorer outcome for both mother and baby, the levels, in themselves, are not useful for clinical decision making.

Renal function is generally maintained in pre-eclampsia until the late stage. Elevated creatinine at presentation should lead to suspicion of an underlying renal problem. In severe disease, rising serum creatinine is associated with a worsening outcome. Renal failure requiring support is now uncommon in pre-eclampsia in the developed world and when it occurs it is usually associated with haemorrhage or sepsis.

Monitoring of clinical signs

■ Blood pressure (see above for details) and pulse rate.

■ Respiratory rate should be measured hourly particularly in women on magnesium.

■ Oxygen saturation should be measured continuously and charted hourly. If oxygen saturation falls then medical review is essential to consider the possible differential diagnosis, with a high index of suspicion of early pulmonary oedema.

- Fluid balance should be monitored very carefully. Detailed input and output recordings should be charted.

- Hourly urine output via an indwelling catheter should be inserted particularly whenever intravenous fluids are given.

- Urine should be tested for proteinuria 4-hourly. If conservative management is planned then a 24-hour assessment of urinary protein is helpful in assessing the disease.

- Temperature should be measured 4-hourly, as women with pre-eclampsia are likely to be in labour or immediately postoperative.

- Optic fundi should be examined to assess for any signs of haemorrhage.

Assessment of the fetus

Antenatal

The fetus is at risk of growth restriction so investigations are aimed at fetal growth and wellbeing. Ultrasound to assess fetal size should consider the abdominal circumference, as often the growth is asymmetrical. This means head growth may be normal but abdominal growth may be reduced.

Reduced liquor volume is also associated with placental insufficiency and fetal growth restriction. Umbilical artery Doppler is a valuable noninvasive test of fetal wellbeing but is gestation dependent and needs careful consideration in the very preterm pregnancy (below 30 weeks). Doppler of fetal vessels can be used but require expert assessment and evaluation.

Cardiotocography (CTG) is the technique most widely used for the initial assessment of fetal wellbeing at that time but it has little predictive value. If the woman is in labour then continuous electronic fetal monitoring would be appropriate.

Antepartum and intrapartum management

Control of blood pressure

The level of blood pressure that requires treatment is still unclear.

Severe hypertension (systolic over 170 mmHg or diastolic 110 mmHg or MAP above 125 mmHg) is generally considered a clear threshold for treatment. The 2000–2002 CEMD report suggests that there should be concern about systolic hypertension and that treatment should be instituted if the systolic blood pressure is over 160 mmHg. At lower levels of blood pressure the evidence is less clear. It was also identified by the CEMD that women with more marginal hypertension and other signs and symptoms may be at risk of blood pressure surges. It is advised to start treatment at lower levels of blood pressure in these women

The aim of therapy should be to stabilise the woman's blood pressure. As a guide, this means:

- maintaining systolic blood pressure at less than 160 mmHg

- reducing diastolic blood pressure by 10 mmHg and bringing it below 105 mmHg in the first instance

- maintaining the blood pressure at or below these levels.

Rapid drops in blood pressure should be avoided, particularly when the fetus is undelivered as this can potentially trigger acute fetal compromise.

Drug treatment

Labetalol

Labetalol is a combined alpha and beta blocker and is less likely to decrease uteroplacental blood flow than beta blockers. It may improve cerebral perfusion, thereby reducing the risk of eclampsia.

Dose

■ Oral

If the woman can tolerate oral therapy, an initial 200 mg dose can be given. This can be done immediately before venous access and so can achieve as quick a result as an initial intravenous dose. This should lead to a reduction in blood pressure in about half an hour. A second oral dose can be given if needed in 1 hour. Over 50% of women requiring antihypertensive treatment can be controlled with oral therapy.

■ Intravenous

If there is no initial response to oral therapy or if it cannot be tolerated, control should be by repeated bolus of labetalol followed by a labetalol infusion. Over 90% of women can be controlled with labetalol alone.

 □ Bolus dose is 50 mg (10 ml labetalol 5 mg/ml) given over at least 1 minute. This should have an effect by 5 minutes and should be repeated if diastolic blood pressure has not been reduced. This can be repeated to a maximum dose of 200 mg. The pulse rate should remain over 60 beats/minute.

 □ Following this or as initial treatment in moderate hypertension, a labetalol infusion should be commenced. An infusion of (neat) labetalol 5 mg/ml at a rate of 4 ml/hour via a syringe pump should be started. The infusion rate should be doubled every half-hour to a maximum of 32 ml (160 mg)/hour until the blood pressure has dropped and then stabilised at an acceptable level.

Vasodilators

As hydralazine and nifedipine are vasodilators, expansion of the circulating blood volume prior to treatment is recommended in many units to reduce the likelihood of decreasing blood pressure too acutely, early signs of which may be signs of fetal distress. This may be achieved with an appropriate volume bolus (e.g. 250-ml bolus of fluid). Plasma volume expander colloid solutions are often used.

Nifedipine

If labetalol is contraindicated or fails to control the blood pressure then nifedipine is an alternative agent. There has been some concern over the interaction between magnesium sulphate and nifedipine. Clinically, this has not been seen to be a problem as, in the MAGPIE study, large numbers of women were treated with nifedipine and magnesium sulphate and no adverse events were reported.

Dose: 10-mg oral tablet (not a slow-release tablet). If this controls blood pressure it should be repeated 6-hourly initially, although the dose may be changed postnatally to a slow-release preparation which lasts 12 hours. Blood pressure should be measured every 10 minutes in the first half-hour after treatment, as often there can be a very marked drop in pressure. The fetal heart rate should be observed carefully after the initial treatment. Oral antihypertensive treatment should be commenced when intravenous treatment has been discontinued.

Hydralazine

Initial dose is 10 mg, slowly, with repeated doses of 5 mg at 20-minute intervals. The drug has effects up to 6 hours.

An infusion of 2 mg/hour can be established for maintenance, increasing by increments of 0.5 mg/hour to a maximum of 20 mg/hour. Eleven percent of women require secondary therapy when treated with hydralazine.

Choice of antihypertensive

A systematic review of hydralazine compared with labetalol identified that hydralazine was associated with more maternal hypotension (OR 3.29, 95% CI 1.50–7.13), more caesarean sections (OR 1.30, 95% CI 1.08–1.59), more placental abruption (OR 4.17, 95% CI 1.19–14.28), more maternal oliguria (OR 4.0, 95% CI 1.22–12.50) and more adverse effects on fetal heart rate (OR 2.04, 95% CI 1.32–3.16). When compared with labetalol, there were more maternal adverse effects (OR 1.5, 95% CI 1.16–1.94) with less neonatal bradycardia (OR –0.24, 95% CI –0.42 to –0.06). It was suggested that, although the results were not robust, they did not support hydralazine as a first-line treatment. However, there is a large experience with the use of hydralazine and it remains in use in many units.

Fluid management prior to delivery

Once a decision has been made to deliver, the major concern is to avoid fluid overload, particularly when intravenous fluids are being given.

Total intravenous input should be limited to 80 ml/hour (approximately 1 ml/kg/hr). If Syntocinon® is used, it should be at high concentration via a syringe driver. The hourly volume of fluid should include magnesium sulphate and or Syntocinon in the total input.

During labour, oliguria should not precipitate any specific intervention except to ensure progress to delivery is being achieved. As women with pre-eclampsia are at high risk of caesarean section, oral intake should be limited appropriately.

Anaesthesia and fluids

Women with significant pre-eclampsia tend to maintain their blood pressure, despite regional blockade. However, it is appropriate to consider the effects of a vasodilator regional block on the blood pressure and therefore on the uterine blood supply and the fetal perfusion. Women suffering from moderate or severe pre-eclampsia may have a relatively reduced intravascular circulating volume and it may be appropriate to consider fluid loading prior to establishing a regional block.

> **Fluid loading in pre-eclampsia should never be done prophylactically or routinely and should always be considered and controlled.**

In general, anaesthetists may be a little overenthusiastic about fluid loading and should be appropriately restrained. Factors to consider prior to fluid loading include:

- previous fluid balance, in particular whether the obstetric team has recently given a fluid load (e.g. prior to administering an antihypertensive treatment)
- examination of the woman looking for signs of severe fluid overload or cardiac dysfunction (e.g. pulmonary oedema)

- degree of vasodilatation likely to be achieved by the block: a cautious low-dose technique for labour should cause little haemodynamic disturbance and fluid load may be unnecessary and may complicate fluid balance

- fetal monitoring as an indicator of adequate perfusion to the placenta.

Controlled fluid loading can be achieved either by use of a pump to control volume or by the simple precaution of using only small bags of intravenous fluids. In this way, an accidental litre of crystalloid cannot run in during the anaesthetic procedure.

Hypotension, if it occurs, can be controlled with very small doses of a vasopressor.

Seizure prophylaxis

Even for women with severe pre-eclampsia, the risk of eclampsia is low, at around 1%. The MAGPIE trial, designed to establish the clinical efficacy of magnesium sulphate in pre-eclampsia, has shown that women treated with magnesium sulphate had a 58% lower risk of seizures. Overall, 11/1000 fewer women had seizures when treated with magnesium sulphate. There was a trend towards a reduction in mortality with a relative risk of 0.55 (95% CI 0.26–1.14). Overall, the number needed to treat (NNT) to prevent a seizure was 63 (range 38–181) with severe pre-eclampsia and 109 (range 72–225) without. In countries with a low perinatal mortality rate, the NNT may be over 300. Adverse effects were more common with magnesium sulphate (25% versus 8%) but were mostly mild; the intravenous route gave fewer problems.

In the UK, decisions have to be made about whether women should be given prophylactic treatment with magnesium sulphate, in terms of risk–benefit and cost. As the drug is relatively cheap, the main cost is the closer observation required during the infusion period. For women already being cared for on a high-dependency basis there is little extra cost to magnesium sulphate. It would seem logical to use it in these circumstances.

Magnesium sulphate protocol

Clinicians need to be aware that there are two concentrations of magnesium sulphate to avoid confusion over dosing in their own unit. Magnesium sulphate is given as a loading dose followed by a continuous infusion for 24 hours or until 24 hours after delivery, whichever is the later. In cases where it is used for prophylaxis, it may be discontinued before 24 hours if all the other features of pre-eclampsia have settled.

Important observations

When magnesium sulphate is in progress, assessment of the patient needs to occur before each new dose. The following observations should be performed:

- continuous pulse oximetry

- hourly urine output

- hourly respiratory rate

- deep tendon reflexes.

Every 5 hours, the observations should show the following before commencing the next dose.

Stop magnesium sulphate infusion if:

- urine output is less than 100 ml in 4 hours

  or if

- patellar reflexes are absent (assuming this is not due to a regional block)

  or if

- respiratory rate is less than 16 breaths/minute

  or if

- oxygen saturation is less than 90%.

Ninety-seven percent of magnesium is excreted in the urine and therefore the presence of oliguria can lead to toxic levels. If the above criteria are not met then further administration of magnesium sulphate should be withheld. If magnesium is not being excreted then the levels should not fall and no other anticonvulsant is needed. Magnesium should be re-introduced if urine output improves.

Adverse effects

Motor paralysis, absent tendon reflexes, respiratory depression and cardiac arrhythmia (increased conduction time) can all occur (Table 16.3) but will be at a minimum if magnesium is administered slowly and the patient closely observed.

The antidote is 10 ml 10% calcium gluconate given slowly intravenously.

There is no need to measure magnesium levels with the following protocol if urine output is maintained.

Dose

If using 20% magnesium:

- **loading dose:** 4 g slow infusion over 10–20 minutes (20 ml magnesium sulphate 20%) according to local protocol

- administer via a syringe pump over 20 minutes (needs an infusion rate of 60 ml/hour).

- **maintenance dose:** 1 g/hour intravenously for 24 hours; 50 ml magnesium sulphate 20% 5 ml/hour via a syringe pump at an infusion and repeat.

If using 50% magnesium:

- **loading dose:** 4 g slow infusion over 10–20 minutes: 8 ml magnesium sulphate 50% added to 12 ml physiological saline (= 20 ml) according to local protocol

- administer via a syringe pump over 20 minutes (needs infusion rate of 60 ml/hour).

- **maintenance dose:** 1 g/hour intravenously for 24 hours

- add 50 ml magnesium sulphate 50% to 250 ml physiological saline

- draw 60 ml out of the bag and administer via a syringe pump at an infusion rate of 12 ml/hour and repeat.

Table 16.3. Levels of magnesium sulphate at which adverse effects occur

Symptoms	MgSO$_4$ level (mmol/l)
Feeling of warmth, flushing, double vision, slurred speech	3.8–5.0
Loss of tendon reflexes	>5.0
Respiratory depression	>6.0
Respiratory arrest	6.3–7.0
Cardiac arrest	>12.0

Antenatal steroids

If the pregnancy can be prolonged in excess of 24 hours, steroids may help to mature the fetal lungs.

RCOG guidelines on the use of antenatal corticosteroid therapy, published in 1996, recommended that 'every effort should be made to initiate antenatal corticosteroid therapy in women between 24 and 36 weeks of gestation in any condition requiring elective preterm delivery'. However, updated guidelines (December 1999) looked at the effectiveness of antenatal steroids: 'While it is accepted that antenatal corticosteroid therapy reduces the incidence of respiratory distress syndrome (RDS), an analysis of the 'number needed to treat' suggests that after 34 weeks, 94 women will need to be treated to prevent one case of RDS, while before 31 weeks one case of RDS is prevented by every five women treated'.

Use of antenatal corticosteroid therapy between 34 and 36 weeks is a grey area and clinicians are asked to refer to the RCOG guidelines and to decide for themselves if antenatal corticosteroid therapy is indicated.

Maximum benefit of steroid therapy is probably at 48 hours after administration. Since the benefits to the fetus peak between 48 hours and 6 days, further consideration should be given to delivery after 48 hours; further delay may not be advantageous to the baby or mother.

Planning delivery

> ## 'Planned delivery on the best day in the best way'

The delivery should be well planned, done on the best day, performed in the best place, by the best route and with the best support team. Timing affects the outcome for both mother and baby. If the mother is unstable then delivery is inappropriate and increases risk. Once stabilised with antihypertensive drugs and magnesium sulphate if required then a decision should be made regarding timing and route of delivery. In the absence of convulsions or other major complications, prolonging the pregnancy may be possible to improve the outcome of a premature fetus but only if the mother remains stable. Continued close monitoring of mother and baby is needed.

It seems ideal to achieve delivery, particularly of premature infants, during normal working hours.

Mode of delivery

The mode of delivery should be discussed with the consultant obstetrician.

Fetal wellbeing and the likelihood of successful labour are important in determining mode of delivery.

The mode of delivery is not necessarily by caesarean section but if gestation is under 32 weeks this is preferable. After 34 weeks, vaginal delivery should be considered in a cephalic presentation. Vaginal prostaglandins will increase the chance of success.

Antihypertensive treatment should be continued throughout assessment and labour.

If vaginal delivery is planned then the second stage should be short with consideration given to elective operative vaginal delivery.

The third stage should be managed with 5 units intravenous Syntocinon. Ergometrine or Syntometrine should not be given in any form because of the risk of precipitating a rapid rise in blood pressure.

Epidural anaesthesia may be helpful in preventing any further rises in blood pressure caused by labour pains.

Appropriate thromboprophylaxis should be given to all women who are immobilised.

Organisation and transfer

Even a few hours' warning of imminent delivery may be helpful if it allows the neonatal unit to be more organised or to transfer a reasonably stable mother to a place where a cot is available.

If a maternity unit does not have access to HDU/ICU, is unable to cope with maternal complications or is unable to cope with preterm babies, it may be appropriate to consider antenatal transfer of the mother.

Maternal safety must not be jeopardised and her condition should be stable before transfer. In some cases it is safer to deliver the mother and then consider the need for transfer of mother and/or child.

Stabilisation before transfer

The following need to be in place for transfer:

- blood pressure should be stabilised at an acceptable level

- all basic investigations should have been performed and the results clearly recorded in the accompanying notes or telephoned through as soon as available

- fetal wellbeing has been assessed to be certain that transfer is in the fetal interest before delivery; steroids should be given if the woman is preterm (see below)

- appropriate personnel are available to transfer the woman; this will normally mean at least a senior midwife with medical staff as appropriate

- transfer has been discussed with appropriate consultant medical staff and all the relevant people at the receiving unit: the neonatal unit and neonatal medical staff, the resident obstetrician, the midwife in charge of delivery suite, intensive care and the intensive care anaesthetist (where appropriate).

Postpartum fluid management

In the immediate post-delivery phase, women will often have a degree of oliguria. Women with severe pre-eclampsia should have controlled fluid in order to wait for the natural diuresis, which occurs sometime around 36–48 hours following delivery. At this time, there is a risk of iatrogenic fluid overload so careful fluid balance is needed. The total intravenous fluid that should be given is approximately 80 ml/hour (1 ml/kg/hour): Hartmann's solution or equivalent plus other infusions of drugs. Urine output should be recorded hourly. It is not necessary to be aggressive in maintaining urine output.

Yorkshire postpartum fluid protocol (as an example of postpartum fluid management)

No response occurs to significant oliguria over an 8-hour period:

▇ the urine output is measured in 4-hour blocks and recorded on the observation chart

▇ each 4-hour block has a target total in excess of 80 ml

▇ if two consecutive blocks fail to achieve 80 ml, further action is taken.

Only 2% of women develop this degree of oliguria and the rate of renal compromise in this group is no higher than in the women without oliguria.

▇ If there are 8 hours with significant oliguria then input and output are compared.

▇ If input is more than 750 ml in excess of output since delivery or in the last 24 hours (whichever is the shorter) then 20 mg furosemide (frusemide) is given intravenously.

▇ If total input is less than 750 ml in excess of output since delivery or in the last 24 hours (whichever is the shorter) then an infusion of 250 ml of gelofusine over 20 minutes is given.

▇ The urine output is then watched until the end of the next 4-hour block.

▇ If the urine output is still low then 20 mg of frusemide is given intravenously. If, after the furosemide, a diuresis in excess of 250 ml occurs in the next hour, the fluid should be replaced with 250 ml of gelofusine in addition to baseline fluids.

▇ If the urine output fails to respond to furosemide in either situation then a discussion with a regional centre is advised.

If there is persisting oliguria requiring fluid challenge or furosemide then the electrolytes need to be carefully assessed and should be checked 6-hourly. If there is concern over a rising creatinine and or potassium the case should be discussed with a renal physician or regional centre.

If the woman has a falling level of SaO_2 it may be due to pulmonary oedema, which may be contributed to by fluid overload. Input and output should be assessed, together with either clinical or invasive assessment of the fluid balance. The chest should be carefully examined and chest X-ray should be performed. Appropriate treatment may include furosemide and oxygen. If there is no diuresis and the oxygen saturation does not rise then intensive care/renal referral should be considered.

Indications for central venous pressure monitoring

CVP monitoring is usually not necessary and may be misleading. This is because pulmonary oedema can occur in the presence of a low CVP because of left ventricular dysfunction and increased pulmonary interstitial fluid.

CVP may be indicated:

▇ at caesarean section, particularly if blood loss is excessive

▇ if blood loss is excessive or if delivery is complicated by other factors such as placental abruption.

Cases requiring large volumes of colloid such as fresh frozen plasma, blood or platelets can lead to fluid overload. Women with significant haemorrhage or HELLP syndrome need to be managed by someone with plenty of experience. It is never difficult putting more fluid in but getting it out can be a real problem.

The 2000–2002 CEMD report suggested a lower threshold for central monitoring. In cases where close fluid balance measurements are likely to be inaccurate owing to the difficulties of measuring blood loss, early recourse to CVP monitoring would be appropriate. This should be a multi-disciplinary decision and the consultant anaesthetist and obstetrician should be involved.

Management of imminent eclampsia or eclampsia

Controlling convulsions

Management should follow the basic principles of Airway, Breathing and Circulation.

Do not leave the woman alone but call for help, including appropriate personnel such as the senior midwife, anaesthetist and senior obstetrician.

Aim to prevent maternal injury during the convulsion.

A   Place the woman in the left lateral position and assess and if necessary maintain the airway.

B   Administer high-flow oxygen and assess breathing. Pulse oximetry is helpful once the fit has stopped. Lungs should always be auscultated after the convulsion has ended to look for evidence of aspiration or pulmonary oedema.

C   Check pulse and blood pressure.

Establish a fluid balance record if this has not already been done, including urinary catheter.

Once the woman is stabilised, plans should be made to deliver the baby but there is no particular hurry. A delay of several hours to stabilise the mother is acceptable assuming there is no acute fetal concern such as a fetal bradycardia.

The mother's condition will always take priority over the fetal condition.

Treatment of seizures

■ Magnesium sulphate is the therapy of choice and diazepam and phenytoin should no longer be used as a first-line treatment.

■ The vast majority of initial seizures are self-limiting.

■ The intravenous route is associated with fewer adverse effects than the intramuscular route.

■ Dosage: see section above on seizure prophylaxis.

■ Treatment is currently maintained for 24 hours after the last seizure (a trial in Bangladesh has shown no significant reduction in recurrent seizures when using only a loading dose as opposed to the standard regimen. The seizure rates were 3.96% in loading versus 3.51% in standard regimen, $P > 0.05$).

There is debate about whether drugs such as diazepam should be given to control the initial seizure. This is not usually necessary and it would only be necessary with a prolonged seizure or recurrent seizures not responding to magnesium sulphate. There is also the risk that multiple drugs increase the risk of respiratory arrest.

Management of recurrent seizures

In the Collaborative Eclampsia Trial, a further bolus of 2 g or 4 g of magnesium sulphate was administered, depending on maternal weight. The larger dose is appropriate for women over 70 kg. An alternative is to increase the rate of infusion of magnesium sulphate to 1.5 g/hour or 2 g/hour.

If there are repeated seizures then alternative agents such as diazepam or thiopentone may be used, the latter by an anaesthetist in conjunction with intubation. If convulsions persist, intubation is likely to be necessary to protect the airway and maintain oxygenation.

Transfer to intensive care facilities with intermittent positive pressure ventilation is appropriate in these circumstances.

Women with recurrent seizures may have had another or additional cerebral event and neuro-imaging may be helpful in excluding other pathology.

Eclampsia box

It has been recommended that each maternity unit should have an 'emergency box' for eclampsia, based on the treatment packs that were available for the Collaborative Eclampsia Trial. This will ensure that appropriate drugs are readily available. Equipment to secure the airway and venous access are dealt with in other chapters. The box should be regularly checked to keep drugs in date (Table 16.4).

HELLP syndrome

HELLP is a syndrome comprising haemolysis, elevated liver enzymes and low platelets. It occurs in 4–12% of women with severe pre-eclampsia. Severe hypertension is not always a feature and the degree of hypertension rarely reflects overall disease severity. It is more common in multi-parous women as well as primigravidae and is associated with a high perinatal mortality rate.

HELLP can present with vague symptoms of nausea, vomiting and epigastric/right upper-quadrant pain and, because of this, there is often a delay in diagnosis. Severe epigastric pain not relieved by antacids should raise the index of suspicion. One unique feature (somewhat late) of HELLP syndrome is 'Coca Cola urine', where small amounts of dark black urine are produced.

The management of HELLP, as for severe pre-eclampsia, is to evaluate the severity, stabilise and deliver. The postnatal course for these women is often more complicated, with oliguria and a slow recovery of biochemical parameters. High-dose corticosteroids may be beneficial but probably only in terms of biochemical recovery rather than preventing morbidity. The risk of recurrence of the HELLP syndrome is approximately 20%.

Postpartum care and follow-up

Severe pre-eclampsia or eclampsia can occur in the postpartum period. Up to 44% of eclampsia has been reported to occur postnatally. Women delivered with severe pre-eclampsia (and/or eclampsia) should have continued close observation postnatally. As eclampsia has been reported up to 4 weeks postnatally, the optimum length of inpatient postnatal stay is unclear but the incidence of eclampsia and severe pre-eclampsia falls after the fourth postpartum day. Women should stay in hospital until their general condition has improved, hypertension is controlled and proteinuria and any other biochemical abnormalities are improving.

Table 16.4. Contents of emergency box for eclampsia

Equipment	Quantity
Drugs	Magnesium sulphate 50%, 5 g in 10-ml ampoule × 10 ampoules (or magnesium sulphate 20%)
	Calcium gluconate 10%, 8.9 mg in 10-ml ampoule × 2 ampoules
	Labetalol 200 mg in 20-ml ampoule × 1 ampoule
	Nifedipine 10 mg orally
	Hydralazine 20 mg in 1-ml ampoule × 2 ampoules
	Sodium chloride 10-ml ampoule × 10 ampoules
Intravenous fluids	250-ml bag of sodium chloride × 2

Antihypertensive therapy should be continued after delivery; although initially the blood pressure may fall, it usually rises again at around 24 hours postpartum. A reduction in antihypertensive therapy should be made in a stepwise fashion. There is no reason why the woman cannot go home on treatment to be weaned off therapy as an outpatient. The blood pressure can take up to 3 months to return to normal. During this time blood pressure should not be allowed to exceed 160/110 mmHg.

Suggested further reading

Altman D, Carroli G, Duley L, Farrell B, Moodley J, Neilson J, *et al.* Do women with pre-eclampsia, and their babies, benefit from magnesium sulphate? The Magpie Trial: a randomised placebo-controlled trial. *Lancet* 2002;359:1877–90.

Douglas KA, Redman CW. Eclampsia in the United Kingdom. *BMJ* 1994;309:1395–400.

Duley L. Magnesium sulphate regimes for women with eclampsia: messages from the Collaborative Eclampsia trial. *Br J Obstet Gynaecol* 1996:103:103–5.

Eclampsia Trial Collaborative Group. Which anticonvulsant for women with eclampsia? Evidence from the Collaborative Eclampsia Trial. *Lancet* 1995:345:1455–63.

Lewis G, editor. *Why Mothers Die 2000–2002. Sixth Report on Confidential Inquiries into Maternal Deaths in the United Kingdom.* London: RCOG Press; 2004.

Magee LA, Cham C, Waterman EJ, Ohlsson A, von Dadelszen P. Hydralazine for treatment of severe hypertension in pregnancy: meta-analysis. *BMJ* 2003;327:955–60.

Magee LA, Ornstein MP, von Dadelszen P. Fortnightly review: management of hypertension in pregnancy. *BMJ* 1999;318:1332–6.

Milne F, Redman C, Walker J, Baker P, Bradley J, Cooper C, *et al.* The pre-eclampsia community guideline (PRECOG): how to screen for and detect onset of pre-eclampsia in the community. *BMJ* 2005;330;576–80.

Royal College of Obstetricians and Gynaecologists. *The Management of Severe Pre-eclampsia/Eclampsia.* Guideline No. 10(A). London: RCOG; 2006.

Tuffnell DJ, Jankowicz, D, Lindow SW, Lyons G, Mason GC, Russell IF, *et al.* Outcomes of severe pre-eclampsia/eclampsia in Yorkshire 1999/2003. *BJOG* 2005;112:875–80.

Algorithm 17.1 Massive obstetric haemorrhage

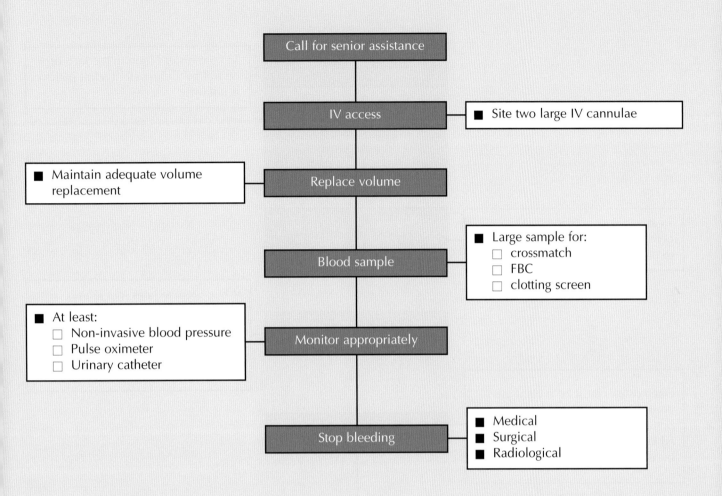

Algorithm 17.2 Patients declining blood and blood products

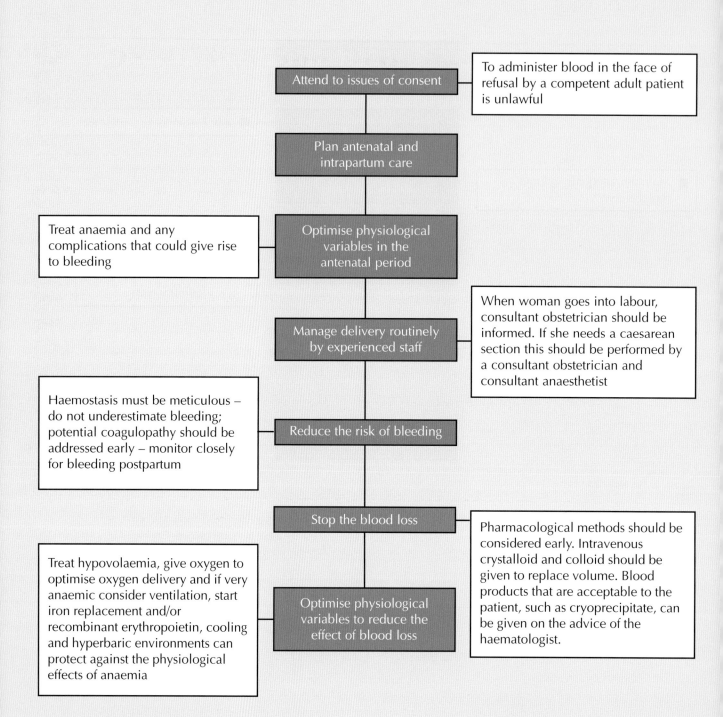

Attend to issues of consent

To administer blood in the face of refusal by a competent adult patient is unlawful

Plan antenatal and intrapartum care

Optimise physiological variables in the antenatal period

Treat anaemia and any complications that could give rise to bleeding

Manage delivery routinely by experienced staff

When woman goes into labour, consultant obstetrician should be informed. If she needs a caesarean section this should be performed by a consultant obstetrician and consultant anaesthetist

Reduce the risk of bleeding

Haemostasis must be meticulous – do not underestimate bleeding; potential coagulopathy should be addressed early – monitor closely for bleeding postpartum

Stop the blood loss

Pharmacological methods should be considered early. Intravenous crystalloid and colloid should be given to replace volume. Blood products that are acceptable to the patient, such as cryoprecipitate, can be given on the advice of the haematologist.

Optimise physiological variables to reduce the effect of blood loss

Treat hypovolaemia, give oxygen to optimise oxygen delivery and if very anaemic consider ventilation, start iron replacement and/or recombinant erythropoietin, cooling and hyperbaric environments can protect against the physiological effects of anaemia

Chapter 17

Massive obstetric haemorrhage

Objectives

On successfully completing this topic you will be able to:

■ understand the definition and causes of major obstetric haemorrhage

■ recognise and manage maternal collapse caused by obstetric haemorrhage

■ understand the pharmacological and surgical options for the treatment of major obstetric haemorrhage

■ make a plan to facilitate optimum management in your environment

■ understand the issues to be discussed with a woman declining blood and blood products during pregnancy

■ consider the management options in individual cases where blood and blood products are delivered.

Introduction

Major haemorrhage remains a leading cause of maternal mortality despite modern improvements in obstetric practice and transfusion services. Complications of haemorrhage associated with first-trimester bleeding due to miscarriage or ectopic pregnancy have not been considered, although most general principles will apply.

Maternal mortality and incidence of major haemorrhage

The 2000–2002 report on Confidential Enquiries into Maternal Deaths in the United Kingdom details a rise in mortality rate from 3.3/million maternities in 1997–99 to 8.5/million maternities in 2000–2002. Concern remains that care is not always optimal, especially in cases where the problems could have been anticipated. Issues of limited training time, obstetric only practitioners and reduced working hours are mentioned in this report. Regular skills update and fire drills are recommended for all staff working in a delivery unit.

Mortality statistics give no data on the incidence of major haemorrhage or on the maternal and fetal morbidity associated with haemorrhage and transfusion. Specific complications include transfusion-related reactions and infections, genital tract trauma, loss of fertility following hysterectomy and the rare Sheehan's syndrome (hypopituitarism).

Definition and epidemiology

Major obstetric haemorrhage has been variously defined as the loss of more than 1000 ml or 1500 ml blood as either antepartum or postpartum loss. This definition is used as a marker for audit or to mobilise additional resources reserved for such emergencies. Considerable problems are recognised in the accurate measurement of blood loss and a definition based on volume alone has some shortcomings. Both visual and measured loss can be highly inaccurate and loss from placental abruption or uterine rupture may be partially or completely concealed. Under-estimation of blood loss may delay active steps being taken to prepare for or prevent further bleeding.

Major causes of obstetric haemorrhage (primary or secondary)

Resulting initially in hypovolaemia:

- uterine atony (multiple causes)
- placenta praevia
- retained or adherent placenta or products of conception
- genital tract injury including broad ligament haematoma
- uterine rupture
- uterine inversion
- uterine anatomical abnormalities e.g. multiple fibroids
- ectopic pregnancy.

Associated with coagulation failure:

- placental abruption
- pre-eclampsia
- septicaemia/intrauterine sepsis
- retained dead fetus
- amniotic fluid embolus
- incompatible blood transfusion
- existing coagulation abnormalities.

Other outcomes may help in the audit of major haemorrhage and could be used to identify problem areas requiring reorganisation or staff training. Auditing records of women requiring more than two units of blood may still underestimate mothers with a blood loss of 1000–1500 ml. A mother with an antenatal Hb of 12 g/dl and a 2000-ml blood loss, replaced with colloid other than blood, might have a postnatal Hb of 8 g/dl or above. This could be treated expectantly with oral iron. This mother would not appear in a review of haemorrhage based on transfusion practice, despite falling within the definition by volume of major obstetric haemorrhage.

In a large series from California, 27 of 16 462 (0.16%) women delivering in one hospital in 1988 received more than two units of blood products. Only 11 of 27 (41.0%) women had conditions that would have led to antenatal warning of major haemorrhage, largely women with a placenta praevia. In a study from Vancouver in 1985–86, 40 of 7731 (0.58%) of women delivering received more than two units of blood. Again these transfusions were described as unpredictable in 27 of 40 (67.5%) cases. Overall rates of transfusion in this series were 48 of 6049 (0.8%) for vaginal births and 52 of 1682 (3.1%) for caesarean delivery.

Guidelines for the management of major haemorrhage

The development of a multidisciplinary massive haemorrhage guideline has been strongly recommended by the 2000–2002 CEMD report. Each unit will have its own problems, depending on staff availability and the geography of the hospital. A management protocol should be agreed by the clinical and laboratory staff and will provide a focus for regular audit. This should include details of senior staff to be contacted in obstetrics, anaesthetics and haematology. The guideline should be readily available and introduced to all staff working on the labour ward.

Summary of audit points

■ Incidence of measured blood loss greater than 1000 ml or 1500 ml.

■ Incidence and indication for transfusion of blood products.

■ Postnatal Hb fall of greater than 3 g/dl in women who have not been transfused. This may identify women with unrecognised significant loss at the time of delivery.

■ Critical incident reporting: a report of difficulties encountered in obtaining staff, equipment or blood products filed by the personnel involved in each critical event for discussion with staff in all disciplines.

■ Morbidity represented by circulatory collapse, organ failure, transfer to the intensive care unit, genital tract trauma and loss of fertility.

Practical management

This involves the identification of a large volume (greater than 1000 ml) blood loss or the recognition of maternal signs of shock in the absence of large visible loss. Either of these should prompt the initiation of the protocol set out in the massive haemorrhage guideline.

The pivotal factor in the management of a major obstetric haemorrhage is the restoration of the circulating blood volume, followed by the prevention of further loss. Failure to maintain adequate tissue perfusion leads to loss of vital organ function and care becomes increasingly more complex.

Maternal signs of shock:

■ tachycardia (on occasions a normal pulse rate or bradycardia can be seen)

■ hypotension

■ tachypnoea

■ poor peripheral perfusion

■ confusion or unresponsive

■ requiring more than two units of colloid to maintain blood pressure

■ oliguria

■ unexplained metabolic acidosis.

Management involves various elements all of which need to be undertaken **simultaneously**:

■ communication and documentation

■ resuscitation

■ monitoring and investigation

■ fluid replacement

■ arresting the bleeding and obstetric intervention

■ anaesthetic management.

Communication and documentation

■ Call senior midwife on duty, obstetric and anaesthetic registrars.

■ Inform consultant obstetrician and anaesthetist.

■ Inform blood bank technician and consultant haematologist.

■ Call porter for delivery of specimens and blood products.

■ Allocate one member of resuscitation team to record events, fluids, drugs and vital signs.

Ongoing communication, written and verbal between senior staff is essential. This may involve the assistance of other specialists such as intensive care specialists, vascular surgeons or radiologists.

Resuscitation

Assess Airway and Breathing. Provide appropriate support.

Administer a high concentration of oxygen (10–15 litres/minute) via a face mask to the mother, regardless of her oxygen saturation. If the baby is undelivered, increasing the maternofetal oxygen gradient may help oxygen transfer, so supranormal values of maternal pO_2 may be valuable. If the airway is compromised (or respiratory effort impaired) owing to obtunded conscious level, anaesthetic assistance should be sought urgently. Usually conscious level and airway control improve rapidly once the circulating volume is restored.

Evaluate the Circulation. Establish two 14-guage intravenous lines and take 20 ml blood for diagnostic tests. Lower limb or femoral access should be avoided. Commence 2 litres of crytalloids intravenously.

Position the mother flat. If she is undelivered, position her in the left lateral position where possible, to minimise the effects of aortocaval compression. Lateral tilt with a wedge (or manual displacement of the uterus by an assistant) is also used when obstetric procedures are in progress. If an epidural is in use, compensatory lower-limb vasoconstriction will be limited, so the effects of positioning may be more marked. Head-down tilt can be used as a short-term measure to improve venous return but this may compromise respiration.

Monitoring and investigation

Diagnostic tests

Table 17.1 shows the blood requirements for diagnostic tests.

Table 17.1. Diagnostic blood tests

Diagnostic tests	Blood required (ml)
Full blood count/platelet count	2.5 (in EDTA)
Coagulation screen (+ fibrinogen assay)	4.5 (in citrate)
Crossmatch 6 units	10–15 (in plain bottle)
FDP/D-dimers	2.0 (in EACA antifibrinolytic agent)

Evaluation of response

Essential monitoring should include pulse, blood pressure (direct or indirect), respiration rate, oxygen saturation and fluid balance. Healthy women can maintain a normal or even high blood pressure while large volumes of blood are lost intra-abdominally. Most, but not all, women will demonstrate a tachycardia if bleeding significantly but paradoxical bradycardia has also been observed. Regular checks of the haematocrit, clotting studies and blood gases will help guide resuscitation.

Insert a catheter to monitor hourly urine output.

A CVP line has been strongly recommended to avoid under-transfusion or fluid overload. Insertion should not delay initial resuscitation. If disseminated intravascular coagulation is suspected, CVP insertion is more hazardous. The antecubital fossa could be considered for CVP access, as this site is more easily compressed.

Simple methods of assessing cardiac output would be useful but these are not readily available for use in the obstetric situation. CVP measurements are usually helpful in assessing filling of the right atrium. The assumption is made that, if the right and left hearts are functioning equally effectively, the right filling pressure reflects filling pressure on the left or systemic side of the circulation. There are occasions when there is left ventricular dysfunction so that the filling pressures on either side of the heart may not be equivalent. This makes interpretation of CVP readings difficult, so that expert advice on further fluid management and appropriate cardiac support may be needed from intensive care specialists.

Conditions where CVP measurement may not be adequate to guide fluid management:

- hypotension unresponsive to fluid therapy
- oliguria despite apparently adequate CVP measurement
- coexisting relevant disease, e.g. cardiac failure
- coexisting severe sepsis
- coexisting severe pre-eclampsia
- management of pulmonary oedema.

Fluid replacement and blood product transfusion

Initial volume replacement should consist of up to 2 litres of physiological saline or Hartmann's solution, followed by plasma expanders until blood is available. If the haemorrhage is life threatening, transfuse uncrossmatched O-negative or group-specific blood.

Fluid therapy – a guide

Crytalloid:	2 litres of physiological saline or Hartmann's solution. Large volumes of crystalloid may be undesirable in view of the relatively low oncotic pressure in pregnancy and can lead to pulmonary oedema.
Colloid:	1–2 litres colloid until blood available.
Blood:	Needed if haemorrhage in excess of 2–3 litres. If life threatening, transfuse uncrossmatched O rhesus-negative blood, otherwise transfuse ABO and rhesus D-compatible blood as soon as feasible.
Fresh frozen plasma:	4 units for every 6 units of red cells or if PT/APTT $> 1.5 \times$ normal.
Platelet concentrates:	If platelet count $< 50 \times 10^9$/l
Cryoprecipitate:	If fibrinogen < 1 g/l

Component blood therapy

There are unresolved dilemmas in deciding the amounts of blood components to be used in situations of haemorrhagic crisis. One option is to transfuse blood components to a formula as suggested in the box above, depending upon the volume of red cells transfused. There is, however, no agreed formula although various guidelines exist. This has the disadvantage that under- or over-transfusion may occur, which may either fail to treat adequately or increase exposure to infection risk and other transfusion complications.

An alternative is to be guided by laboratory results. This has the difficulty of delay in obtaining results while the clinical situation is changing rapidly. In practice, a combination of both approaches is appropriate. Laboratory assistance may be vital where bleeding is persistent.

Blood

Fresh whole blood is not used in adult practice in the UK because release from the blood bank less than 24 hours after collection does not allow completion of a full infection screen. After 48 hours storage, viable platelet numbers and the function of important clotting factors (factors V and VIII) are already reduced. Concentrated red cells are the mainstay of treatment for volume replacement and the restoration of the oxygen-carrying capacity of blood. Each pack contains approximately 220 ml red cells and 80 ml saline-adenine-glucose-mannitol (SAG-M) solution, giving it a shelf life of 35 days. The haematocrit varies from 55% to 70% so a plasma substitute needs to be given in appropriate amounts to provide the additional volume required.

Full crossmatching of blood may take up to 1 hour. In an emergency, group-specific blood should be used. A woman's blood group and presence of abnormal antibodies are usually established during pregnancy, which facilitates the provision of blood when needed. The use of group-specific blood following antibody screening carries a risk of less than 0.1% of a haemolytic transfusion reaction, which rises to 1.0% if group-specific blood is used without antibody screening. In most circumstances, issuing of group- and rhesus-compatible blood should be possible within 5 minutes. Group O Rh-negative blood should be available on the labour ward for dire emergencies but this carries a small risk of sensitisation to 'c' antigen with possible problems for future pregnancies. It should rarely be needed.

In order to reduce the transmission of the CJD virus, the blood is further leucodepleted. At present, there is no specific test to check the blood for this virus.

Defective blood coagulation

In a previously healthy woman, a clotting-factor deficiency is unlikely to occur until around 80% of the original blood volume has been replaced. Large infusions of replacement fluids, such as plasma substitutes, and red cells suspended in additive solutions will dilute further the coagulation factors and platelets, causing a dilutional coagulopathy. This, in combination with hypotension-mediated endothelial injury, may trigger DIC and the downward spiral into coagulation failure. Hypothermia and metabolic acidosis due to poor tissue perfusion all worsen coagulation disorders.

The tests in common use (prothrombin time and activated partial thromboplastin time, platelets, fibrinogen) may be further improved by the use of a measure of whole blood clotting. The ideal tool would involve a rapid testing system for use in the labour ward and operating theatre, which could give real time information to clinicians to aid clinical judgment. The Thromboelastograph® provides information on whole blood clot formation and lysis and has been used in obstetrics. There are training and cost issues to be addressed in the use of this tool.

Clotting factors and platelets

Fresh frozen plasma (FFP) is separated from whole blood within 6 hours of donation and stored for up to 1 year at minus 20 to minus 30°C. It then needs careful defrosting before use. FFP contains clotting factors at physiological levels which will be diluted on addition of anti-coagulants. Methylene blue-treated FFP is also available. This helps to inactivate the CJD virus. The FFP so treated is 10–15 times more expensive than its untreated form.

Cryoprecipitate contains more fibrinogen than FFP but lacks antithrombin III (coagulation inhibitor), which is depleted in obstetric-related coagulopathies. Cryoprecipitate may be useful if the patient develops profound hypofibrinogenaemia.

Platelet packs have a limited shelf life of 5 days. They are rarely indicated above a platelet count of 50×10^9/l but may be required to raise the level to $80–100 \times 10^9$/l if surgical intervention is planned. It is not just numbers but function of platelets that results in effective clot formation. This is difficult to measure in a laboratory but again is included in any tests of whole blood clotting.

Haemostatic agents

In some cases, despite optimal replacement of clotting factors, haemostasis is still inadequate and is not thought to be due to surgical bleeds. This general ooze may be worsened by many factors such as acidosis, hypothermia and less than optimum platelet and clotting factor function.

Recombinant activated factor VII (rfVII or Novoseven®, Novo Nordisk) has been used in such situations in trauma and obstetric haemorrhage. In case reports, it has been successfully used to retrieve very difficult situations of severe bleeding. It is a potent prothrombotic agent so the risk of thromboembolic complications has still to be assessed. In a trauma context, some guidelines have been published suggesting targets of platelet count of greater than 50×10^9/l, fibrinogen levels of 0.5 g/l and pH greater than 7.2 should be achieved before giving rfVIIa.

RfVIIa comes as a freeze-dried preparation needing reconstitution. It needs to be refrigerated and is very expensive. A recommended starting dose is 90 micrograms/kg, repeated as needed. More than one dose may be needed.

Practical additions

Alternatives to homologous blood transfusion

Interest in reducing homologous transfusion has increased in recent years and some alternatives have been tried in obstetric practice.

■ Autologous blood transfusion by antenatal donation (mainly in North America)

This appears to be a safe technique in pregnancy, although its use is likely to be restricted to women who are at high risk of needing a blood transfusion, for example, in placenta praevia, or those for whom blood is not readily available owing to maternal antibodies to blood antigens. Unfortunately, many obstetric transfusions are unexpected, which limits the use of this technique.

■ Cell salvage procedures

A number of techniques exist to recover blood for reinfusion from clean operative sites. Aspirated blood is anticoagulated, filtered, washed and the red cells re-suspended in saline before reinfusion. Potential problems in obstetric practice include possible bacterial contamination from ruptured membranes and the need to avoid contamination with fetal cells or amniotic fluid. There is little information on its use in obstetric practice. Other considerations include the time required for setting up and the cost of disposables. Current equipment has become quicker and easier to use and most anaesthetists and theatre technicians should be familiar with its use.

■ Warmers, filters and high-pressure infusers

All large-volume infusions should be warmed but it is mandatory to avoid infusing cold fluid directly into the heart through a CVP line. High-pressure infusion devices are essential. Hand-inflated pressure bags are effective but labour intensive. More sophisticated high-pressure infusers use pressure from gas cylinders to provide very high flows. Hazards of any high-pressure infusion include fluid overload and air embolism. The patient should also be kept warm, as hypothermia will exacerbate poor peripheral perfusion, acidosis and coagulation abnormalities.

Citrate anticoagulation

Large volumes of citrate anticoagulants are present in stored red blood cells and FFP. Citrate binds to ionised calcium, which may result in hypocalcaemia. This in turn contributes to coagulopathy and to a negative intropic action on the heart. Both effects can be reversed by a slow (20-minute) infusion of Ca^{2+} e.g. 10 mls 10% calcium gluconate with subsequent laboratory checks of serum Ca^{2+}.

Immediate bedside testing of haematocrit

This acts as a good guide to the need for red blood cells or colloid. It is possible to over-enthusiastically transfuse red blood cells, forgetting that these are concentrated red cells, not whole blood, and cannot be used as full replacement for loss on a volume-for-volume basis.

Interventions for the management of haemorrhage

First line:

- Empty uterus:
  - deliver fetus if undelivered
  - remove placenta or retained products of conception.
- Oxytocics: syntocinon, ergometrine.
- Massage and bimanual compression of the uterus following delivery.
- Repair of genital tract injury, e.g. vaginal/cervical lacerations.

Further uncontrolled bleeding:

- Medical options:
  - carboprost
  - misoprostol 1000 micrograms rectally.
- If clotting problems thought to be contributory:
  - tranexamic acid 1 g intravenously
  - aprotonin infusion
  - recombitant factor VIIa.
- Surgical options:
  - uterine tamponade:
    - intrauterine catheter, e.g. Rusch balloon
    - uterine packing.
  - laparotomy:
    - compression of the aorta (temporary to allow catch up resuscitation)
    - uterine haemostatic suture, e.g. B-Lynch suture
    - arterial ligation
    - hysterectomy.
- radiological:
  - selective arterial embolisation
  - internal iliac artery balloon (temporary) to allow surgical haemorrhage control.

Uterotonic drugs

Oxytocin

Drugs used as prophylaxis to maintain a well-contracted uterus include oxytocin (Syntocinon®, Alliance) 5 units intramuscular or intravenous and oxytocin 5 units, ergometrine 0.5 mg (Syntometrine®, Alliance). The BNF recommended dose after caesarean section is 5 units by slow intravenous injection immediately after delivery. Oxytocin has a short duration of action and may be used as an infusion to maintain a contracted uterus (40 units in 500 ml 0.9% saline over 4 hours). Adverse effects include hypotension due to vasodilatation when given as a rapid intravenous bolus and fluid retention. The intramuscular use of ergometrine (0.5 mg intramuscularly) is relatively contraindicated in pre-eclampsia due to its hypertensive action.

A Cochrane systematic review has been carried out on umbilical vein injection for the management of retained placenta. This review suggested that the umbilical vein injection of saline solution with oxytocin appears to be effective in the management of retained placenta. The reviewers suggested that, as the numbers of included trials are small, further research is required in the area.

Prostaglandins

Although prostaglandins appear to be effective in treating postpartum haemorrhage, concerns about safety limit their suitability for routine prophylactic management of the third stage.

Prostaglandin E_2 (PGE_2), prostaglandin F_2 (PGF_2) and its analogue 15-methylprostaglandin F_2 stimulate myometrial contraction and have been used for refractory haemorrhage due to uterine atony.

Use of PGE_2 results primarily in vasodilatation with a fall in systemic and pulmonary vascular resistance and resulting fall in blood pressure. Cardiac output can be maintained by an increase in heart rate and stroke volume. Both severe hypotension following intramyometrial injection and paradoxical severe hypertension following intravenous injection have been reported after the use of this drug. There are reports of PGE_2 pessaries being placed in the uterine or vaginal cavities with good effect. Intrauterine infusions of PGE_2 (7.5 micrograms/ minute) via a Foley catheter have been used successfully without significant reported adverse effects.

Carboprost (Hemabate®, Pharmacia) is a potent synthetic analogue of PGF_2 licensed for use in postpartum haemorrhage via deep intramuscular injection. The dose is 250 micrograms repeated if required at not less than a 15-minute interval, with a total recommended dose of 2 g (i.e. eight injections).

Carboprost has been used successfully following failure of conventional treatment. It is not licensed for intramyometrial use. Failure of carboprost to control haemorrhage has been associated with the presence of both chorioamnionitis and coagulation abnormalities.

Serious adverse effects include bronchospasm, pulmonary oedema and hypertension. An increase in intrapulmonary shunting with an accompanying fall in PO_2 has been described following the use of both PGF_2 and carboprost. Oxygen saturation monitoring should be used for women receiving this drug. It should be used cautiously in women with pre-eclampsia or cardiac problems.

Misoprostol (800 micrograms given rectally) is cheap, stable and has been shown to be more effective than Syntometrine and oxytocin infusion for primary postpartum haemorrhage in a randomised controlled trial.

Obstetric interventions

Tone, tissue, trauma, thrombin

When a uterus fails to contract in response to oxytocic agents, there may be retained tissue or trauma to the genital tract. Once initial resuscitation is effective the vagina, cervix and uterine cavity need to be explored urgently. Further interventions will depend on the cause found if any.

Uterine tamponade

Uterine packing has been reported with successful outcomes in the management of haemorrhage from an atonic uterus where conservative measures have failed. A ribbon gauze (bandage rolls securely tied to each other) is inserted into the uterus and snugly packed in a zigzag fashion. Poor packing or insufficient length of gauze can compromise this simple technique. This technique can also be used at caesarean section when faced by sustained atonicity. The pack should be removed after 24 hours under the cover of intravenous antibiotics and a Syntocinon drip.

The use of a hydrostatic balloon is now advocated as a simpler and less time-consuming alternative method for controlling haemorrhage. The inflated Rusch balloon can conform to the contour of the uterine cavity and provides effective tamponade. In a developing country, an inflated condom attached to a Foley's catheter appears to be a cheaper alternative.

Laparotomy

At laparotomy, the following techniques may be undertaken:

Compression of the aorta

In life-threatening situations, compression of the aorta can be a simple, temporary but effective manoeuvre to allow time for the resuscitating team to catch up with volume replacement and the surgical team to clear the operative field.

Arterial ligation

Bilateral uterine artery ligation:	By decreasing the arterial flow pressures and correcting coagulation a hysterectomy may be avoided. The ureters should be identified prior to ligation.
Bilateral internal iliac artery ligation:	Recognised complications of this procedure include ligation of the external iliac artery, trauma to the iliac veins, ureteric injury and retroperitoneal haematoma. Internal iliac arterial ligation is best done by a vascular surgeon or one with equivalent experience.

Stepwise uterine devascularisation

Step 1	Unilateral uterine artery ligation at the upper part of the lower segment.
Step 2	Bilateral uterine artery ligation at the upper part of the lower segment.
Step 3	Lower uterine vessel ligation after mobilisation of the bladder and ureter.
Step 4	Unilateral ovarian vessel ligation.
Step 5	Bilateral ovarian vessel ligation.

Steps 1 and 2 have been reported as being effective in over 80% of cases.

Uterine haemostatic sutures

A variety of haemostatic suture methods have been described which might be appropriate once it has been established that direct bimanual compression of the uterus arrests the haemorrhage.

B-Lynch suture

The B-Lynch suture is a brace-type suture that mimics the effect of bimanual compression. A stitch is passed through the anterior wall of the uterus at the level of the uterine incision, over the right cornu, horizontally through the lower posterior wall, over the left cornu, back through the anterior wall at the right side of the uterine incision and tied in front (Figure 17.1). An assistant needs to manually compress the uterus as the suture is tightened.

Modified B-Lynch suture

'Multiple simple brace' sutures are inserted to control bleeding. This does not require the uterus to be opened.

Hysterectomy

If the haemorrhage cannot be adequately controlled by reasonable measures, a hysterectomy may be required.

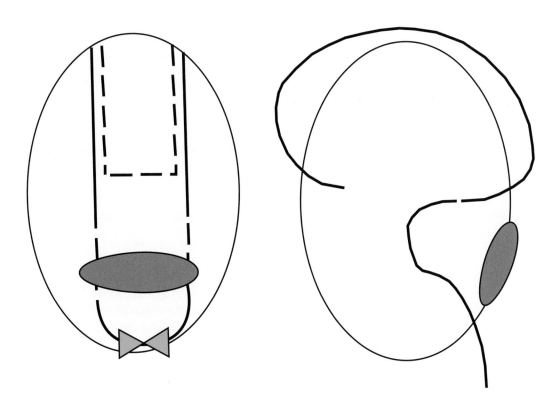

Figure 17.1 B-Lynch brace suture

Radiological measures

Arterial embolisation

There are a number of reports of this technique in obstetric practice. Access is obtained via the femoral artery, from where the bleeding point is identified by contrast injection. The feeder artery is catheterised and embolised with absorbable gelatin sponge (Gelfoam®, Upjohn), usually resorbed in 10 days. This procedure seems to be a useful addition to the management of obstetric haemorrhage in centres with suitably trained staff.

Internal iliac balloon catheters

Appropriately sited catheters in the internal iliac arteries have been positioned preoperatively in women at very high risk, such as in cases of placenta accreta. In women who subsequently bleed, the inflation of the balloons allows control of haemorrhage giving a much better surgical field and reducing blood loss.

Specific situations leading to obstetric haemorrhage

- Bleeding associated with caesarean section (see Chapter 18)
- Placenta praevia (see Chapter 24)
- Placental abruption.

Placental abruption

The incidence of antepartum haemorrhage is 3%: 1% from placenta praevia, 1% from abruption and 1% from other causes.

An abruption results from the separation of the placenta from the uterine wall and blood being driven into the myometrium, with resulting damage and release of thromboplastins and bleeding into the myometrial layers (Couvelaire uterus). This damage interferes with uterine contractility, causing atony predisposing to postpartum haemorrhage. Alongside this, there may also be a coagulopathy.

Signs of abruption are sudden onset of severe abdominal pain and tenderness, shock and a hard, woody uterus. However, with a posterior abruption (i.e. with a posterior placenta), the abdomen may be soft. Fetal heart sounds may be muffled or absent: abdominal ultrasound is often necessary to establish the presence or absence of a fetal heart.

Small abruptions are often difficult to diagnose, usually based on clinical suspicions, an ultrasound is not diagnostic in the early stages although these cases may develop large retroplacental collections.

If there is a fetal death in association with abruption then the abruption is major and represents significant maternal blood loss. The blood loss may be without any vaginal loss (concealed) and may be compensated for in the maternal circulation by the shutting down of the blood supply to the fetoplacental unit. It is therefore frequently underestimated. As a rule of thumb, an abruption resulting in fetal death requires maternal transfusion.

Abruption and intrauterine death are both causes of DIC, further predisposing to postpartum haemorrhage. Early delivery protects against the severity of DIC, which is due in part to the massive release of thromboplastins from the damaged uterus.

Initial management is:

- A B C

- send blood samples for tests, including Kleihauer

- deliver the fetus

- treat coagulopathy.

If significant haemorrhage has occurred and the fetus is viable, consider immediate delivery by caesarean section if necessary. The method of delivery is almost always caesarean section unless the cervix has dilated rapidly and the fetal heart trace is very good. With the contractions of labour, the abruption is likely to worsen with increasing separation of the placenta from the uterine wall: a fetal scalp clip is essential.

If the fetus is dead, induction aiming toward a vaginal delivery is usually considered. Monitor for hypovolaemia during labour and consider caesarean section if the woman does not labour fairly quickly.

Expect massive postpartum haemorrhage. The underestimation of blood loss antepartum makes the effect of further bleeding less well tolerated and significant cardiovascular compromise can occur, together with further exacerbation of DIC secondary to more blood loss and blood transfusion.

Consider CVP monitoring, involve senior staff and arrange for high-dependency care postoperatively.

There is a possibility of caesarean hysterectomy. Senior staff should be involved.

Important points to remember

- Haemorrhage is concealed and therefore can be grossly underestimated.

- The mother protects her own circulation from the effects of hypovolaemia by shutting down the supply to the fetoplacental unit, so signs of blood loss are not reflected in maternal signs but in fetal distress as picked up on the CTG. Principles of ABC apply and resuscitation of the mother is paramount in spite of dramatic CTG changes and should be undertaken without delay.

- Fetal death is a sign of a major abruption.

- Delay in delivery makes DIC more likely.

- Expect postpartum haemorrhage because the uterus is atonic and there may be DIC.

- The effect of postpartum haemorrhage is greater in the patient who is already hypovolaemic because the antepartum haemorrhage has been underestimated.

Placenta accreta/increta and percreta
See Chapter 24.

Anaesthetic management for obstetric haemorrhage

The general approach should be the same regardless of the aetiology of the haemorrhage. The anaesthetist needs to be able to assess the patient quickly, to initiate or continue to resuscitate to restore the intravascular volume and provide safe anaesthesia.

Important points in the assessment will include:

- previous medical, obstetric and anaesthetic history

■ a working diagnosis

■ current vital signs and laboratory results

■ an examination of the cardiovascular and respiratory systems

■ an assessment of the upper airway as regards ease of intubation for rapid sequence induction of anaesthesia.

Prophylaxis against acid aspiration is recommended for all patients.

Regional or general anaesthesia

The presence of cardiovascular instability is a relative contraindication to regional blockade. The accompanying sympathetic blockade has the potential to worsen hypotension due to haemorrhage. There are no controlled data comparing techniques in the context of haemorrhage for either maternal or fetal outcomes. Choice for each case will depend on discussion with both the mother and surgeon involved.

If cardiovascular stability has been achieved and there is no evidence of coagulation failure, regional anaesthesia can be used. This may be particularly appropriate for elective cases or where a working epidural has been in place during labour. Continuous epidural block is preferred to a single-injection spinal technique, to allow better control of blood pressure and for prolonged surgery. Adequate quantities of blood, equipment, intravenous lines and monitoring must be available to cope with further bleeding. The height of the block needs to be well maintained to allow intra-abdominal handling of viscera without discomfort.

When bleeding is torrential and cardiovascular stability cannot be achieved, rapid sequence induction of general anaesthesia is more appropriate. Induction agents with minimal peripheral vasodilator action, such as ketamine 1–2 mg/kg (Ketalar®, Parke-Davis) or etomidate 100–300 micrograms/kg (Hypnomidate®, Janssen-Cilag) should be considered and in extreme circumstances adrenaline and atropine should be ready in case of cardiovascular collapse on induction. Ventilation with high concentrations of oxygen may be needed until bleeding is controlled.

Volatile agents have been associated with increased blood loss due to their relaxant effects on uterine muscle. Anaesthesia should be maintained with intravenous agents if uterine atony is a problem. If uterine relaxation is specifically required (e.g. evacuation of retained placenta or uterine inversion) volatile agents and beta-adrenergic drugs have been used. More recently, nitroglycerin has been successfully used both intravenously and as a sublingual spray, with the major advantage of rapid onset and short duration of action.

Anaesthetic consideration for placenta praevia

A woman with a placenta praevia has a considerable risk of haemorrhage at some time during pregnancy or delivery. Anaesthetic considerations for caesarean section include the position of the placenta and the likelihood of placenta accreta. A posteriorly positioned placenta should not require surgical access to the uterus through the placental bed and therefore blood loss is usually reduced. The presence of the placental bed in the lower uterine segment results in less effective uterine contraction, so these women are at increased risk of postpartum haemorrhage. Regional anaesthesia may be used.

In all cases, preparations for major haemorrhage should be made, including immediate availability of crossmatched blood. Similar preparation should be made for women taken to theatre for vaginal examination to evaluate a possible low-lying placenta.

Regional anaesthesia has been used successfully in cases of both anterior and posterior placenta praevia where cardiovascular stability can be maintained.

Patients declining blood and blood products

Issues of consent

Patients may decline blood and blood products because of their religious commitment or other personal belief. Jehovah's Witnesses believe that blood transfusion is forbidden. This is a deeply held core value and they regard a nonconsensual transfusion as a gross physical violation. Jehovah's Witnesses wish to be treated with effective non-blood alternatives. For all patients, doctors are obliged to deliver the best care in keeping with the patient's wishes. If they feel unable to comply with the patient's wishes they should refer the patient to a sympathetic colleague. A list of consultants with experience in treating patients without recourse to blood is available from the local Hospital Liaison Committee for Jehovah's Witnesses. The legal position is that any adult patient (i.e. 16 years of age and over) who has the necessary mental capacity to do so is entitled to refuse treatment, even if it is likely that refusal will result in the patient's death. No other person is legally able to consent to treatment for that adult or to refuse treatment on that person's behalf.

Witnesses view Scripture as ruling out the transfusion of whole blood, packed red blood cells, white blood cells, plasma and platelets. However, when it comes to derivatives of blood components (for example, albumin, coagulation factors, immunoglobulins, etc.) the use of these products is viewed as a matter of personal choice. Specific products must be discussed.

There is also variation as to which blood-saving techniques are acceptable. Jehovah's Witnesses may accept reinfusion of their own blood where equipment is arranged in a circuit which is constantly linked to the patient's own circulatory system. This involves bleeding off approximately 500 ml of blood into a bag containing anticoagulant (this can be obtained from the hospital blood bank), which remains in contact with the patient's circulation before the start of surgery. The volume is replaced by infusing clear fluid. When the patient bleeds intraoperatively they are then losing 'diluted' blood. When haemostasis has been achieved the blood that is contained in the bag can be reinfused. Some Witnesses may find this technique unacceptable. Cell salvaging with leucocyte depletion filters may be acceptable. Witnesses usually do not usually accept preoperative storage of their own blood but, in the UK, this is not a technique that is usually available from the blood transfusion services.

Obtaining consent

Obtain from the patient a clear statement of what products and techniques she will accept and what she refuses.

Explain the risk of refusal of allogenic blood frankly but not dramatically. Discuss earlier surgical intervention, including the possibility of an earlier decision to proceed to caesarean hysterectomy in uncontrolled postpartum haemorrhage. In the case of antepartum haemorrhage, discuss with the paediatrician the balance between delayed and immediate delivery and present these facts to the mother. If she continues to refuse blood products in the face of life-threatening haemorrhage, proceed to caesarean section. If she maintains her refusal to accept blood or blood products, her wishes should be respected.

Most Jehovah's Witnesses will carry with them a clear Advance Directive prohibiting blood transfusions and including information relating to the patient's view of blood products and autologous transfusion procedures. The Advance Directive should be lodged with the patient's GP, as well as with family and friends. If the patient is not in a condition to give or withhold consent but has expressed a wish at an earlier date (Advanced Directive or Healthcare Advance Directive), respect the patient's instructions in the Advance Directive or Healthcare Advance Directive.

If such instructions do not specifically apply to the patient's current condition, if the patient's instructions are vague and open to interpretation or if there is good reason to believe that the patient has had a change of heart since making the declaration, the doctor's duty is to exercise good medical judgement and treat the patient in her best interests as determined by a responsible body of medical opinion.

Allow the patient the opportunity to speak with the Hospital Liaison Committee for Jehovah's Witnesses and, if requested, join their discussion.

Ensure that the patient has had the opportunity to speak with the obstetrician in privacy. The doctor must be satisfied that the woman is not being subjected to pressure from others. It is reasonable to ask the accompanying persons to leave the room for a while so that the doctor (with a midwife or other colleague) can ask her whether she is making her decision of her own free will.

Keep a clear record of the discussion and particular aspects of consent. Note precisely which products and treatments she refuses and which she would accept. Complete a 'no blood' consent form (featured as an appendix in the Royal College of Surgeons Code of Practice for The Surgical Management of Jehovah's Witnesses: www.rcseng.ac.uk).

Have discussion and take and document consent in the presence of a witness. The person witnessing the discussion should sign a record of the discussion and consent as made and signed by the doctor.

A verbally expressed change of mind should be honoured. Again, it should be given in the presence of a witness and recorded in the notes.

Plan antenatal and intrapartum care

Massive obstetric haemorrhage is often unpredictable and can become life threatening in a short time. Delivery should be planned in a unit that has the facilities to cope with massive obstetric haemorrhage to include appropriate surgical expertise, interventional radiology and the option of cell salvage. Management should be geared to anticipating, e.g. identifying the placental site, preventing or stopping bleeding.

If any complications are noted during the antenatal period, the consultant obstetrician must be informed.

Optimise physiological variables in the antenatal period

The woman's blood group and antibody status should be checked in the usual way and the haemoglobin and serum ferritin should be checked regularly. Haematinics should be given throughout pregnancy to maximise iron stores. Treat any complications that could give rise to bleeding.

Manage delivery routinely by experienced staff

The consultant obstetrician should be informed when a woman who will refuse blood transfusion is admitted in labour. Consultants in other specialties need not be alerted unless complications occur.

The labour should be managed routinely by experienced staff.

Oxytocics should be given when the baby is delivered. The woman should not be left alone for at least an hour after delivery and there should be early intervention to stem postpartum bleeding.

If caesarean section is necessary, the operation should be carried out by a consultant obstetrician with a consultant anaesthetist.

When the mother is discharged from hospital, she should be advised to report promptly if she has any concerns about bleeding during the puerperium.

Reduce the risk of bleeding

The patient should be monitored closely for bleeding postpartum. Blood loss should not be underestimated, as potential coagulopathy should be addressed early.

Stop the blood loss

Pharmacological and surgical treatment is described in greater detail earlier in this chapter. Recombinant factor VII is an option.

The principle of management of haemorrhage in these cases is to avoid delay. Rapid decision making may be necessary, particularly with regard to surgical intervention.

If unusual bleeding occurs at any time during pregnancy, labour or the puerperium, the consultant obstetrician should be informed and the standard management should be commenced promptly. The threshold for intervention should be lower than in other patients. Extra vigilance should be exercised to quantify any abnormal bleeding and to detect complications, such as clotting abnormalities, as promptly as possible.

Consultants in other specialties, particularly anaesthetics and haematology, are normally involved in the treatment of massive haemorrhage. When the patient is a woman who has refused blood transfusion, the consultant anaesthetist should be informed as soon as possible after abnormal bleeding has been detected. The consultant haematologist should also be informed particularly if the patient is suffering from disseminated intravascular coagulation. Intensive care may need to be warned.

Surgery

Hysterectomy is normally the last resort in the treatment of obstetric haemorrhage but with such women delay may increase the risk. The woman's life may be saved by timely hysterectomy, although even this does not guarantee success.

When hysterectomy is performed, the uterine arteries should be clamped as early as possible in the procedure. Subtotal hysterectomy can be just as effective as total hysterectomy, as well as being quicker and safer. In some cases there may be a place for internal iliac artery ligation.

The timing of hysterectomy is a decision for the consultant on the spot. Survival without hysterectomy has been recorded with a haemoglobin concentration of 4.9 g/dl.

Optimise physiological variables to reduce the effect of blood loss

Treat hypovolaemia with non-blood products and use vasopressors to maintain blood pressure if necessary. Give oxygen to optimise oxygen delivery and, if very anaemic, consider ventilation to deliver oxygen maximally. Start iron replacement and/or recombinant erythropoietin. Cooling and hyperbaric environments can protect against the physiological effects of anaemia.

Suggested further reading

Please refer to the references at the end of the **Care plan for women in labour refusing a blood transfusion** on pages 190–1.

Care plan for women in labour refusing a blood transfusion

Reproduced with permission from the Hospital Information Services for Jehovah's Witnesses.

This document has been prepared as an aid for medical staff and midwives who are managing a Jehovah's Witness or other patient who refuses a blood transfusion and is at risk of, or experiencing, postpartum haemorrhage. We urge clinicians to plan in advance for blood loss, which includes correction of antenatal anaemia (see: Management of postpartum anaemia, second bullet point, italicised note). This should be discussed with the patient in keeping with her wishes that blood or blood products will not be used. Readiness to act promptly to prevent or stop bleeding is paramount.

Consider booking high-risk patients into a unit with facilities such as interventional radiology, cell salvage and surgical expertise.[1]

Please ensure that the consultant obstetrician and anaesthetist are aware that a Jehovah's Witness has been admitted in labour.

All such patients should have the third stage of labour actively managed with oxytocic drugs together with early cord clamping and controlled cord traction after placental separation. Do not leave the patient alone for the first hour after delivery.

Risk factors predisposing to postpartum haemorrhage

If the patient has any of the risk factors below, an intravenous infusion of oxytocin (Syntocinon) should be considered after delivery of the baby.

- Previous history of bleeding, ante or postpartum haemorrhage
- Prolonged labour (especially when augmented with oxytocin)
- Abnormal placentation
- Large baby (over 3.5 kg) and/or polyhydramnios
- Increased maternal age (over 40 years)
- Fibroids/myomectomy scars
- More than three children
- Maternal obesity
- Multiple pregnancy.

Management of active haemorrhage

First steps

- Involve obstetric, anaesthetic and haematology consultants.
- Establish intravanous colloid infusion (e.g. gelofusine).
- Give oxytocic drugs first, then exclude retained products of conception or trauma (this could save time).
- Proceed with bimanual uterine compression.
- Give oxygen.
- Catheterise and monitor urine output.

Obstetric emergencies

■ Consider central venous pressure line. Aortic compression against the spine, using a fist just above the umbilicus, may buy time in an emergency.[2]

■ Slow but persistent blood loss requires action. Anticipate coagulation problems.

■ Keep patient fully informed.

Next steps

Proceed with following strategies if bleeding continues:

■ Ergometrine with oxytocin (Syntometrine) is marginally more effective than oxytocin alone. If patient is hypertensive, use oxytocin 10 units (not 5 units) by slow intravenous injection (in postpartum haemorrhage, benefits of the higher dose outweigh the risks).[3,4]

■ Carboprost (Hemabate) 250 micrograms/ml intramuscularly, can be repeated after 15 minutes. Direct intramyometrial injection is faster (less hazardous at open operation). If not available, use one or two gemeprost pessaries in the uterus.[5]

■ Oral misoprostol (200-microgram tablets) 600 micrograms (three tablets, prostaglandin E_1 analogue), use when unresponsive to oxytocin andergometrine.[6] Intrauterine misoprostol 800 micrograms (four tablets) has been successfully used when refractory to oxytocin, ergometrine and also to carboprost.[7,8] Rectal misoprostol 800 micrograms or 1000 micrograms (five tablets), rapid absorption and control of haemorrhage reported when unresponsive to oxytocin and ergometrine, avoids problems associated with oral administration.[9,10] Misoprostol does not cause hypertension.

■ Recombinant factor VIIa (rFVIIa; NovoSeven) 90 micrograms/kg, provides site-specific thrombin generation. Increasingly used to successfully treat uncontrollable haemorrhage; for example, in placenta accreta/percreta, ruptured uterus, uterine atony and HELLP syndrome[11–17] (in seven of these cases, bleeding was controlled even in the presence of DIC despite the failure of all conventional therapies, including packing of pelvis, arterial ligation and hysterectomy[12–16]). Expert advice on this drug will be available from the local Haemophilia Comprehensive Care Centre or Novo Nordisk 24-hour medical advice line (0845 600 5055; emergency UK-wide delivery available). Some hospitals now hold a small stock of factor VIIa to avoid delivery delay. Aprotinin (Trasylol), 2 000 000 units followed by 500 000 units/hour or tranexamic acid (Cyklokapron) 1 g intravenously three times daily; both are anti-fibrinolytic agents well established for controlling haemorrhage.[18–20] Additionally, consider IV vitamin K.

■ Intrauterine balloon tamponade: stomach balloon of a Sengstaken-Blakemore tube used to control postpartum haemorrhage in 14 of 16 cases, including bleeding from an atonic uterus in nine cases.[21,22] Rüsch urological balloon catheter also used.[23] Consider having a purpose-designed 500 ml tamponade balloon available (J-SOS-100500-Bakri. Cook [UK] Ltd. tel. 01462 473100).[24] Balloon tamponade is able to indicate if bleeding will stop (as measured via catheter drainage shaft; the 'tamponade test'), thus avoiding unnecessary surgery.[21] Systematic uterine packing is also an option.[25]

■ B-Lynch brace suture:[26,27] simple suture technique to control massive haemorrhage. Can be combined with intrauterine balloon catheter if bleeding persists[28] (note: prophylactic insertion of this suture has been used in high-risk caesarean section[29]).

■ Embolisation/ligation of internal iliac arteries or embolisation/bilateral mass ligation of uterine vessels.[27,30]

■ Blood salvage may be life-saving if substantial blood loss anticipated.[31] Check if acceptable to patient. It has been used at caesarean section in at least 400 reported cases, without complications of amniotic fluid embolism or coagulopathy.[32] A cell saver with leucocyte depletion filter together with separate suction (one for amniotic fluid and one for blood salvage) minimises amniotic fluid contamination.[32,33]

■ Hysterectomy: subtotal hysterectomy can be just as effective, also quicker and safer.[34] Clamp uterine arteries as early as possible.

Management of postpartum anaemia

■ For severe anaemia give oxygen and use recombinant human erythropoietin (rHuEPO, NeoRecormon or Eprex) 300 units/kg (not 50 units), three-weekly subcutaneously or intravenously without delay, for accelerated haemoglobin recovery.[35–37] Augment with iron, vitamin B12 and folic acid.

■ Iron supplementation essential with EPO. Oral iron is too slow and unreliable, use intravenous iron sucrose (Venofer) by drip infusion or slow intravenous bolus (200 mg three-weekly).[35,36] This drug is rarely associated with anaphylaxis. (Note: optimisation of antenatal haemoglobin is essential: when unresponsive to oral iron, iron sucrose can be efficacious in reversing iron deficiency.[38,39] The addition of EPO [which does not cross the placenta and is reportedly safely used in pregnancy] enhances the response.[29,31,39,40] Suggested dosages of EPO and intravenous iron as above, but two-weekly[39].)

■ Consider elective ventilation in the intensive care unit. Use microsampling techniques (such as HemoCue haemoglobin analyser).

■ Hyperbaric oxygen therapy is an option in life-threatening anaemia due to postpartum haemorrhage[41] – telephone 0151 648 8000 (24-hours) for available centres.

This document reflects current clinical and scientific knowledge and is subject to change. The strategies are not intended as an exclusive guide to treatment. Good clinical judgement, taking into account individual circumstances, may require adjustments.

Reviewed by consultants in obstetrics and gynaecology, anaesthesia, and haematology (including experts in haemostasis), September 2005.

References

1. Hall MH. Haemorrhage. In: Lewis G, editor. *Why Mothers Die 2000–2002. Sixth Report of the Confidential Enquiries into Maternal Deaths.* London: RCOG Press; 2004.
2. Riley DP, Burgess RW. External abdominal aortic compression: a study of a resuscitation manoeuvre for postpartum haemorrhage. *Anaesth Intensive Care* 1994;**22**:571–5.
3. Scottish Obstetric Guidelines and Audit Project. *The Management of Postpartum Haemorrhage.* SPCERH 6. June 1998. Guideline Update prepared March 2002 [www.sign.ac.uk/guidelines/sogap/sogap4.html].
4. Choy CMY, Lau WC, Tam WH, Yuen PM. A randomised controlled trial of intramuscular syntometrine and intravenous oxytocin in the management of the third stage of labour. *BJOG* 2002;109:173–7.
5. Barrington JW, Roberts A. The use of gemeprost pessaries to arrest postpartum haemorrhage. *Br J Obstet Gynaecol* 1993;100:691–2.
6. El-Refaey H, O'Brien P, Morafa W, Walder J, Rodeck C. Use of oral misoprostol in the prevention of postpartum haemorrhage. *Br J Obstet Gynaecol* 1997;104:336–9.
7. Oboro VO, Tabowei TO, Bosah JO. Intrauterine misoprostol for refractory postpartum hemorrhage. *Int J Gynecol Obstet* 2003;80:67–8.
8. Adekanmi OA, Purmessur S, Edwards G, Barrington JW. Intrauterine misoprostol for the treatment of severe recurrent atonic secondary postpartum haemorrhage. *BJOG* 2001;108:541–2.
9. Lokugamage AU, Sullivan KR, Niculescu I, Tigere P, Onyangunga F, El Refaey H, et al. A randomized study comparing rectally administered misoprostol versus Syntometrine combined with an oxytocin infusion for the cessation of primary post partum hemorrhage. *Acta Obstet Gynecol Scand* 2001;80:835–9.
10. O'Brien P, El-Refaey H, Gordon A, Geary M, Rodeck CH. Rectally administered misoprostol for the treatment of postpartum hemorrhage unresponsive to oxytocin and ergometrine: a descriptive study. *Obstet Gynecol* 1998;92:212–14.
11. Branch DW, Rodgers GM. Recombinant activated factor VII: a new weapon in the fight against hemorrhage. *Obstet Gynecol* 2003;101:1155–6.
12. Moscardó F, Pérez F, de la Rubia J, Balerdi B, Lorenzo JI, Senent ML, et al. Successful treatment of severe intra-abdominal bleeding associated with disseminated intravascular coagulation using recombinant activated factor VII. *Br J Haematol* 2001;114:174–6.
13. Zupancic Salek S, Sokolic V, Viskovic T, Sanjug J, Simic M, Kastelan M. Successful use of recombinant factor VIIa for massive bleeding after caesarean section due to HELLP syndrome. *Acta Haematol* 2002;108:162–3.

17

Obstetric emergencies

14. Bouwmeester FW, Jonkhoff AR, Verheijen RHM, van Geijn HP. Successful treatment of life-threatening postpartum hemorrhage with recombinant activated factor VII. *Obstet Gynecol* 2003;101:1174–6.

15. Segal S, Shemesh IY, Blumenthal R, Yoffe B, Laufer N, Ezra Y, L *et al.* Treatment of obstetric hemorrhage with recombinant activated factor VII (rFVIIa). *Arch Gynecol Obstet* 2003;268:266–7.

16. Price G, Kaplan J, Skowronski G. Use of recombinant factor VIIa to treat life-threatening non-surgical bleeding in a post-partum patient. *Br J Anaesth* 2004;93:298–300.

17. Ahonen J, Jokela R. Recombinant factor VIIa for life-threatening post-partum haemorrhage. *Br J Anaesth* 2005;94:592–5.

18. Valentine S, Williamson P, Sutton D. Reduction of acute haemorrhage with aprotinin. *Anaesthesia* 1993;48:405–6.

19. Gai M-Y, Wu L-F, Su Q-F, Tatsumoto K. Clinical observation of blood loss reduced by tranexamic acid during and after caesarian section: A multicenter, randomized trial. *Eur J Obstet Gynecol Reprod Biol* 2004;112:154–7.

20. As AK, Hagen P, Webb JB. Tranexamic acid in the management of postpartum haemorrhage. *Br J Obstet Gynaecol* 1996;103:1250–1.

21. Condous GS, Arulkumaran S, Symonds I, Chapman R, Sinha A, Razvi K. The "tamponade test" in the management of massive postpartum hemorrhage. *Obstet Gynecol* 2003;101:767–72.

22. Katesmark M, Brown R, Raju KS. Successful use of a Sengstaken-Blakemore tube to control massive postpartum haemorrhage. *Br J Obstet Gynaecol* 1994;101:259–60.

23. Johanson R, Kumar M, Obhrai M, Young P. Management of massive postpartum haemorrhage: use of a hydrostatic balloon catheter to avoid laparotomy. *BJOG* 2001;108:420–2.

24. Bakri YN, Amri A, Abdul Jabbar F. Tamponade-balloon for obstetrical bleeding. *Int J Gynecol Obstet* 2001;74:139–42.

25. Maier RC. Control of postpartum hemorrhage with uterine packing. *Am J Obstet Gynecol* 1993;169:317–23.

26. B-Lynch C, Coker A, Lawal AH, Abu J, Cowen MJ. The B-Lynch surgical technique for the control of massive postpartum haemorrhage: an alternative to hysterectomy? Five cases reported. *Br J Obstet Gynaecol* 1997;104:372–5.

27. Dildy GA III. Postpartum hemorrhage: new management options. *Clin Obstet Gynecol* 2002;45:330–44.

28. Danso D, Reginald P. Combined B-Lynch suture with intrauterine balloon catheter triumphs over massive postpartum haemorrhage. *BJOG* 2002;109:963.

29. Kalu E, Wayne C, Croucher C, Findley I, Manyonda I. Triplet pregnancy in a Jehovah's Witness: recombinant human erythropoietin and iron supplementation for minimising the risks of excessive blood loss. *BJOG* 2002;109:723–5.

30. Drife J. Management of primary postpartum haemorrhage. *Br J Obstet Gynaecol* 1997;104:275–7.

31. de Souza A, Permezel M, Anderson M, Ross A, McMillan J, Walker S. Antenatal erythropoietin and intra-operative cell salvage in a Jehovah's Witness with placenta praevia. *BJOG* 2003;110:524–6.

32. Catling S, Joels L. Cell salvage in obstetrics: the time has come. *BJOG* 2005;112:131–2.

33. Waters JH, Biscotti C, Potter PS, Phillipson E. Amniotic fluid removal during cell salvage in the caesarean section patient. *Anesthesiology* 2000;92:1531–6.

34. Johanson R, Cox C, Grady K, Howell C. *Managing Obstetric Emergencies and Trauma: The MOET Course Manual.* London: RCOG Press; 2003.

35. Busuttil D, Copplestone A. Management of blood loss in Jehovah's Witnesses. Recombinant human erythropoietin helps but is expensive. *BMJ* 1995;311:1115–16.

36. Breymann C, Richter C, Hüttner C, Huch R, Huch A. Effectiveness of recombinant erythropoietin and iron sucrose vs. iron therapy only, in patients with postpartum anaemia and blunted erythropoiesis. *Eur J Clin Invest* 2000;30:154–61.

37. Rizzo JD, Lichtin AE, Woolf SH, Seidenfeld J, Bennett CL, Cella D, *et al.* Use of epoetin in patients with cancer: evidence-based clinical practice guidelines of the American Society of Clinical Oncology and the American Society of Hematology. *Blood* 2002;100:2303–20.

38. Perewusnyk G, Huch R, Huch A, Breymann C. Parenteral iron therapy in obstetrics: 8 years experience with iron-sucrose complex. *Br J Nutr* 2002;88:3–10.

39. Breymann C, Visca E, Huch R, Huch A. Efficacy and safety of intravenously administered iron sucrose with and without adjuvant recombinant human erythropoietin for the treatment of resistant iron-deficiency anemia during pregnancy. *Am J Obstet Gynecol* 2001;184:662–7.

40. Sifakis S, Angelakis E, Vardaki E, Koumantaki Y, Matalliotakis I, Koumantakis E. Erythropoietin in the treatment of iron deficiency anemia during pregnancy. *Gynecol Obstet Invest* 2001;51:150–6.

41. McLoughlin PL, Cope TM, Harrison JC. Hyperbaric oxygen therapy in the management of severe acute anaemia in a Jehovah's Witness. *Anaesthesia* 1999;54:891–5.

Algorithm 18.1 Prerequisites for caesarean section

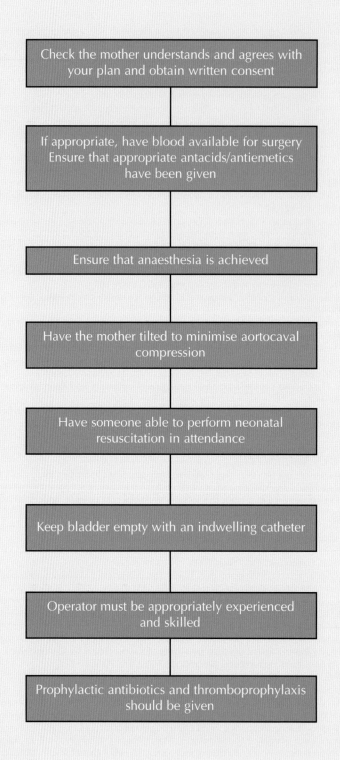

Check the mother understands and agrees with your plan and obtain written consent

If appropriate, have blood available for surgery
Ensure that appropriate antacids/antiemetics have been given

Ensure that anaesthesia is achieved

Have the mother tilted to minimise aortocaval compression

Have someone able to perform neonatal resuscitation in attendance

Keep bladder empty with an indwelling catheter

Operator must be appropriately experienced and skilled

Prophylactic antibiotics and thromboprophylaxis should be given

Algorithm 18.2 **Avoiding problems during key surgery**

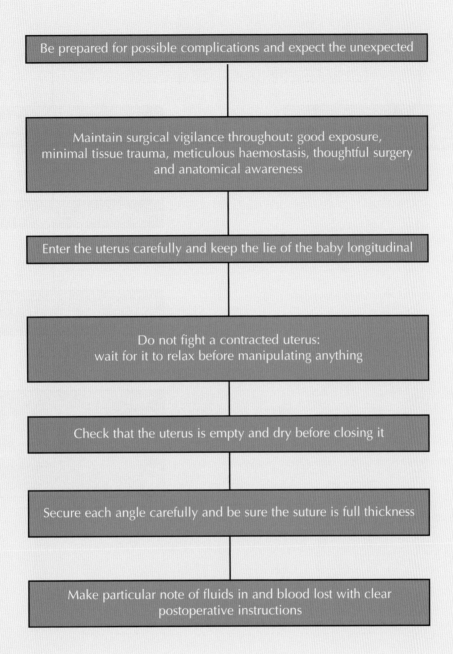

Algorithm 18.3 Rules for safe use of intravenous GTN to relax the uterus and aid delivery of the impacted head at caesarean section

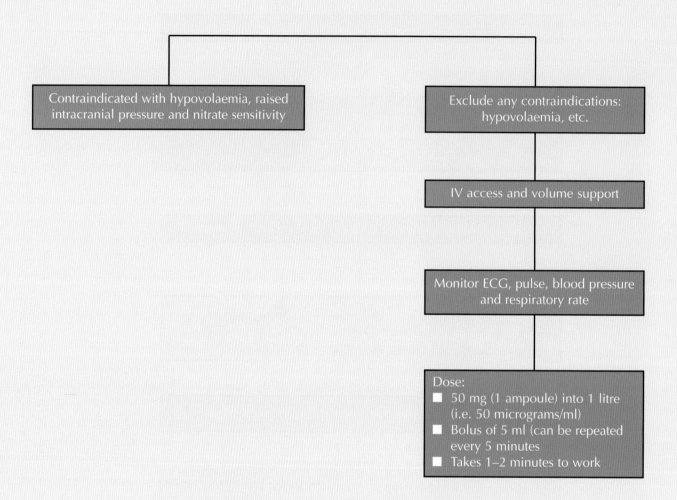

Contraindicated with hypovolaemia, raised intracranial pressure and nitrate sensitivity

Exclude any contraindications: hypovolaemia, etc.

IV access and volume support

Monitor ECG, pulse, blood pressure and respiratory rate

Dose:
- 50 mg (1 ampoule) into 1 litre (i.e. 50 micrograms/ml)
- Bolus of 5 ml (can be repeated every 5 minutes
- Takes 1–2 minutes to work

Chapter 18

Caesarean section

Objectives

On successfully completing this topic you will understand:

■ how to anticipate and to some extent avoid difficulties encountered at caesarean section

■ the techniques which can help you cope with such difficulties.

Introduction

Caesarean section is the process of delivering a baby abdominally. It is required if it is unsafe for the baby to be delivered vaginally. Rates vary enormously, not only between countries but also between hospitals, but trends are generally increasing worldwide. In the UK, the National Sentinel Caesarean Section Audit Report published in 2001 identified a rate of 21.5% from a 3-month period in the previous year. The rate has risen slightly since then but remains an approximation, as subsequent national data collection has been incomplete.

The decision to perform a caesarean section can be obvious in some circumstances while in others it can be extremely difficult. This decision-making skill in terms of timing and mode of delivery is acquired over many years with experience and clinical judgement. Caesarean section should never be seen as the easy option and all risks of caesarean section, as opposed to those of proceeding with an attempt at labour and vaginal delivery, should be considered and balanced in each individual circumstance, taking into account both maternal and fetal interests.

This chapter is not designed to list the indications or arguments for caesarean section, nor to give intricate detail into surgical technique, but rather to highlight the difficulties that can be encountered (both anticipated and unexpected) and to suggest ways in which they can be dealt with in the acute situation.

Prerequisites for caesarean section

■ The woman should understand the indications for the procedure and agree to it, giving written informed consent.

■ Anaesthesia should be achieved (either regional or general).

■ The operating table should be tilted laterally 30 degrees, to minimise aortocaval compression during the procedure.

■ The bladder should be kept empty with a urethral catheter.

■ Someone should be in attendance who is capable of performing neonatal resuscitation.

■ The operator must have appropriate experience and competence.

195

■ Prophylactic antibiotics and appropriate thromboprophylaxis should be used.

■ Blood should either be grouped and saved or crossmatched, depending on the clinical situation at hand and local arrangements.

Anticipating problems in specific circumstances

Before embarking on any surgery, rehearse the principals of good and safe surgical technique:

■ Maintain a sterile operative field.

■ Achieve good exposure with an appropriate incision.

■ Keep tissue handling to a minimum and avoid unnecessary dissection and trauma.

■ Treat the tissues with respect.

■ Achieve meticulous haemostasis.

■ While operating, positively think of and avoid the common problems that can otherwise turn what should have been a straightforward procedure into a complex one.

Incision

A low transverse skin incision is usually adequate for all uterine incisions except the true high classical incision extending up to the fundus.

Make sure that the incision used affords adequate access.

Entry

Entry to the peritoneal cavity should be careful and safe. Special care is needed if there has been previous surgery (bowel can be tethered or bladder can be high).

The operator and the assistant should avoid hooking fingers under the rectus muscle (between the rectus muscle and the peritoneum), as this can seriously threaten the inferior epigastric vascular bundle.

Before extending the peritoneal incision, check there are no adhesions hidden from view: the tearing which is done at this stage of surgery can be frighteningly vicious – be gentle.

Assess the lower uterine segment

The uterovesical peritoneal reflexion identifies the upper limit of the lower uterine segment and is invaluable in planning the uterine incision in difficult circumstances such as caesarean section at full dilatation, preterm delivery or abnormal lie situations.

Always check the degree of uterine rotation and correct it or allow for it prior to making the uterine incision.

Exposure

Make sure the peritoneum is reflected well clear of the proposed angles of the uterine incision as failure to do this can compromise access, haemostasis and closure of the angles if they have extended during delivery.

Uterine incision

Do not do this until you have either checked and confirmed that there is a presenting part in the pelvis or you have felt for the fetal lie and made a plan with your assistant regarding how to conduct the delivery.

In making the uterine incision, always try to leave membranes intact, as this will make it less likely that you will cut the baby (the membranes can then be carefully nicked just prior to delivery).

Remember that the thicker the uterine segment (preterm, placenta praevia or abnormal lies) the less space it affords you in terms of access to the baby – make sure the incision is big enough.

Be careful during this stage of the surgery to get your assistant to keep the lie of the baby longitudinal – this is especially important if the lower segment is poorly formed or full of fibroid or placenta – the last thing you need in this difficult situation with compromised space is for the baby to drift off into an oblique or transverse lie.

Delivery

At caesarean section, the baby's head delivers into the wound in the occipitotransverse position by lateral flexion. This procedure should be conducted gently and slowly to avoid trauma to and extension of the uterine angles (see 'Difficulty with delivery of the head').

Fundal pressure during the delivery should be sustained and should follow the distal end of the fetus on its way out (like squeezing toothpaste from a tube).

Placenta

While the placenta is attached, the placental site will not bleed and there is no need to hurry this process. Wait for separation to occur rather than precipitating a problem. If there is bleeding then Green-Armytage clamps can be placed on the bleeding sinuses or angles as needed.

Check that all placenta and membranes have been removed.

Check the patency of the internal cervical os and that it is not covered with membrane.

Closure of uterus

Both uterine angles need to be secured carefully and accurately, with each stitch passing full thickness into the uterine cavity (failure to achieve this full thickness can leave a bleeding vessel within the cavity which will remain hidden from the surgeon's view and produce vaginal bleeding later).

If there are placental bed bleeders (commonly seen with placenta praevia) then attention should be given to these before closing the uterus (as once closed such bleeding is hidden from the surgeon's view). These can be dealt with by systemic uterotonics but may also need either an under-running suture or local injection of uterotonics (e.g. a solution of Syntocinon 10 units diluted in 20 ml physiological saline).

Routinely, the uterus should be closed in a double layer, as a single layer has a higher rate of future dehiscence and rupture (occasionally the lower segment is so thin that a single layer is all that is possible).

Haemostasis

Once the uterus is closed, the suture line and both angles should be checked for haemostasis while exposed without tension.

Great care should then be taken checking the peritoneal edges, the subrectus space and, if exposed, the inferior epigastric bundles for haemostasis before the sheath is closed. As the peritoneum is no longer routinely closed this process of haemostasis is even more vital than previously, as there is no tamponade effect on bleeding vessels in this layer and massive obstetric haemorrhage occurring due to bleeding from this site has been reported.

Drains

Anyone who claims never to need drains because they 'never close if everything isn't perfectly dry' paints an enviable but rather naïve picture. While haemostasis should always be the aim, very occasionally drains can be useful if there has been extremely difficult surgery with extensive dissection and raw surfaces or if there is likely to be a postpartum clotting problem (fulminating pre-eclampsia, HELLP, DIC, sepsis).

Any drain placed within the peritoneal cavity should be soft and large-bore (such as the Robinson drain) and not suctioned. If a suctioned drain is placed in the rectus space then the peritoneum should be closed (otherwise the drain is effectively intra-abdominal).

Closure

Close the sheath, then check for haemostasis before closing the fat layer (if greater than 2 cm) and skin.

Postoperatively

If the baby is delivered in good condition it should be handed to the mother as soon as possible to encourage skin-skin contact – the midwife can facilitate this during surgery.

After surgery, the uterus should be palpated and the vagina should be swabbed out to check that the uterus has contracted well and there is no continued bleeding. If there is concern at this stage the mother should not leave theatre until the uterus is contracted and the bleeding has stopped.

The swabs and instruments should be counted.

Every aspect of the delivery should be documented but, most particularly, the findings, including the position of the baby's head, should be clearly described, as should any problems encountered.

Prior to leaving theatre, the estimated blood loss, the urine output (and colour) and the amount and type of fluids the anaesthetist has given should all be clearly noted. They can be summarised on a fluid/recovery chart and discrepancies noted and managed.

Supervising a caesarean section

The supervisor is responsible for the quality and safety of the surgery. They must be comfortable that the procedure is within the scope of the trainee and they must be able to stop unsafe hands quickly, effectively and subtly if indicated. Conversation needs to maintain calm and demonstrate control, and frank feedback must wait until after the procedure is over.

During the delivery of the head, there needs to be communication as to whether progress is being made or not. This is usually what trainees find most difficult and talking them through the process of rotation and flexion of the fetal head, followed by lateral flexion into the wound, can be helpful.

Specific difficulties encountered at caesarean section

Difficulty delivering the head in advanced labour

Caesarean section in the second stage of labour is associated with high maternal morbidity and can be extremely difficult. In the UK there have been some instances of severe fetal trauma caused by difficulty in delivering an impacted fetal head at caesarean section. There is some work that suggests that this is due to decreasing skill in effecting instrumental vaginal delivery, making caesarean section necessary when forceps or ventouse would have been more appropriate and successful previously. Caesarean section at full dilatation is not straightforward and should be decided and conducted or supervised by a senior obstetrician (Year 4/5 SpR or a consultant).

Do not fight the uterus: if the head is deeply impacted in the pelvis in advanced labour, then once the uterus is opened at caesarean section and the hand inserted into the pelvis a uterine contraction will follow. This can be felt as huge pressure on the operator's hand, which is rendered ischaemic. Struggling to manipulate the fetal head against uterine activity in this situation should be avoided – it will prolong the uterine contraction and is highly likely to fail or will cause extension of the uterine angles. Wait with the hand unmoving until the contraction eases off and the hand no longer feels so squashed. Then proceed with disimpaction/ flexion/ rotation/lateral flexion and delivery, which can usually be achieved gently without force.

Pushing the head up from below or pushing up on the fetal shoulder is common practice but if the uterus is contracting this can also be unhelpful and patience awaiting uterine relaxation is the key. Equally, trying to apply one blade of the forceps to try to scoop the head up is illogical and potentially dangerous.

In the rare circumstances when, despite doing the above, the head still cannot be disimpacted then the uterus can be further relaxed by the anaesthetist administering a tocolytic (for example, an intravenous tocolytic of either 250 micrograms terbutaline or 250 micrograms glyceryl trinitrate – with circulatory support and intensive monitoring – see Algorithm 18.2).

Uterine incision extension (either in an inverted T or a J) can improve access if the problem is one of inadequate access.

Access to the uterine cavity

When performing a caesarean section in the second stage of labour, the lower segment will have stretched and its upper limit can extend much higher than initially thought. The danger in this situation is to enter the 'lower segment' too low and inadvertently go straight into the vagina. Such inadvertent laparoelytrotomies have been reported and, to avoid this, the uterovesical fold should be positively identified and then the uterine incision should be made approximately 3 cm below it.

Fibroids can seriously hamper access to the uterine cavity and antenatal ultrasound scans, however descriptive of the fibroids, are not conducted with surgical access in mind. For this reason, an ultrasound scan performed immediately before surgery, by the surgeon, can check the thickness of the anterior wall over the proposed incision site and the relative positions of the fibroids to this and to the fetal lie. This can be of enormous benefit in planning the most accessible route of entry and how best to conduct the delivery.

Access to the baby

Babies with an unstable or abnormal lie can cause problems with delivery at caesarean section. The question 'why is this baby lying abnormally' should be asked and answered prior to surgery. An experienced surgeon should be present in all such 'unexplained' cases in nulliparous women, as the technical problems encountered, if they are due to amniotic bands or uterine anomaly, can be demanding.

Placenta praevia

Access to the uterine cavity and the baby is hampered by a thick vascular lower segment as well as by the placenta itself. The assistant should maintain the longitudinal lie of the baby while the uterus is being incised and not get distracted by the bleeding. Interrupting the continuous pressure on the abdomen can allow the baby to drift away from a longitudinal lie if the placenta is filling the lower segment.

Anterior placenta

Depending on where the placenta is lying, it may be possible to incise the uterus down to the placenta and then separate it from uterine wall to expose membranes without dividing the placenta itself. Planning this preoperatively is aided by an ultrasound scan by the surgeon just prior to surgery (to decide which direction to work towards). Sometimes it is necessary to go through the placenta, however, and in such cases the cord should be clamped as soon as possible on delivering the baby to minimise any fetal blood loss. The neonatologist in attendance should also be warned that this is what is expected so they are prepared in case the baby does show signs of acute haemorrhage.

Breech

Many obstetricians believe the breech is much more at risk of being cut by the scalpel at uterine incision than with a cephalic baby but studies have shown no difference with a rate of around 1% and this reiterates the previous advice – always take care and try to leave the membranes intact until the uterine incision is complete.

Make the incision big enough and all the principles of vaginal breech delivery hold true at caesarean section. Pressure from above (do not pull) and do not lift the body till the nape of the neck is visible. In most cases, manipulation can be kept to a minimum if the initial incision is adequate.

A trapped fetal head during a breech delivery at caesarean section is particularly stressful for the obstetrician and it can be helpful if the anaesthetist administers a uterine relaxant.

In anticipation of an entrapment, always ensure that both abdominal and uterine incisions are adequate. If problems are still encountered and tocolysis does not resolve the problem, consider converting the incision to a 'J' incision by extending upwards from the angle of the incision.

Wrigley's forceps can be applied to assist in the delivery of the breech head at caesarean section but care still needs to be taken in avoiding hyperflexion during the application of the blades and then the direction of traction must flex the neck.

Shoulder presentation

If a fetal arm is prolapsed through the vagina, consider Patwardhan's procedure, which involves delivering the fetal breech first.

Usually, a transverse incision in the uterus is adequate, although the incision can be extended by converting it to a 'J' shape. The operator's hand is passed upwards until a leg is reached and either the leg or the breech is delivered. The rest of the delivery is as for a caesarean breech delivery. This technique can also be used if the head is deeply engaged and disimpaction is unsuccessful.

Premature infant

A premature infant in the transverse or breech position with absent liquor may best be managed with a vertical incision in the uterus.

Uterine trauma

The uterine incision may extend into the broad ligament, tearing the uterine artery and leading to brisk bleeding. After consultation with the anaesthetist, if the woman is awake, it may be helpful to exteriorise the uterus so that the posterior aspect of the uterus and broad ligament can be examined. In addition, traction to elevate the uterus may slow the blood loss and help to identify the bleeding areas requiring attention. The proximity of the ureter must be borne in mind and an effort made to sweep the bladder down and with it the ureter. This will enable better access to the uterine vessels. If bleeding is heavy it may be very difficult to identify the ureter. The first priority is to control haemorrhage and subsequent expert urological help should always be requested if damage is suspected.

Troublesome haemorrhage from the angle of the uterine incision may be controlled by the insertion of a suture to control the uterine artery. Again every effort should be made to identify the ureter.

Audit standards

The following should be audited routinely (RCOG 2005):

- rates of caesarean section, especially in different groups of women (e.g. Robson groups)

- incidence of massive blood loss associated with caesarean section

- returns to theatre

- wound infections

- standard of documentation (including operative findings).

Suggested further reading

Althabe F, Belizan JM, Villar J, Alexander S, Bergel E, Ramos S, *et al*. Mandatory second opinion to reduce rates of unnecessary caesarean sections in Latin America: a cluster randomised controlled trial. *Lancet* 2004;363:1934–40.

Bujold E, Bujold C, Hamilton EF, Harel F, Gauthier RJ. The impact of a single-layer or double-layer closure on the uterine rupture. *Am J Obstet Gynecol* 2002;186:1326–30.

Cetin A. Superficial wound disruption after cesarean delivery: effect of the depth and closure of subcutaneous tissue. *Int J Gynecol Obstet* 1997;57:17–21.

Clark AS. Nonclosure of peritoneum at surgery. *Br J Obstet Gynaecol* 1997;104:1099–200.

Department of Health. NHS Maternity Statistics Bulletin 2005/10. www.dh.gov.uk/PublicationsAnd Statistics/Publications/fs/en

Haaz DM, Ayres AW. Laceration injury at cesarean section. *J Matern Fetal Neonatal Med* 2002;11:196–8.

Murphy DJ, Liebling RE, Patel R, Verity L, Swingler R. Cohort study of operative delivery in the second stage of labour and standard of obstetric care. *BJOG* 2003;110:610–15.

Murphy DJ, Liebling RE, Verity L, Swingler R, Patel R. Early maternal and neonaatal morbidity associated with operative delivery in second stage of labour: a cohort study. *Lancet* 2001;358:1203–8.

Murphy DJ, Pope C, Frost J, Liebling RE. Women's views on the impact of operative delivery in the second stage of labour: qualitative interview study. *BMJ* 2003;327:1132–5.

National Collaborating Centre for Women's and Children's Health. *Caesarean Section*. Clinical Guideline. London: RCOG Press; 2004.

Olah KS. Reversal of the decision for casesarean section in the second stage of labour on the basis of consultant vaginal assessment. *J Obstet Gynaecol* 2005;25:115–16.

Peleg D, Perlitz Y, Pansky S, Levit A, Ben-Ami M. Accidental delivery through a vaginal incision (laparoelytrotomy) during caesarean section in the second stage of labour. *BJOG* 2001;108:659–60.

Porter S, Paterson-Brown S. Avoiding inadvertent laparoelytrotomy. *BJOG* 2003;110:91–2.

Royal College of Obstetricians and Gynaecologists Clinical Effectiveness Support Unit. *The National Sentinel Caesarean Section Audit Report.* London: RCOG Press; 2001.

Wiener JJ, Westwood J. Fetal lacerations at caesarean section. *J Obstet Gynaecol* 2002;22:23–4.

Algorithm 19.1 Sepsis

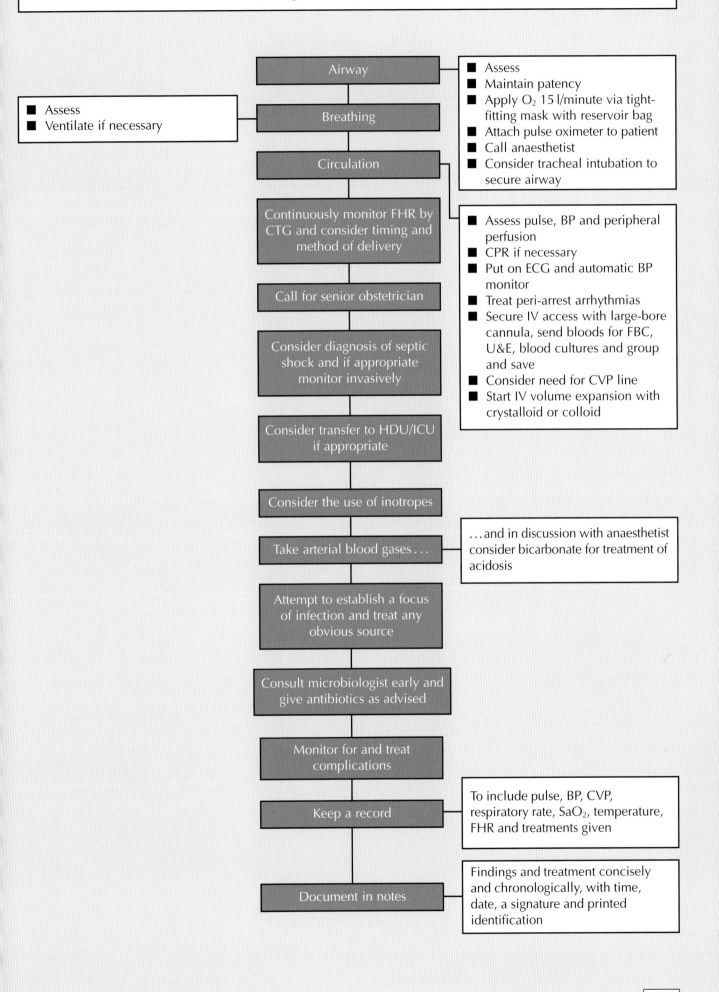

Airway

Breathing

Circulation

- Assess
- Ventilate if necessary

- Assess
- Maintain patency
- Apply O₂ 15 l/minute via tight-fitting mask with reservoir bag
- Attach pulse oximeter to patient
- Call anaesthetist
- Consider tracheal intubation to secure airway

Continuously monitor FHR by CTG and consider timing and method of delivery

Call for senior obstetrician

- Assess pulse, BP and peripheral perfusion
- CPR if necessary
- Put on ECG and automatic BP monitor
- Treat peri-arrest arrhythmias
- Secure IV access with large-bore cannula, send bloods for FBC, U&E, blood cultures and group and save
- Consider need for CVP line
- Start IV volume expansion with crystalloid or colloid

Consider diagnosis of septic shock and if appropriate monitor invasively

Consider transfer to HDU/ICU if appropriate

Consider the use of inotropes

Take arterial blood gases...

...and in discussion with anaesthetist consider bicarbonate for treatment of acidosis

Attempt to establish a focus of infection and treat any obvious source

Consult microbiologist early and give antibiotics as advised

Monitor for and treat complications

Keep a record

To include pulse, BP, CVP, respiratory rate, SaO₂, temperature, FHR and treatments given

Document in notes

Findings and treatment concisely and chronologically, with time, date, a signature and printed identification

Chapter 19

Sepsis

Objectives

On successfully completing this topic you will be able to:

- discuss the pathophysiology of sepsis
- identify the septic patient
- commence supportive management
- arrange appropriate investigations and referral.

Introduction and incidence

Sepsis is a major cause of mortality, killing approximately 1400 people worldwide every day. In addition, data in the literature suggest that the incidence of severe sepsis is going to double over the next 25–30 years; so the implications for resource allocation and use are enormous. Despite the projected increase in the number of people with sepsis in the future, there are specific opportunities to improve the management of the condition. Improvements can be made by the earlier identification of patients through the use of globally accepted definitions, treating with the most appropriate medication and adopting agreed standards of care. All these initiatives will assist in reducing mortality.

The rapid diagnosis and management of sepsis is critical to successful treatment. Mortality rates and recovery can be improved by early accurate diagnosis and treatment of patients who develop sepsis.

Clinical trials involving new therapeutic interventions have demonstrated, for the first time in 20 years, improved survival in patients with severe sepsis and septic shock.

Terminologies

Different terminologies have been used to describe the various manifestations of sepsis; a brief account of these will help in understanding the syndrome. Sepsis, severe sepsis and septic shock are terms used to identify the continuum of the clinical response to severe infection (Figure 19.1).

Sepsis is one of the five major causes of maternal morbidity and mortality worldwide. It accounts for 10% of maternal mortality in the developed world. This figure is higher in the developing world, as septic abortions are seen more frequently.

Unlike other causes of direct deaths, the rate of maternal deaths from sepsis has changed very little in recent CEMD reports. Sepsis was the fifth direct cause of maternal mortality in the 2000–2002 report, with 13 deaths directly attributable to genital tract sepsis. Substandard care was identified in ten of the 13 deaths, which accounts for 77% of the fatalities.

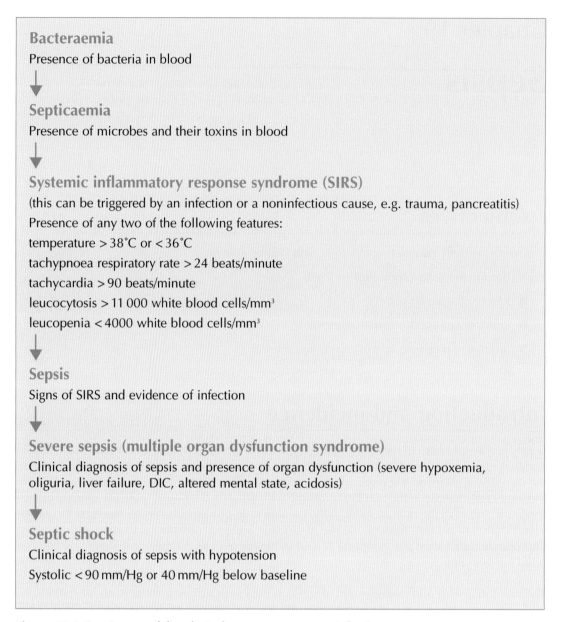

Bacteraemia

Presence of bacteria in blood

↓

Septicaemia

Presence of microbes and their toxins in blood

↓

Systemic inflammatory response syndrome (SIRS)

(this can be triggered by an infection or a noninfectious cause, e.g. trauma, pancreatitis)

Presence of any two of the following features:

temperature > 38°C or < 36°C

tachypnoea respiratory rate > 24 beats/minute

tachycardia > 90 beats/minute

leucocytosis > 11 000 white blood cells/mm³

leucopenia < 4000 white blood cells/mm³

↓

Sepsis

Signs of SIRS and evidence of infection

↓

Severe sepsis (multiple organ dysfunction syndrome)

Clinical diagnosis of sepsis and presence of organ dysfunction (severe hypoxemia, oliguria, liver failure, DIC, altered mental state, acidosis)

↓

Septic shock

Clinical diagnosis of sepsis with hypotension

Systolic < 90 mm/Hg or 40 mm/Hg below baseline

Figure 19.1 Continuum of the clinical response to severe infection

The report identified some necessary improvements to reduce deaths caused by sepsis, including education to front line staff and encouragement to call for senior help early to reduce deaths from sepsis.

Important causes of sepsis in obstetric patients

Pyelonephritis

Chorioamnionitis

Postpartum endometritis

Wound infection

Pneumonia

Acute appendicitis

Acute cholecystitis

Pancreatitis

Necrotising fasciitis

Microbiology

Pregnant women tend to be young and healthy. Only 0–4% of pregnant women who develop bacteraemia develop septic shock and, of these, 2–3% die. The most common microbes responsible for sepsis in UK include streptococcus groups A, B and D, followed by *Escherischia coli*. Other organisms that can cause sepsis include obligate anaerobic bacteria, *Fusobacterium necrophorum* and *Staphylococcus aureus.*

Pathophysiology of sepsis

Sepsis represents the body's response to an insult, be it an infection or an injury. The initial response involves the release of primary mediators, interleukin-1 and tumour necrosis factor alpha. These are cytokines produced from activated macrophages. The primary mediators stimulate the production of secondary mediators, which in turn activate coagulation and complement cascades. This is followed by the expression of anti-inflammatory mediators, which help to contain the inflammation locally. This is the period during which there is immunoparesis. As with many other regulatory processes, there is a fine balance between the pro- and anti-inflammatory mediators.

In situations where the bacterial load is high or there is an imbalance between pro- and anti-inflammatory mediators, inflammation becomes generalised, resulting in severe sepsis. There is growing evidence that this fine balance is genetically controlled.

At a cellular level, the inducible form of nitric oxide synthase is stimulated. This causes overproduction of nitric oxide from endothelial cells, macrophages and muscle cells. Nitric oxide is the major mediator of vasodilatation and myocardial dysfunction, which results in hypotension. Superoxide radicals also react with nitric oxide to form peroxynitrate, which causes direct cellular injury.

Clinical manifestations

Haemodynamic alterations

There is a decrease in arteriolar and venous tone. This causes venous pooling of blood and a drop in vascular resistance, resulting in hypotension. In the initial stages of sepsis, there is hypotension with reduced cardiac output and low filling pressures. With fluid resuscitation, cardiac output increases, resulting in a hyperdynamic circulation, but there is not much change in blood pressure owing to a reduced vascular resistance. There is an increase in pulmonary vascular resistance, resulting in raised pulmonary arterial pressures. The changes in the vascular tone differ in different vascular beds, resulting in the maldistribution of blood volume and flow. There is evidence to suggest that the ability of tissues to extract oxygen is impaired due to mitochondrial dysfunction. This encourages anaerobic metabolism in tissues, promoting lactic acidosis.

Other clinical manifestations

Sepsis is a complex syndrome that is difficult to define, diagnose and treat. Some of the signs and symptoms are rather vague and there is an overlap with other clinical conditions. Many women with pelvic sepsis present with diarrhoea, vomiting and abdominal pain. These symptoms are often attributed to gastroenteritis.

Sepsis has a range of clinical conditions caused by the body's systemic response to an infection, which, if it develops into severe sepsis, is accompanied by single or multiple organ dysfunction or failure leading to death. Tachypnoea, tachycardia and altered mental state are early manifestations of sepsis, frequently preceded by fever and hypotension. Some patients with sepsis may not have a fever and, in a state of shock, may even be hypothermic. Isolated thrombocytopenia with no evidence of DIC is seen in more than 50% of patients. Other complications include DIC,

ARDS, renal failure and hepatic failure, seen in 30–50% of patients with severe sepsis. One-third of patients who die, do so early, because of refractory hypotension and the rest, who succumb late, die because of multiple organ failure.

A high index of suspicion and close surveillance will help in identifying women with early sepsis. In the antenatal period, avoidance of unnecessary vaginal examinations may reduce the incidence of sepsis. Close surveillance and assessment of postnatal mothers, especially those with prolonged rupture of membranes, ragged membranes or possibly incomplete delivery of placenta and women with uterine tenderness or enlargement, will help to identify women developing serious infection.

Management

Infection should never be underestimated, as it continues to be an important cause of maternal mortality. Puerperal sepsis can be insidious in onset and can progress rapidly to fulminating sepsis and death. Treatment of underlying infection goes hand in hand with supporting failing organ functions. A woman with single-organ failure that is not responding to simple measures needs to be cared for in a high-dependency unit. Two or more organ failures and/or respiratory failure needs admission to an intensive care unit.

Initial management of patients with sepsis should be aimed at maintaining adequate Airway, Breathing and Circulation.

Appropriate monitoring in the early stages of sepsis includes temperature, pulse, respiratory rate, blood pressure, arterial saturation (SaO_2) and hourly urine output. Baseline blood investigations required include full blood count, coagulation profile, urea and electrolytes, liver function tests, serum lactate and blood cultures. Senior clinicians should be involved at an early stage.

Airway and breathing

Maintenance of adequate oxygenation is an important step in the resuscitation of women with sepsis. This includes a patent airway with adequate breathing and supplemental oxygen. Most patients in shock will ultimately need intubation and ventilation because of increased difficulty in breathing, development of ARDS or for primary underlying disease.

Circulation

Hypovolaemia is present in almost all patients with septic shock and fluid resuscitation is the mainstay of treatment.

Should patients not respond to simple measures of resuscitation, CVP monitoring should be instituted to guide further fluid replacement. In severe sepsis, early goal-directed therapy of fluid resuscitation and aggressive haemodynamic management to predefined end points has been shown to reduce mortality. Two essential features of early goal-directed therapy include:

- maintaining an adequate central venous pressure to carry out other haemodynamic adjustments

- maximising mixed or central venous oxygen saturation (derived from blood gas analysis of a blood sample drawn from the central line).

Appropriate levels of vascular filling should be achieved to provide an optimal cardiac function. A target CVP of around 8 mmHg in self-ventilating patients and around 12–15 mmHg in ventilated patients is recommended. Achieving a central venous oxygen saturation value of 70% has been shown to reduce mortality in patients with persistent elevation of serum lactate above 4 mmol/l, despite early fluid resuscitation. This is attempted initially with further fluid challenge with recourse to vasopressors and blood as necessary.

In most patients with septic shock, a haemoglobin of 8 g/dl may be appropriate. However, in patients with ischaemic heart disease and those with persistent lacatataemia, a target haemoglobin of 10 g/dl is desirable.

In patients who remain hypotensive despite adequate fluid resuscitation, early recourse to vasopressor therapy with or without inotropes is recommended. Evidence supports the use of norepinephrine (noradrenaline) as the vasopressor and dobutamine as the inotrope, both of which have the least detrimental effects on splanchnic circulation. Other agents used include epinephrine (adrenaline), dopamine and dopexamine. Sensitivity to catecholamines is significantly altered in septic patients and they require much higher doses than in other clinical situations.

The endpoints with any treatment include a normal or above normal cardiac output to help optimise oxygen delivery to the tissues. Despite aggressive management of septic shock, mortality is around 40%. During the course of sepsis, it is not uncommon for different organs to fail. The most common include kidneys, haematological, liver and gastrointestinal systems. These failing organs need support during this critical period; however, predicted mortality increases with increasing number of failed organs, approaching 85–100% with three or more organ failures.

Control of infection

Septic shock carries high morbidity and mortality and it is therefore important to prevent infections. There is good evidence for the use of prophylactic antibiotics in preventing postoperative infection following caesarean sections.

In the 2000–2002 CEMD report, substandard care with regards to treating infections was reported in a number of cases.

A microbiology consultation must be sought at an early stage to manage patients who are systemically ill. This helps in the collection of appropriate specimens and instituting the correct antibiotic therapy. Choice of antibiotic therapy depends on the clinical suspicion, local flora and culture information if available.

Urgent blood, urine, high vaginal, endocervical and other appropriate cultures must be obtained before starting antibiotics. This should help in identifying the offending microbe. Systemically ill patients require prompt broad-spectrum, intravenous antibiotics even before culture reports are available. Empirical treatment should include cover for Gram-negative and anaerobic organisms. Gram-positive cover is necessary if the likelihood of this infection is high.

Closed-space infections need surgical drainage including evacuation of retained products of conception. In women with endometritis not responding to antibiotics, septic pelvic thrombosis should be considered. These patients may require heparin, together with antibiotics. Patients not responding appropriately to the above measures are likely to have myometrial necrosis and/or abscess, which continue to seed the bloodstream. In these cases, early surgical intervention with possible recourse to hysterectomy could save lives. Necrotising fasciitis is another condition that requires early surgical intervention with fasciotomy and aggressive antibiotic therapy.

Specific therapies

Steroids

Data published from a multicentre randomised trial from France has shown a better survival in patients given small dose steroid supplementation. Preliminary data from a Cochrane meta-analysis considering 15 randomised controlled trials of low- and high-dose corticosteroids in 2022 patients with septic shock gives further support for using hydrocortisone in septic shock.

The number needed to treat with low-dose corticosteroids to save one additional life was nine (95% CI 5–33). The dose recommended is 200–300 mg administered three to four times in divided doses.

Activated protein C

The inflammatory response in severe sepsis is integrally linked to procoagulant activity and endothelial activation. The inflammatory response in sepsis is procoagulant in the early stages. In a large, multicentre randomised controlled trial, the PROWESS trial (Recombinant Human Activated Protein C Worldwide Evaluation in Severe Sepsis) recombinant activated protein C (rhAPC), an endogenous anticoagulant with anti-inflammatory properties, has been shown to improve survival in patients with sepsis-induced organ dysfunction.

Drotrecogin alfa (activated), recombinant activated protein C, is recommended in patients with two or more organ failure at high risk of death and no absolute contraindication related to bleeding risk or relative contraindication that outweighs the potential benefit of rhAPC.

Insulin

Evidence from a single-centre randomised controlled trial supports the early use of insulin infusion to keep the blood glucose under 8.3 mmol/l to improve morbidity and mortality from severe sepsis. It remains an open question whether the benefits are brought about directly by the infused insulin *per se* or by the prevention of hyperglycaemia, as both occurred concomitantly.

Surviving Sepsis Campaign

Spearheaded by the ESICM (European Society of Intensive Care Medicine), ISF (International Sepsis Forum) and SCCM (Society of Critical Care Medicine), the Surviving Sepsis Campaign is aimed at improving the diagnosis, survival and management of patients with sepsis by addressing the challenges associated with it.

The 28-day mortality rate in sepsis patients is comparable to the 1960s hospital mortality rate in patients of acute myocardial infarction. Over recent years, there has been an improvement in the awareness and management of acute myocardial infarction, resulting in a decline in mortality, while sepsis remains an unacknowledged killer.

The Surviving Sepsis programme aims to:

- increase awareness, understanding and knowledge
- change perceptions and behaviour
- increase the pace of change in patterns of care
- influence public policy
- define standards of care in severe sepsis
- reduce the mortality associated with sepsis by 25% over the next 5 years.

The Surviving Sepsis Campaign, in collaboration with the Institute of Healthcare Improvement, has developed 'Sepsis change bundles' to improve the outcomes in sepsis. A 'bundle' is a group of interventions related to a disease process that, when executed together, result in better outcomes than when implemented individually. Two care bundles have been developed, the first to be instituted within 6 hours and the second within 12 hours of diagnosing sepsis.

Six-hour severe sepsis bundle

- Serum lactate measured

- Blood cultures obtained prior to antibiotic administration

- Broad-spectrum antibiotics administered within 3 hours of presentation

- In the event of hypotension (systolic blood pressure less than 90 mmHg, mean arterial pressure greater than 70 mmHg) or lactate greater than 4 mmol/l, begin initial fluid resuscitation with 20–40 ml crystalloid (or colloid equivalent)/estimated kg bodyweight

- Vasopressors employed for hypotension during and after initial fluid resuscitation

- In the event of septic shock or lactate greater than 4 mmol/l, central venous pressure and central venous oxygen saturation or mixed venous oxygen saturation measured.

- In the event of septic shock or lactate greater than 4 mmol/l, central venous pressure maintained at 8–12 mmHg.

- Inotropes (and/or packed red blood cells if haematocrit ≤ 30%) delivered for central venous oxygen saturation less than 70% or mixed venous oxygen saturation less than 65% if central venous pressure ≥ 8 mmHg.

Twelve-hour severe sepsis bundle

- Glucose control maintained less than 150 mg/dl (8.3 mmol/l).

- Drotrecogin alfa (activated) administered in accordance with hospital guidelines.

- Steroids given for septic shock requiring continued use of vasopressors for ≥ 6 hours.

- Adoption of a lung-protective strategy with plateau pressures ≤ 30 cmH$_2$O for mechanically ventilated patients.

Suggested further reading

Astiz ME, Rackow EC. Septic shock. *Lancet* 1998;351:1502–5.

Faro S. Sepsis in obstetric and gynecology patients. *Curr Clin Top Infect Dis* 1999;19:1–82.

Hollenberg SM, Ahrens TS, Annane D, Astiz ME, Chalfin DB, Dasta JF, *et al*. Practice parameters for hemodynamic support of sepsis in adult patients: 2004 update. *Crit Care Med* 2004;32:1928–48.

Ledger WJ, Norman M, Gee C, Lewis W. Bacteremia in obstetric-gynaecologic service. *Am J Obstet Gynecol* 1975;121:205–12.

Lewis G, editor. *Why Mothers Die 2000–2002. Sixth Report on Confidential Inquiries into Maternal Deaths in the United Kingdom.* London: RCOG Press; 2004.

Parrillo JE, Parker MM, Natanson C, Suffredini AF, Danner RL, Cunnion RE, *et al*. Septic shock in humans. Advances in the understanding of pathogenesis, cardiovascular dysfunction, and therapy. *Ann Intern Med* 1990;113:227–42.

Rackow EC, Falk JL, Fein IA, Siegel JS, Packman MI, Haupt MT, *et al*. Fluid resuscitation in circulatory shock: a comparison of the cardiorespiratory effects of albumin, hetastarch, and saline solutions in patients with hypovolemic and septic shock. *Crit Care Med* 1983;11:839–50.

Task Force of American College of Critical Care Medicine. Practice parameters for haemodynamic support of sepsis in adult patients in sepsis. *Crit Care Med* 1999;27:639–56.

Chapter 20

Cardiac disease in pregnancy

Objectives

On successfully completing this topic you will:

■ know about serious cardiac problems which can affect pregnant women

■ understand important aspects of service provision for women with heart disease.

Incidence

The 2000–2002 Confidential Enquiries into Maternal Deaths reported a total of 44 deaths from heart disease related to pregnancy. This was an increase from the previous triennia when 35 deaths were reported. Cardiac disease is now the second most common cause of maternal death after psychiatric causes and more common than the most frequent direct cause of maternal death, thromboembolism.

Some degree of substandard care was present in 40% of cases.

Cardiac disease can be divided into congenital heart disease and acquired heart disease. Pulmonary hypertension is the main cause of death in women with congenital heart disease and cardiomyopathy, myocardial infarction and aortic dissection the main causes of death in the women with acquired heart disease.

Congenital heart disease

Congenital heart disease accounted for 20% of all cardiac deaths. Almost 50% of the deaths from congenital heart disease were attributable to pulmonary hypertension, reflecting the 30–50% maternal mortality rate associated with severe pulmonary vascular disease.

Women with surgically corrected congenital heart disease are still at risk, as there may be a residual defect. Women with significant congenital heart disease should be closely monitored by a cardiologist with expertise in the care of adult congenital heart disease during and after pregnancy.

Echocardiograms in women at risk of developing pulmonary hypertension from their congenital heart disease should be repeated during the pregnancy. In women with Eisenmenger syndrome, right to left shunting increases during pregnancy because of systemic vasodilatation. This decreases pulmonary blood flow and increases cyanosis.

Prepregnancy counselling should include a frank discussion of the risks to enable a woman to make an informed choice about whether to embark on pregnancy or not.

Acquired heart disease

Ischaemic heart disease

Although coronary artery dissection is rare in the nonpregnant population, it is a recognised complication of pregnancy and the puerperium. It can lead to coronary artery occlusion and myocardial infarction. There should be a low threshold for angiography when myocardial infarction occurs in pregnancy or the puerperium, since demonstration of dissection allows the possibility of intervention.

Aortic aneurysm dissection

Of the disorders affecting the aorta during pregnancy Marfan syndrome and Ehlers Danlos syndrome type IV are the most important. Approximately 80% of women with Marfan syndrome have some cardiac involvement, the majority having mitral valve prolapse. Women with Marfan syndrome should have regular echocardiograms during pregnancy.

Risk of aortic dissection:

- aortic root diameter less than 4 cm   1%

- aortic root diameter greater than 4 cm   10%

The risk is lower for pregnancy following elective aortic root replacement for aortic root diameters of 4.7 cm and over. If the aortic root is 4.5 cm or larger, delivery should be by elective caesarean section. The time of greatest risk is in labour and immediately postpartum period, when cardiac output is increased.

Women with Ehlers Danlos syndrome type IV are known to be at risk of aortic dissection even if the aortic root is of normal size.

Consider the diagnosis in women with

- central crushing chest pain not due to pulmonary embolism

- interscapular pain

- family history (Marfan syndrome and Ehlers Danlos syndrome type IV are autosomal dominant).

Cardiomyopathy

There are different types of cardiomyopathy: peripartum, dilated and hypertrophic. Peripartum cardiomyopathy typically presents either as a woman approaches term or in the first few weeks after delivery, although it can occur up to 5 months postpartum. While it is more common in older women, obese women or hypertensive women and those of Afro-Caribbean origin, it can present in women with no risk factors who have previously been well. Unexplained breathlessness, tachycardia, gross oedema or supraventricular tachycardia should prompt echocardiography. There is a high risk of recurrence in future pregnancies.

If dilated cardiomyopathy is present, anticoagulation should be instigated.

Hypertrophic cardiomyopathy (HOCM) is an autosomal dominant condition, which shows anticipation (gets worse in each subsequent generation). Usually pregnancy outcome is good unless there is severe diastolic dysfunction. Output may be compromised by:

- bleeding – prevent/treat blood loss aggressively

- tachycardia – consider betablockers to prolong diastole and allow adequate ventricular filling

- vasodilatation – avoid nifedipine as a tocolytic

- arrhythmias – treat arrhythmia and consider anticoagulation.

Valve disease

Regurgitant valve disease

Although cardiac output increases in pregnancy, the reduction in systemic vascular resistance compensates in part for this, and pregnancy is generally well tolerated.

Stenotic valve disease

Increased cardiac output across the stenosed valve will increase the transvalvular gradient and pregnancy may be poorly tolerated. The onset of functional worsening occurs most frequently during the second trimester.

Prosthetic valves

Women with mechanical prostheses require anticoagulation throughout pregnancy. There is debate as to which anticoagulant regime to use. Low molecular weight heparin does not cross the placenta and is therefore safer for the fetus but it may be associated with a higher risk of valve thrombosis. Whatever the anticoagulation regimen, pregnancy in a woman with a mechanical prosthesis is associated with a maternal mortality of 1–4% and is mainly due to valve thrombosis.

Service provision for women with heart disease

Preconceptual care

For all of the above conditions, prepregnancy counselling should ideally be provided jointly by an obstetrician and a cardiologist and should include:

■ a frank discussion of the risks involved, to enable the woman to make an informed choice as to whether to embark on pregnancy

■ optimising cardiac function (medically, e.g. control arrhythmias, or surgically, e.g. valvotomy)

■ review and adjust medication, avoiding teratogens

■ contraception advice if the woman decides against embarking on pregnancy

■ contact numbers to facilitate early referral once pregnant.

Women undergoing assisted conception often have additional risk factors such as increased age, the risk of ovarian hyperstimulation and multiple pregnancy.

Early pregnancy

Ideally, women with heart disease should be referred to a joint obstetric and cardiac clinic. There should be:

■ easy access to facilitate prompt referral

■ a frank discussion of the risks involved to enable the woman to make an informed choice as to whether to continue with the pregnancy

■ a professional interpreter (if needed) to ensure that relevant history is disclosed. Interpreters from within the family should not be used, as, in the family's desire to help the woman to have a successful pregnancy, risks may not be accurately relayed to her

■ easy access to termination of pregnancy in a hospital that can care for a woman with heart disease, for women who choose not to continue the pregnancy (infection, bleeding and the need for anaesthesia are recognised complications of termination but may pose a more significant risk to a woman with cardiac disease).

> **Recognition of relevant history, important signs and symptoms that may prompt referral to a cardiologist**
>
> ▪ Unexplained breathlessness
>
> ▪ Isolated systolic hypertension
>
> ▪ Interscapular pain
>
> ▪ Severe chest pain not due to thromboembolism
>
> ▪ Polycythaemia
>
> ▪ Tachycardia

Routine cardiac examination

Since rheumatic valve disease or undiagnosed valve disease is rare in Western Europe it may engender complacency and it may be missed in first-generation immigrants, simply because a routine cardiac examination has not been performed.

Recurrence of disease in subsequent pregnancies may be more severe or the woman may have less cardiac reserve. Some women may become complacent after one successful pregnancy and disregard the risks.

Protocols to enable recognition of risk factors at the time of the initial antenatal visit and facilitate appropriate referral

The appropriate pattern of care should be initiated, which would ideally be hospital-based care with a joint cardiac and obstetric clinic for women at a high risk.

Follow up of women with heart disease who do not attend for care.

Multidisciplinary management of women with heart disease to plan delivery or to facilitate prompt attention if their condition deteriorates.

> **Appropriate response to cardiac arrest**
>
> ▪ Knowing how to call the arrest team for an obstetric patient.
>
> ▪ Efficient bleep system to ensure that the appropriate people, including an obstetrician and a paediatrician, are called.
>
> ▪ Resuscitation training and drills specifically directed at cardiac arrest in a pregnant woman; for example, ALSO, MOET courses.
>
> ▪ Well-maintained equipment with which staff are familiar.

Inherited cardiac disease

Family members may also be at risk of cardiac disease and may need to be screened (for example, Marfan syndrome, HOCM and possibly sudden adult death syndrome).

Fetal echocardiography may be indicated if either parent had congenital heart disease.

The 22q11 deletion in either parent would increase the risk of congenital heart disease in the fetus.

Obstetric emergencies

Multidisciplinary working

A joint obstetric and cardiac clinic should enable plans to be made for the place, timing and mode of delivery. Liaison with other professionals is necessary to optimise the care of women with heart disease, for example:

- midwives and cardiac nurses
- obstetric and cardiac anaesthetists
- geneticists
- paediatricians
- haematologists
- dentists
- cardiac surgeons.

Contraception

Appropriate contraceptive advice must be provided after any pregnancy. This allows time for reassessment of cardiac function and treatment to improve function (for example, valvotomy). One successful pregnancy must not engender complacency. Some conditions, such as peripartum cardiomyopathy, have a high recurrence risk. Other conditions would worsen with age and in each subsequent pregnancy the risks would be higher.

Summary

- Appropriate support by a multidisciplinary team can optimise the care of women with heart disease in pregnancy.

Suggested further reading

Elkayam U, Tummala PP, Rao K, Akhter MW, Karaalp IS, Wani OR, *et al*. Maternal and fetal outcomes of subsequent pregnancies in women with peripartum cardiomyopathy. *New Engl J Med* 2001;344:1567–71.

Hameed A, Karaalp IS, Tummala PP, Wani OR, Canetti M, Akhter MW, *et al*. The effect of valvular heart disease on maternal and fetal outcome of pregnancy. *J Am Coll Cardiol* 2001;37:893–9.

Hanania G. Management of anticoagulants during pregnancy. *Heart* 2001;86:125–6.

Lewis G, editor. *Why Mothers Die 2000–2002. The Sixth Report of the Confidential Enquiries into Maternal Deaths in the United Kingdom*. London: RCOG Press; 2004.

Lewis G, editor. Why Mothers Die 1997–1999. *Fifth Report of the Confidential Enquiries into Maternal Deaths in the United Kingdom*. London: RCOG Press; 2001.

Lipscomb KJ, Smith JC, Clarke B, Donnai P, Harris R. Outcome of pregnancy in women with Marfan syndrome. *Br J Obstet Gynaecol* 1997;104:201–6.

Pearson GD, Veille JC, Rahimtoola S, Hsia J, Oakley CM, Hosenpud JD, *et al*. Peripartum Cardiomyopathy National Heart, Lung, and Blood Institute and Office of Rare Diseases (National Institutes of Health) Workshop Recommendations and Review. *JAMA* 2000;283:1183–8.

Rossiter JP, Repke JT, Morales AJ, Murphy EA, Pyeritz RE. A prospective longitudinal evaluation of pregnancy in the Marfan syndrome *Am J Obstet Gynecol* 1995;173:1599–606.

Task Force on the Management of Cardiovascular Diseases during Pregnancy of the European Society of Cardiology. Expert consensus document on management of cardiovascular diseases during pregnancy. *Eur Heart J* 2003;24:761–81.

Weiss BM, Hess OM. Pulmonary vascular disease and pregnancy: current controversies, management strategies, and perspectives. *Eur Heart J* 2000;21:104–15.

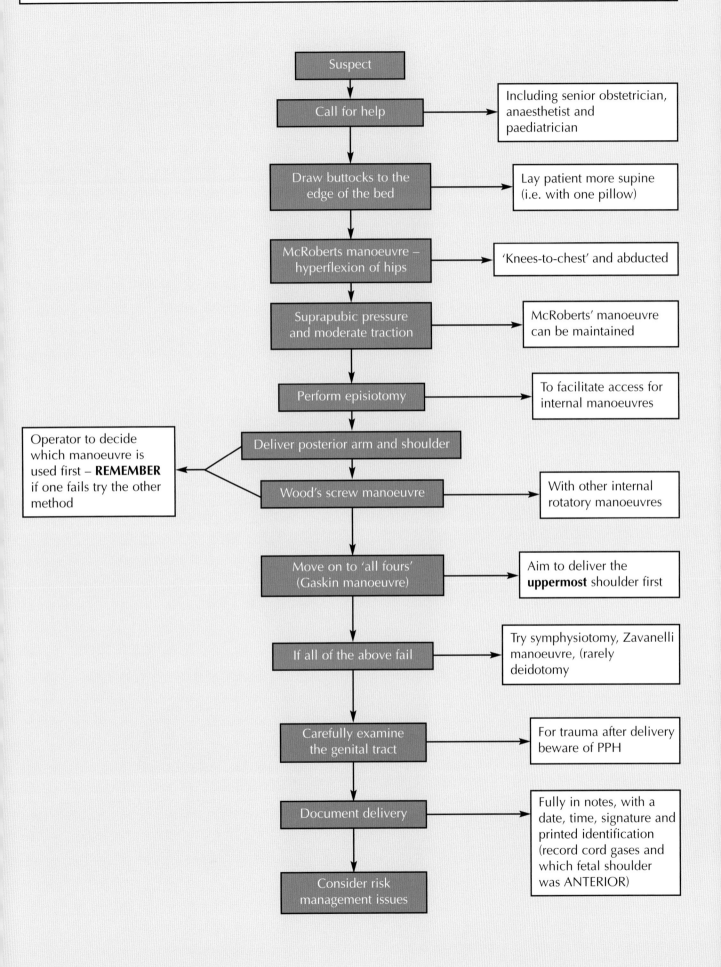

Algorithm 21.1 Management of shoulder dystocia

Suspect

Call for help → Including senior obstetrician, anaesthetist and paediatrician

Draw buttocks to the edge of the bed → Lay patient more supine (i.e. with one pillow)

McRoberts manoeuvre – hyperflexion of hips → 'Knees-to-chest' and abducted

Suprapubic pressure and moderate traction → McRoberts' manoeuvre can be maintained

Perform episiotomy → To facilitate access for internal manoeuvres

Operator to decide which manoeuvre is used first – **REMEMBER** if one fails try the other method ←

Deliver posterior arm and shoulder

Wood's screw manoeuvre → With other internal rotatory manoeuvres

Move on to 'all fours' (Gaskin manoeuvre) → Aim to deliver the **uppermost** shoulder first

If all of the above fail → Try symphysiotomy, Zavanelli manoeuvre, (rarely deidotomy

Carefully examine the genital tract → For trauma after delivery beware of PPH

Document delivery → Fully in notes, with a date, time, signature and printed identification (record cord gases and which fetal shoulder was ANTERIOR)

Consider risk management issues

Chapter 21

Shoulder dystocia

Objectives

On successfully completing this topic, you will:

■ understand aetiology and complications of shoulder dystocia

■ understand the risk factors for shoulder dystocia

■ be aware of strategies tried to prevent shoulder dystocia

■ be confident in understanding the variety of obstetric manoeuvres used to overcome shoulder dystocia.

Introduction

Shoulder dystocia remains one of the most dreaded obstetric complications and one that is often unanticipated. It is one of the primary causes of perinatal mortality and morbidity, maternal morbidity and a costly source of litigation. In this chapter, a number of issues will be addressed.

Methodology

This chapter is an abbreviated update of a previous review of the subject. In order to review current publications on shoulder dystocia, a review of the literature was carried out using Medline and Embase online databases. Older references were sought through previous reviews and chapters on the subject.

Definition and incidence

The term has been used to describe a range of difficulties encountered with delivering the shoulders after delivering the head. Discrepancies in the definition, the degree of difficulty and the variation in manoeuvres used, have resulted in differences in the reported incidence of this obstetric emergency.

Many attempts have been made to standardise the definition. One author suggested defining shoulder dystocia as prolonged head-to-body delivery time (more than 60 seconds) or the need for ancillary obstetric manoeuvres. The latter part of this definition agreed with Resnik's 1980 definition of shoulder dystocia as 'a condition requiring special manoeuvres to deliver the shoulders following an unsuccessful attempt to apply downward traction'. A further suggestion gives a more descriptive definition to the condition but with no reference to the degree of the difficulty. Shoulder dystocia is defined as 'arrest of spontaneous delivery due to impaction of the anterior shoulder against the symphysis pubis'. Another definition defined three degrees of shoulder dystocia varying from 'slight difficulty' with the shoulders associated with a normal mechanism of rotation, through to severe, bilateral dystocia with both shoulders stuck above the brim. Standardising the definition will not only make it easier to report the incidence but also will make it possible to compare the effectiveness of the different manoeuvres. We propose here to keep the definition of Resnik.

The reported incidence of shoulder dystocia varies between 0.15% and 2% of all vaginal deliveries. It has been suggested that better treatment of diabetes mellitus should result in a reduced incidence.

Fetal mortality and morbidity

Shoulder dystocia is still a significant cause of term fetal mortality. In the Confidential Enquiry into Stillbirths and Deaths in Infancy (CESDI) Annual Report for 1993, shoulder dystocia was responsible for 8% of all intrapartum fetal deaths. Although, on the whole, fetal mortality from shoulder dystocia has improved over the last 30 years, there is no room for complacency. Indeed, the Fifth Annual CESDI Report (1998) published the discussions of an expert focus group which looked critically at 56 cases of death associated with shoulder dystocia: 47% had died despite delivery within 5 minutes. In 37 (66%) cases, the level of substandard care offered by professionals was graded at 'level 3' (i.e. a different management would have likely resulted in an improved outcome). Although 65% of babies were delivered by midwives, approximately one-third were delivered by medical staff, emphasising the need for all professionals involved in delivery to be aware of appropriate drills. Although the CESDI reports have produced interesting and pertinent findings, the data are difficult to quantify because of the lack of adequate denominator data.

Fetal morbidity

- Cerebral hypoxia
- Cerebral palsy
- Fracture clavicle and/or humerus
- Brachial plexus injuries

Following delivery of the head, the umbilical cord pH falls by 0.04 unit/minute. As a result, delay in completing the delivery may result in asphyxia and, if the interval between head and trunk delivery is prolonged, permanent neurological deficit may occur. Delivery should occur within 5 minutes and permanent injury is progressively more likely with delays above 10 minutes. One study found abnormal CNS signs and convulsions in two of 70 babies who suffered shoulder dystocia (2.9%). In another study, shoulder dystocia was responsible for 7.5% of all term infants who suffered neonatal seizures in the first 72 hours of their lives. Owing to the poor association between the parameters used to define birth asphyxia (pH, Apgar score, etc.) it is difficult to ascertain the incidence of permanent CNS deficit resulting from shoulder dystocia.

Brachial plexus injuries are common in shoulder dystocia. Erb's palsy is the most common presentation. Erb's palsy presents as internal rotation and adduction of the shoulders and extension and pronation of the elbow. The incidence of brachial plexus injuries varies significantly between different papers but it has been decreasing, from 100% in a series reported in the 1960s to 13% from a series reported in 1995.

It has been suggested that intrauterine maladaptation may play a role in brachial plexus impairment, implying that brachial plexus impairment should not be taken as *prima facie* evidence of birth process injury. The mechanism of damage may not always be clear, as brachial plexus injury has also been reported at caesarean section, in the opposite arm to the trapped shoulder and also without any recorded dystocia. One case series found that only 50% of cases of Erb's palsy were associated with shoulder dystocia. The relative risk of developing Erb's palsy was 4.7 times higher after a precipitate second stage. The authors implied that the prevention of many cases of Erb's palsy was outwith the attendant's control. It has been suggested that the use of more 'invasive' means of treating shoulder dystocia (i.e. removing the posterior arm) were not associated with an increased risk of brachial plexus injury compared with more benign 'external' manouevres (such as suprapubic pressure): 21/158 versus 27/127. A study in 2000 found 62 cases of brachial plexus injury in 13 366 deliveries (incidence 0.46%); 22 recovered completely within a month, while a further 23 had delayed but complete recovery. Of 17 with residual paresis, 11 underwent surgery but only three had severe paresis. The most significant marker to predict the likelihood of 'non-recovery' was birth weight greater than 4000 g (OR 51).

Musculoskeletal injuries in the form of fractured clavicle or humerus can also happen. These fractures usually heal quickly and have a good prognosis.

Maternal morbidity

Postpartum haemorrhage is common following shoulder dystocia. Vaginal and perineal lacerations are also common following delivery of shoulder dystocia. Uterine rupture may also happen, especially if undue abdominal force is used.

The issues that lend themselves for discussion are:

■ How specific and sensitive are our methods to predict macrosomia?

■ What is the right course of action if macrosomia is predicted?

Antenatal risk factors

It seems that most of the antenatal risk factors are so common that they lack sensitivity and specificity. Moreover the majority of cases of shoulder dystocia occur without any risk factors. A retrospective analysis of 12 532 deliveries concluded that most of the 'traditional' risk factors for shoulder dystocia have no predictive value. Thus, although it is clear that there is a strong correlation between fetal weight and shoulder dystocia, all professionals need to be prepared for unexpected shoulder dystocia at all deliveries.

Intrapartum risk factors

Secondary arrest and slow progress in the first stage were associated with increased incidence of shoulder dystocia. McFarland *et al.* (1995) reviewed 276 cases of shoulder dystocia and compared them to 600 deliveries in the same period. They concluded that labour abnormalities were comparable in the shoulder dystocia and in the control groups both in the active phase and in the second stage and as a result these labour abnormalities may not serve as clinical predictors for subsequent development of shoulder dystocia. Acker *et al.* (1985) found that, in the birthweight group 4000–4999 g, no specific labour abnormality was clearly predictive of shoulder dystocia but, in birth weights of 5000 g or more, labour arrest heralded a shoulder dystocia in 55% of cases. Langer *et al.* (1991) found that the duration of labour and other labour abnormalities may increase the risk of shoulder dystocia but they did not show how this could predict shoulder dystocia.

Shoulder dystocia is more frequently encountered in assisted vaginal deliveries. Boekhuizen *et al.* (1987) analysed 256 vacuum extractions and 300 forceps deliveries. They found an incidence of 4.6% of shoulder dystocia compared with 0.17% of all cephalic vaginal deliveries. Keller *et al.* (1991) found the use of forceps was clearly associated with increased risk of shoulder dystocia. This emphasises the importance of particularly careful abdominal and vaginal assessment before performing assisted deliveries for clinically macrosomic babies.

Risk factors for shoulder dystocia

Antepartum:

■ fetal macrosomia
■ maternal obesity
■ diabetes
■ prolonged pregnancy
■ advanced maternal age
■ male gender
■ excessive weight gain
■ previous shoulder dystocia
■ previous big baby.

Intrapartum:

■ prolonged first stage
■ prolonged second stage
■ oxytocin augmentation of labour
■ assisted delivery.

How does shoulder dystocia happen?

In the slighter degrees, the cause may be failure of the shoulders to rotate into the anteroposterior diameter as they traverse the pelvic cavity. The posterior shoulder usually enters the pelvic cavity while the anterior shoulder remains hooked behind the symphysis pubis. In the more severe forms of shoulder dystocia, both shoulders do not cross the pelvic brim.

Strategies suggested for prevention and management of shoulder dystocia

■ Identifying risk factors.

■ Training and teaching.

■ Prevention: delivery by caesarean section for macrosomic babies.

■ Early induction of labour to prevent macrosomia.

■ Risk assessment: documentation of risk factors, events and their timings.

■ Early detection: turtle sign.

■ Plan of action

Identifying risk factors

Identify the risk of shoulder dystocia antenatally and recommend clearly in the mother's notes that an experienced obstetrician should be available for the second stage.

Training and teaching

In the CESDI report (1993) it is stated that, 'There should be regular rehearsals of emergency procedures and training sessions in the management of rare or troublesome complications for obstetricians and midwives involved in care. Such complications include obstructed delivery... and shoulder dystocia'.

In one questionnaire survey which involved 120 midwives assessing their training, 80% thought that they did not have any theoretical training in shoulder dystocia and more than 95% thought that they did not have any practical training, more than 98% expressed a need for more theoretical and simulated training to manage shoulder dystocia. More than 60% of midwives involved in this survey said they would use fundal pressure and apply strong traction to the fetal neck, two actions known to increase the incidence of brachial plexus injury and fracture clavicle.

Prevention

Prevention by performing caesarean section for macrosomic infants

Various authors have recommended an elective caesarean section for diabetic mothers with estimated fetal weight of 4250 g and nondiabetic mothers with estimated fetal weight of 4500 g or above. Clearly, the difficulty in complying with the latter recommendation is that it is difficult to obtain an accurate estimate of fetal weight, as indicated above.

A 1995 study found that expectant management of 482 infants with suspected birth weight of 4000 g and above was safe unless there was a reason for caesarean section. In their review, 396 of 482 infants with birth weight of 4000 g and above achieved normal delivery with no single case of birth trauma. It appears that many cases of shoulder dystocia occur in babies of average weight. Equally, most cases of macrosonic fetuses delivered vaginally do not suffer from shoulder dystocia. One series reported that 50% of shoulder dystocia occured in normally grown fetuses and 98% of macrosonic fetuses who were delivered vaginally did not have shoulder dystocia.

In the CESDI (1993) report, there were 29 fetal deaths due to shoulder dystocia and ten of these babies (35%) weighed less than 4 kg. Most cases of shoulder dystocia can be overcome without trauma to mother or baby if proper precautions are taken. Abdominal delivery is not 100% safe to the baby. A case series reported an incidence of 2.6% of birth trauma to babies 4500 g delivered by caesarean section.

Even if it is acceptable to perform a large number of caesarean section operations to reduce the rate of shoulder dystocia by 50–60%, first there needs to be a method for accurately estimating fetal weight at term. The sensitivity and specificity of current methods of diagnosing macrosomia are not satisfactory. Thus, a policy of elective caesarean section for all clinically big babies will not be effective in reducing the incidence of shoulder dystocia and subsequent brachial plexus injuries.

Prevention by induction of labour for suspected macrosomia

Induction of labour has been considered as an option for managing mothers with suspected macrosomic babies to try to reduce the incidence of shoulder dystocia and subsequent birth trauma. A 1995 study reviewed 186 mothers with suspected macrosomic fetuses at term. Labour was induced in 46 cases, 23.9% of them needed caesarean section while, with spontaneous onset of labour in 140 cases, the caesarean section rate was 14%. This difference was statistically significant, regardless of parity or gestational age. The frequencies of shoulder dystocia, 1 minute Apgar score less than 7 and abnormal umbilical blood gas were not different. They concluded that spontaneous labour is associated with a lower chance of caesarean section than induced labour when the birth weight is 4000 g and above.

The situation in women with diabetes is different, for reasons mentioned earlier. Various recommended caesarean section for babies with estimated fetal weight 4000 g or above. Induction of labour is also recommended for women with diabetes at 38 weeks, especially if their diabetic control has not been ideal, to avoid shoulder dystocia and birth trauma.

Risk assessment

Although the conclusion has been reached that most cases of shoulder dystocia are unpredictable, it is recommended documenting in the notes the risk factors, especially if they are multiple. It is also recommended that an experienced clinician is present during the second stage. It is strongly recommended that events, manoeuvres and accurate times are documented in the notes.

Early detection

- ■ 'Head bobbing' (the head coming down towards the introitus with pushing but retracting well back between contractions)
- ■ 'Turtle' sign at delivery (the delivered head becomes tightly pulled back against the perineum).

Have a plan of action

As shoulder dystocia is infrequently predictable, every clinician should be armed with a plan of action; that is, a sequence of manoeuvres. All manoeuvres result from one (or a combination of) the following three mechanisms:

■ increase in the available pelvic diameter

■ narrowing of the transverse (bisacromial) diameter of the shoulders by adduction

■ movement of the bisacromial diameter into a more favourable angle relative to the antero-posterior pelvic diameter (e.g. into the oblique).

Recent literature and expert opinion will be reviewed as part of the course. For the purposes of the MOET course, the plan of action recommended below includes the authors' opinions based on their own experiences.

Plan of action

1. Call for help.

2. Draw buttocks to edge of bed.

3. Episiotomy.

4. McRoberts' manoeuvre + moderate traction.

5. Suprapubic pressure + moderate traction.

6. Deliver posterior arm and shoulder or internal rotational manoeuvres (including Woods' screw manoeuvre).

7. Change of position ('All fours' or 'Gaskin' manoeuvre).

8. If all the above fail, try symphysiotomy, cleidotomy or Zavanelli manoeuvre (? cleidotomy).

9. Ensure comprehensive and contemporaneous written records.

Call for help

This includes calling the most experienced obstetrician available, a paediatrician and an anaesthetist, and other nursing and ancillary staff as available.

Episiotomy

Episiotomy is recommended to allow more room for manoeuvres such as delivering the posterior arm or internal rotation of the shoulders. Although it has been suggested that episiotomy does not affect the outcome of shoulder dystocia, there is strong evidence to suggest that the incidence of vaginal lacerations with shoulder dystocia is high and performing an episiotomy to reduce the chance of having severe lacerations is recommended. The main reason for recommending an episiotomy is to allow the operator more space to use the hollow of the sacrum to perform the different internal manoeuvres.

McRoberts' manoeuvre (with or without moderate traction)

Both thighs are sharply flexed, abducted and rotated outwards. The legs should not be in lithotomy poles, as this would limit the amount of flexion obtained. This position serves to straighten the sacrum relative to the lumbar vertebrae and causes cephalic rotation of the pelvis to occur, which helps to free the impacted shoulder. One study tested McRoberts' position with laboratory maternal pelvic and fetal models. Their findings showed that this manoeuvre reduced the amount of traction needed and the likelihood of subsequent brachial plexus injuries or fractured clavicle. For this reason patients should be put in McRoberts' before applying

Obstetric emergencies

appropriate traction on the fetal neck. Another study also used models to measure objectively the degree of clinician-applied load in routine and difficult shoulder dystocia deliveries. The average combined force for a normal delivery was 84 newtons (N), with a 473 newtons/cm² (N-cm) neck-bending moment. For a shoulder dystocia delivery, the equivalent average forces were 163 N and 700 N-cm. Clavicular fracture can occur at peak force magnitudes around 100 N. Lurie *et al.* (1994) reviewed 76 cases of shoulder dystocia and found that McRoberts' manoeuvre was sufficient to achieve delivery of the impacted shoulder in 67 cases (88%). McRoberts' manoeuvre is associated with the least neonatal trauma.

Suprapubic pressure (with moderate traction)

Suprapubic pressure is applied to adduct and internally rotate the anterior shoulder and thus reduce the bis-acromial diameter and push the anterior shoulder underneath the symphysis pubis. A 'cardiac massage' grip is used, with pressure applied to the posterior aspect of the shoulder with the heel of the hand. It is important to know where the fetal back lies so that pressure is applied in the right direction. At this stage only moderate traction is applied. Strong traction, as well as fundal pressure, should be avoided. If continuous pressure is not successful, a 'rocking' movement may be tried. This is also known as the 'Rubin I' manoeuvre. It has been stated that increased traction on the head was associated with the greatest degree of neonatal trauma. Fundal pressure should also be avoided. Strong pushing may have similar effects and we recommend that maternal efforts should be discouraged until shoulder displacement is achieved, as these could increase the impaction of the shoulders and increase the neurological and orthopaedic complications.

Deliver posterior arm and shoulder

The hand of the operator should be passed up to the fetal axilla and the shoulder hooked down. There is always more room in the hollow of the sacrum. Traction on the posterior axilla usually enables the operator to bring the posterior arm within reach.

The posterior arm can then be delivered or, if the cubital fossa is within reach, backward pressure on it will result in disengagement of the arm, which will then be brought down. This is achieved by getting hold of the hand and sweeping it across the chest and fetal face. This process is similar to the Pinard method for bringing down a leg in breech presentation. This procedure is usually successful.

Internal rotatory manoeuvres

Internal rotatory manoeuvres, such as Rubin II, Woods' screw and reverse Woods' screw, are often confused with each other and are often incorrectly described in the literature.

Rubin II

The operator inserts the fingers of one hand vaginally, positioning the fingertips **behind** the anterior shoulder. The shoulder is pushed towards the fetal chest (adducting the shoulders and rotating the bisacromial diameter into the oblique). If unsuccessful, this can then be combined with the Woods' screw manoeuvre.

Woods' screw

This manoeuvre was described by Woods in 1943. The fingers of the opposite hand are inserted vaginally to approach the posterior shoulder from the **front** of the fetus, aiming to rotate the shoulder towards the symphysis pubis. The Rubin II and Woods' screw can be combined to rotate the shoulders through 180 degrees ('like a thread on a screw'). It is important not to twist the fetal head or neck.

Reverse Woods' screw

If the above fail, the fingers of the hand used for the Rubin II manoeuvre are placed on the posterior shoulder from behind and an attempt is made to rotate in the opposite direction to the original Woods' screw. If successful, the shoulders will rotate 180 degrees in the opposite direction and deliver.

All-fours position ('Gaskin' manoeuvre)

The maternal weight lies evenly on the four limbs and this increases the anteroposterior diameter of the inlet and facilitates other manoeuvres. The posterior shoulder (with respect to the maternal pelvis) may be delivered first in this position. Midwives will often use this manoeuvre early in the management of shoulder dystocia. In a series of 82 cases of shoulder dystocia amongst 4452 deliveries (incidence 1.8%), all babies were delivered successfully with this manoeuvre in a mean time of 2.3 (range 1–6) minutes. There were no cases of mortality and no cases of brachial plexus injury. One baby suffered a fractured humerus. Obstetricians should consider the merits of this alternative approach.

Other measures

Zavanelli manoeuvre

This method has been named after the physician who first performed the manoeuvre in 1978. It describes reversal of the delivery process by rotating, flexing and reinserting the head into the vagina, followed by caesarean section; that is, after failure of all manoeuvres to overcome shoulder dystocia, restitution and neck extension are reversed and the head recoils into the vagina.

A study reported 59 women who underwent cephalic replacement. All but six were successfully replaced and delivered by caesarean section without excessive maternal or fetal morbidity. The study described the need for a tocolytic and used 0.25 mg subcutaneous terbutaline, depressing the posterior wall and using firm and constant pressure on the head. Those who have had experience of applying this technique have reported very good outcomes.

Descriptions in the literature report an almost automatic ease in performance of the Zavanelli manoeuvre and a complication-free procedure. However, it has been reported how difficult the process can be. One author reported three cases of hysterectomies necessitated because of uterine rupture during the procedure. There have also been cases of severe perinatal hypoxia, which ultimately resulted in brain damage and/or death. It has been recommended that it should be used as a last resort.

Symphysiotomy

Symphysiotomy requires inserting a urethral catheter to move the urethra to one side. Two assistants support the legs after taking them out off the stirrups. An incomplete midline cut in the symphyseal joint is made. This, in addition to an episiotomy, will increase the space available and facilitate the delivery of the shoulders. The danger of performing this uncommon procedure in an emergency situation by an operator who has never performed it before must carry a considerable risk. However, the successful use of the technique has been described. The importance of supporting the woman's legs when the incision is made must be emphasised, in order to prevent sudden abduction.

Intentional fracture of the clavicle

This is really a manoeuvre of last resort.

Approaches advocated by other authors

Several authors have advocated the use of similar systematic approaches to the hands-on management of shoulder dystocia. They vary in the order in which manoeuvres may be recommended but the more important principle of having an orderly, logical and calm approach is advocated by all. Two examples are given below, both of which use mnemonics as an aid to memory.

The Advanced Life Support in Obstetrics (ALSO) approach uses the mnemonic 'HELPERR' (the order of manoeuvres is not mandatory):

H   Help (call for plenty)

E   Evaluate for episiotomy

L   Legs (McRoberts' manoeuvre)

P   Pressure (suprapubic)

E   Enter (rotational manoeuvres)

R   Remove the posterior arm

R   Roll (Gaskin manoeuvre)

Another mnemonic approach is **'PALE SISTER'**:

P   Prepare – have a plan

A   Assistance

L   Legs (McRoberts' manoeuvre)

E   Episiotomy

S   Suprapubic pressure

I   Internal rotation (Wood's)

S   Screw (Reverse Wood's)

T   Try recovering posterior arm

E   Extreme measures

R   Repair, record and relax.

Guidelines may differ at the point where internal manoeuvres are required. Should one 'enter and rotate (the shoulders)' first or 'enter and remove' (the posterior arm) first? It has been clearly stated that there is no scientific evidence on which to base this choice. Therefore, it should be left to the attending professional to use the manoeuvre with which they are most familiar and most comfortable. In a survey of obstetricians, it was found that 56% would attempt delivery of the posterior arm first and 36% the internal rotatory manoeuvres first. For the purposes of the MOET course, where the majority of attendees are obstetricians, the course manual suggests removal of the posterior arm first. However, it is recommended that candidates should be familiar with the rotatory movements as well.

Medico-legal aspects

Courts have found in favour of the professionals involved, when the allegations have been that shoulder dystocia 'should have been predicted' and caesarean section offered in order to avoid the complication. It was accepted that the majority of cases are unpredictable and that professionals could not be expected to predict this catastrophe antenatally. However, in many cases, there were no departmental guidelines available for the management of shoulder dystocia once it had occurred. Inappropriate manoeuvres such as excessive lateral traction and fundal pressure would not be acceptable and, indeed, would be difficult to defend in present-day practice.

Units should continually review and revise their management guidelines with reference to changing, evidence-based practice. It is accepted that it is not possible to produce Grade A (randomised controlled trial) evidence in this field. Therefore, the manoeuvres recommended by 'expert' opinion will be the basis of best practice. These opinions will be reviewed later and the approach recommended by MOET will be presented. There are other equally acceptable approaches that could also be followed.

Summary

Although shoulder dystocia is usually an unpredictable obstetric emergency, having guidelines and a plan of action plus being vigilant to the possibility of shoulder dystocia should minimise the fetal and maternal trauma.

■ It is important that every institution has a guideline, with which all staff are familiar and comfortable.

■ The setting up of mock 'fire-drills' has been recommended by CESDI and many of the authors cited in this chapter.

■ Confidence with this rare emergency can be enhanced with the use of fire drills and by completing structured skills-training courses.

Suggested further reading

Allan RH, Bankoski BR, Butzin CA, Nagey DA. Comparing clinician-applied loads for routine, difficult and shoulder dystocia deliveries. *Am J Obstet Gynecol* 1994;171:1621–7.

Baxley EG, Gobbo RW. Shoulder dystocia (ALSO series). *Am Fam Physician* 2004;67:1707–14 [www.aafp.org/afp/20040401/1707.pdf].

Boyd M, Usher R, McLean FH. Fetal macrosomia: prediction, risks, proposed management. *Obstet Gynecol* 1983;61:715–22.

Confidential Enquiry into Stillbirths and Deaths in Infancy. *Annual Report 1 January – 31 December 1993*. London: Maternal and Child Health Research Consortium; 1995.

Diani F, Moscatelli C, Toppano B, Turinetto A. [Fetal macrosomia and mode of delivery]. *Minerva Ginecol* 1995;47:77–82. Italian.

Focus Group: Shoulder dystocia. In: Confidential Enquiries into Stillbirths and Deaths in Infancy. *5th Annual Report*. London: Maternal and Child Health Research Consortium; 1998. p.73–9.

Friesen CD, Miller AM, Rayburn WF. Influence of spontaneous labor on delivering macrosomic fetus. *Am J Perinatol* 1995;12:63–6.

Gherman RB, Chauhan S, Ouzounian JG, Lerner H, Gonik B, Goodwin TM. Shoulder dystocia: the unpreventable obstetric emergency with empiric management guidelines. *Am J Obstet Gynecol* 2006;195:657–72.

Gurewitsch ED, Donithan M, Stallings SP, Moore PL, Agarwal S, Allen LM, *et al.* Episiotomy versus fetal manipulation in managing severe shoulder dystocia: a comparison of outcomes. *Am J Obstet Gynecol* 2004;191:911–16.

Hartfield VJ. Symphysiotomy for shoulder dystocia. *Am J Obstet Gynecol* 1986;155:228.

Leigh TH, James CE. Medicolegal commentary: shoulder dystocia. *Br J Obstet Gynaecol* 1998;105:815–17.

Lerner H. Shoulder dystocia. 2004 (web-based text) [http://shoulderdystociainfo.com/index.htm].

Obstetric emergencies

Magowan B. Shoulder dystocia: In: Magowan B. *Churchill's Pocketbook of Obstetrics and Gynaecology*. 2nd ed. Edinburgh: Churchill Livingstone; 2000. p. 99–5.

Moses S. Shoulder dystocia management. In: Family Practice Notebook.com 2000 (web-based text with regular updates) [www.fpnotebook.com/OB112.htm].

O'Leary J. Cephalic replacement for shoulder dystocia: present status and future role of Zavanelli manoeuvre. *Obstet Gynecol* 1993;82:847–55.

Resnik R. Management of shoulder girdle dystocia. *Clin Obstet Gynecol* 1980;23:559–64.

Royal College of Obstetricians and Gynaecologists. *Shoulder Dystocia*. Guideline No. 42. London: RCOG; 2005 [www.rcog.org.uk/index.asp?PageID=1317].

Sandmire HF, DeMott RK. Erb's palsy: concepts of causation. *Obstet Gynecol* 2000;95:941–2.

Shoulder dystocia (stuck shoulders). In: World Health Organization, Department of Reproductive Health and Research. *Managing Complications in Pregnancy and Childbirth: Guidelines for Midwives and Doctors*. Geneva: WHO; 2003. p. S83–5 [www.who.int/reproductive-health/impac/Symptoms/Shoulder_dystocia_S83_S85.html].

Wolf H, Hoeksma AF, Oei SL, Bleker OP. Obstetric brachial plexus injury: risk factors related to recovery. *Eur J Obstet Gynecol Reprod Biol* 2000;88:133–8.

Algorithm 22.1 Umbilical cord prolapse management plan

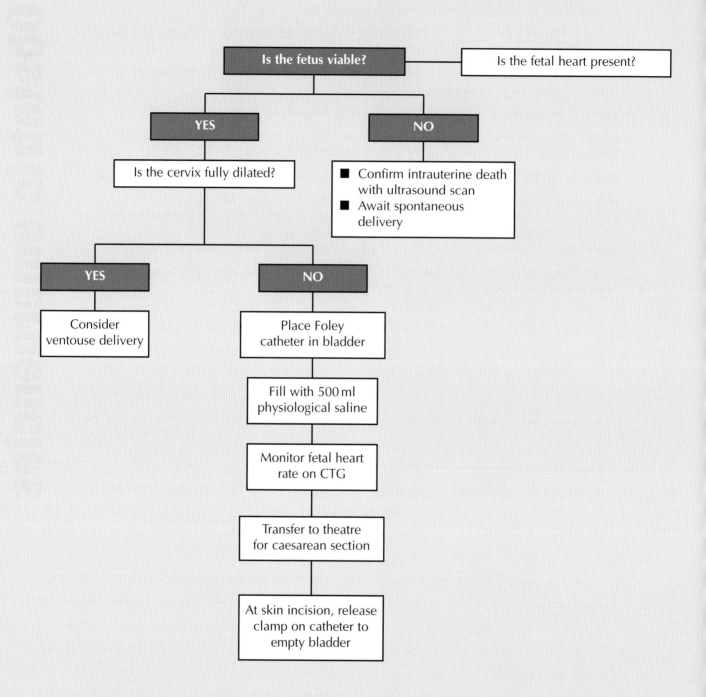

Chapter 22

Umbilical cord prolapse

Objectives

On successfully completing the topic you will be able to:

■ manage prolapse of the umbilical cord to improve perinatal outcome

■ safely and efficiently manage umbilical cord prolapse to minimise maternal risk.

Definition and incidence

A loop of umbilical cord is below the presenting part and the membranes are ruptured. Umbilical cord prolapse occurs in approximately 0.2% of all births.

A high percentage of mothers are multiparous. The incidence of prolapsed cord was 0.6% of all births in 1932 and the reduction in frequency of the complication probably reflects changes in obstetric practice, with increased use of elective and intrapartum caesarean section for a non-cephalic or an unengaged presenting part and a more active approach to intrapartum management of the very preterm fetus.

Significance

In cord prolapse, the fetal perinatal mortality has been as high as 25–50% from asphyxia due to:

■ mechanical compression of the cord between the presenting part and bony pelvis

■ spasm of the cord vessels when exposed to cold or manipulations.

The perinatal mortality rate associated with umbilical cord prolapse has also fallen. Rates reported as high as 375/1000 between 1924 and 1948 have fallen to 36–162/1000 within the past few decades. The cause of death for infants born after umbilical cord prolapse now seems to be related more to the complications of prematurity and low birth weight than to intrapartum asphyxia as such.

It is considered that part of the fall in perinatal mortality is due to the more rapid and frequent use of caesarean section once prolapsed cord has been diagnosed. However, given the association between umbilical cord prolapse and preterm birth, improvements in neonatal intensive care are probably more important.

Aetiology

The presenting part does not remain in the lower uterine segment due to:

■ fetal causes

- malpresentations (e.g., complete or footling breech, transverse and oblique lie):
  - ☐ prematurity
  - ☐ polyhydramnios
  - ☐ multiple pregnancy
  - ☐ anencephaly
- maternal causes:
  - ☐ contracted pelvis
  - ☐ pelvic tumours
- low-grade placenta praevia
- long cord
- sudden rupture of membranes in polyhydramnios.

Risk factors

In one series, obstetric interventions (such as amniotomy, scalp electrode application, intra-uterine pressure catheter insertion, attempted external cephalic version, expectant management of premature rupture of membranes) preceded 47% of umbilical cord prolapse.

Diagnosis

Vaginal examination

If the cord is prolapsed it is necessary to detect whether it is pulsating; that is, whether the fetus is alive or dead.

Ultrasound

An ultrasound scan is performed in order to confirm a fetal heartbeat, if this facility is rapidly available. In addition, it can occasionally diagnose cord presentation. Colour flow Doppler sonography can diagnose cord presentation that is likely to be the harbinger of cord prolapse, and, in turn, its potential complications may be avoided. This is only recommended if there is reason to suspect cord presentation and if clinically indicated.

Obstetric management of umbilical cord prolapse

Obstetric management of umbilical cord prolapse has largely been unchanged since the 1950s. The approach if the baby is alive and of a viable gestation continues to be elevation of the presenting part and rapid delivery, usually by caesarean section.

Early diagnosis is important and continuous electronic fetal monitoring may be of assistance as fetal heart rate changes frequently recur.

A management plan is shown in Algorithm 22.1.

A number of manoeuvres are described to reduce the risk of cord compression, including manual elevation of the presenting part off the cord, tocolysis, bladder filling, placing the patient in the knee–chest position and funic reduction.

Traditionally, management of umbilical cord prolapse has included knee–chest or Trendelenburg positioning and manual elevation of the presenting part of the fetus above the pelvic inlet, to relieve cord compression. Provided that delivery is not imminent and the fetus is viable, this traditional management occurs while preparations for emergency caesarean section are made.

At this time, an absence of audible fetal heart tones and a nonpulsatile cord may be noted. Increasing the intravenous fluid rate, administering oxygen by facemask and discontinuing the oxytocin infusion are indicated. If the umbilical cord protrudes through the introitus, it may need to be moistened with sterile gauze soaked in warm, physiological saline. The importance of prompt ultrasound assessment in a woman presenting with the absence of cord pulsation and inaudible fetal heart tones has been demonstrated: fetal heart movements can be visualised, even in the absence of cord pulsation and inaudible heart tones.

Vigorous attempts to accomplish a safe vaginal delivery after the diagnosis of umbilical cord prolapse have been reported. Barrett manually replaced the prolapsed cord in the uterine cavity in six cases where the patient was remote from delivery. Of these, five had successful 'funic reduction', followed by a normal vaginal delivery. This potentially beneficial management needs further evaluation in larger studies.

An advance in the management of umbilical cord prolapse has been the development of bladder filling. Bladder filling was first proposed by Vago in 1970 as a method of relieving pressure on the umbilical cord. Bladder filling raises the presenting part of the fetus off the compressed cord for an extended period of time, thereby eliminating the need for an examiner's fingers to displace the presenting part. A number-16 Foley catheter is placed into the urinary bladder. The bladder is filled via the catheter with physiological saline by a standard infusion set. The quantity to be instilled has varied from 400 ml to 750 ml in different reports. The quantity of saline needed is determined by the appearance of the distended bladder above the pubis, with 500 ml usually being sufficient. The balloon is then inflated, the catheter is clamped and the drainage tubing and urine bag are attached and secured.

Bladder filling has an additional advantage in that the full bladder may decrease or inhibit uterine contractions. In a series by Chetty and Moodley, there were no cases of perinatal mortality. All the babies had Apgar scores of 6 or more and the mean elapsed time from diagnosis to delivery was 69 minutes. Eight women in their study delivered after an elapsed time of 80 minutes or more.

Caspi et al. and Katz et al. found no perinatal deaths when bladder filling was used to manage umbilical cord prolapse.

Given that there is no evidence of fetal distress, it may be reasonable to proceed with a regional block. The bladder is emptied by unclamping the catheter before opening the peritoneal cavity for caesarean delivery. Some authors have suggested the continuous usage of betasympathomimetic drugs to inhibit uterine contractions, such as terbutaline sulphate.

Umbilical cord prolapse at full dilatation with a live viable fetus is one of only two situations where the vacuum extractor may be used with an unengaged head. This is discussed in the section on instrumental vaginal delivery.

The evidence suggests that the interval between diagnosis and delivery is significantly related to stillbirth and neonatal death, although Prabulos and Philipson, in their review of 65 cases of cord prolapse, suggest that the time from diagnosis to delivery may not be the only critical determinant of neonatal outcome, particularly with frank cord prolapse. This was further supported by a retrospective study of 132 cases examining the mortality and morbidity associated with cord prolapse. Neonatal condition, as assessed by Apgar scores and cord blood gas analysis, was not obviously influenced by the time interval between diagnosis of cord prolapse and delivery. Fetal mortality was attributed to prematurity and congenital anomalies, rather than birth asphyxia.

In a study by Critchlow et al., in 709 cases of cord prolapse there were only three who presented with an intrauterine death. Although the risk factors already discussed are important, the majority of babies in this study were of normal birth weight and at term with cephalic presentation.

Tchabo reported that approximately 25% of umbilical cord prolapses occur outside the hospital. Indeed, in the Oxford study, the only baby that died was the first of twins where the cord prolapse occurred at home; the woman was transferred to the hospital and subsequent delivery took 100 minutes. Dare reported an incidence of cord prolapse of 76.7% in unbooked women, with a perinatal mortality rate as high as 86.4% in the unbooked women. This suggests that umbilical cord prolapse occurring at home carries a worse prognosis.

Summary

■ Obstetricians assume a dual role in the provision of health care for both mother and fetus during labour.

■ Umbilical cord prolapse continues to be associated with poor perinatal outcome in some cases, despite emergency delivery in a modern high-risk obstetric unit.

■ It is important that staff are fully aware of the procedures to be followed, which will ensure that they are carried out as efficiently and successfully as possible.

Suggested further reading

Barrett JM. Funic reduction for the management of umbilical cord prolapse. *Am J Obstet Gynecol* 1991;165:654–7.

Caspi E, Lotan Y, Schreyer P. Prolapse of the cord: reduction of perinatal mortality by bladder instillation and caesarean section. *Isr J Med Sci* 1983;19:541–5.

Chetty RM, Moodley J. Umbilical cord prolapse. *S Afr Med J* 1980;57:128–9.

Critchlow CW, Leet TL, Beneditti TJ, Daling JR. Risk factors and infant outcomes associated with umbilical cord prolapse: a population-based case-control study among births in Washington State. *Am J Obstet Gynecol* 1994;170:613–18.

Dare FO, Owolabi AT, Fasubaa OB, Ezechi OC. Umbilical cord prolapse: a clinical study of 60 cases seen at Obafemi Awolowo university teaching hospital. *East Afr Med J* 1998;75:308–10.

Driscoll JA, Sadan O, Van Gelderen CJ, Holloway GA. Cord prolapse: can we save more babies? *Br J Obstet Gynaecol* 1987;94:594–5.

Fenton AN, d'Esopo DA. Prolapse of the cord during labor. *Am J Obstet Gynecol* 1951;62:52–64.

Ferrara TB, Hoekstra RE, Gaziano E, Knox GE, Couser RJ, Fangman JJ. Changing outcome of extremely premature infants (< 26 weeks' gestation and < 750 gm): survival and follow-up at a tertiary center. *Am J Obstet Gynecol* 1989;161:1114–18.

Goldthorp WO. A decade in the management of prolapse and presentation of the umbilical cord. *Br J Clin Pract* 1967;21:21–26.

Koonings PP, Paul RH, Campbell K. Umbilical cord prolapse: a contemporary look. *J Reprod Med* 1990;35:690–2.

Griese ME, Prickett SA. Nursing management of umbilical cord prolapse. *J Obstet Gynecol Neonatal Nurs* 1993:311–15.

Katz Z, Shoham Z, Lancet M, Blickstein I, Mogilner BM, Zalel Y. Management of labor with umbilical cord prolapse: a 5 year study. *Obstet Gynecol* 1994;94:278–81.

Mesleh T, Sultan M, Sabagh T, Algwiser A. Umbilical cord prolapse. *J Obstet Gynecol* 1993;13:24–28.

Murphy DJ, MacKenzie IZ. The mortality and morbidity associated with umbilical cord prolapse. *Br J Obstet Gynaecol* 1995;102:826–30.

Panter KR, Hannah ME. Umbilical cord prolapse: so far so good? *Lancet* 1996;347:74.

Prabulos AM, Philpson EH. Umbilical cord prolapse: so far so good. *J Reprod Med* 1998;43:129–32.

Raga F, Osborne N, Ballister MJ. Color flow Doppler: a useful instrument in the diagnosis of funic presentation. *J Natl Med Assoc* 1996; 88:94–6.

Tchabo JG The use of the contact hysteroscope in the diagnosis of cord prolapse. *Int Surg* 1988;73:57–8.

Usta IM, Mercer BM, Sibai BM. Current obstetrical practice and umbilical cord prolapse. *Am J Perinatol* 1999;16:479–84.

Vago T. Prolapse of the umbilical cord. A method of management. *Am J Obstet Gynecol* 1970;107:967–9.

Yla-Outinen A, Heinonen PK, Tuimala R. Predisposing and risk factors of umbilical cord prolapse. *Acta Obstet Gynecol Scand* 1985;64:567–70.

Algorithm 23.1 Uterine inversion

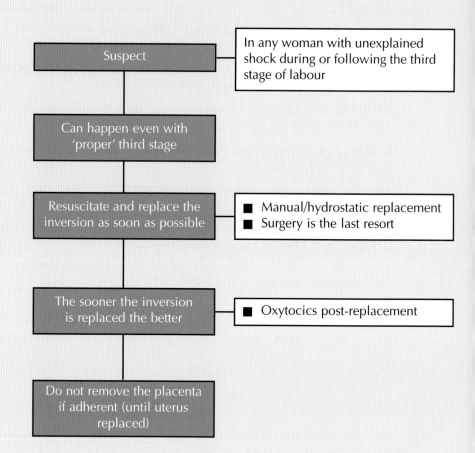

Chapter 23

Uterine inversion

Background

Reported incidence ranges from 1/2000 to 1/6400. Although it has often been thought to be related to mismanagement of the third stage, uterine inversion was found even in an institution that did not use the Crede's manoeuvre, where they strongly discourage vigorous cord traction and where oxytocin was not given until after placental separation. Brar *et al.* found a fundal placenta in the majority of women. Other associated obstetric conditions include a short cord, a morbidly adherent placenta and uterine anomalies.

Inversion of the uterus can be puerperal and nonpuerperal. However, chronic nonpuerperal uterine inversions are rare. In a study by Mwinyoglee *et al.*, only 77 cases were reported; 75 (97.4%) were tumour-produced and 20% of these tumours were malignant.

Puerperal uterine inversions can follow normal vaginal delivery or occur at caesarean sections. Usual causes at caesarean section are short umbilical cord and fundal insertion of placenta. Prompt understanding and repositioning by manual replacement will prevent further complications.

Immediate nonsurgical measures are successful in the vast majority of cases of uterine inversion. The pooled experience of Brar *et al.* and Watson demonstrated only three laparotomies requiring surgical reposition out of a total of 102 uterine inversions.

Recognition

Early recognition of uterine inversion is vital to enable prompt treatment and to reduce morbidity and mortality.

Symptoms and signs include:

■ severe lower abdominal pain in the third stage

■ haemorrhage (present in 94% of cases)

■ shock that is out of proportion to the blood loss, owing to vagal stimulation

■ placenta may or may not be in place

■ uterine fundus not palpable per abdomen (in milder degrees there may be a dimple in the fundal area)

■ pelvic examination showing a mass in the vagina (in milder degrees) or outside the introitus.

Prevention

Mismanagement of the third stage should be avoided and cord traction should not be applied until the signs of placental separation are apparent.

Management

1. Call for help (experienced obstetrician/anaesthetist/midwives).

2. Arrange replacement of uterus concurrently to anti-shock measures, as resuscitation may not be successful until the inversion is corrected. Sometimes the delivering attendant may be successful at immediate replacement within seconds of delivery.

3. Insert two wide-bore cannulae.

4. Collect blood for full blood count, coagulation studies and group and cross match (4–6 units).

5. Start fluid replacement immediately (colloids and crystalloids).

6. Continuously monitor blood pressure, pulse, respiratory rate, urine output, O_2 saturation.

7. Arrange appropriate analgesia.

8. Transfer to theatre.

9. Attempt to reposition the uterus; the earlier the restoration, the more likely the success.

10. **If the placenta is still attached, it should be left alone until after repositioning. Attempts to remove the placenta may result in major bleeding, as there will be no uterine muscular contraction to constrict blood vessels in the placental bed.**

Replace the uterus using one of the following techniques:

■ manual replacement (the Johnson manoeuvre)

■ hydrostatic repositioning (O'Sullivan's technique)

■ medical approach

■ surgery (laparotomy and Haultain's procedure or Huntingdon's operation)

Manual replacement

Manual replacement should be performed preferably under general anaesthesia. The uterus may require relaxation for manual replacement to succeed.

Hydrostatic repositioning (O'Sullivan's technique)

Uterine rupture must be excluded first.

Infuse warm saline into the posterior fornix of the vagina (via a rubber tube held 2 metres above the patient) while the vaginal orifice is blocked by an assistant. The water distends the posterior fornix of the vagina gradually so that it stretches. This relieves cervical constriction and results in correction of the inversion.

Another technique involves attaching the intravenous giving set to a silicone ventouse cup inserted in the vagina, which tends to produce a better seal.

A hard, black, rubber anaesthetic facemask can be used, which may fit over the vulva. The oxygen inlet allows access for fluid input.

Medical approach

Drugs are used to relax the cervical ring to facilitate replacement.

Agents include:

- magnesium sulphate 2–4 g infused intravenously over 5 minutes
- ritodrine 0.15 mg intravenous bolus
- terbutaline 0.25 mg intravenously
- nitroglycerine 100 mg intravenously.

Surgery

Surgery is only used if all other attempts fail.

In **Huntingdon's procedure**, Allis forceps are placed within the dimple of the inverted uterus and gentle upward traction is exerted on the clamps, with a further placement of forceps on the advancing fundus.

Haultain's technique involves incising the cervical ring posteriorly (where the incision is least likely to involve the bladder or uterine vessels) with a longitudinal incision and facilitates uterine placement by Huntingdon's method. After replacement has been completed the hysterotomy site is repaired.

Oxytocics should be administered after repositioning to keep the uterus contracted and prevent recurrence. The attendant's hand should remain in the uterine cavity until a firm contraction occurs.

Suggested further reading

Abouleish E, Ali V, Joumaa B, Lopez M, Gupta D. Anaesthetic management of acute puerperal uterine inversion. *Br J Anaesth* 1995;75:486–7.

Brar HS, Greenspoon JS, Platt LD, Paul RH. Acute puerperal uterine inversion. New approaches to management. *J Reprod Med* 1989;34:173–7.

Clark S. Use of ritodrine in uterine inversion. *Am J Obstet Gynecol* 1984;151:705.

Dayan SS, Schwalbe SS. The use of small dose nitroglycerine in a case of uterine inversion. *Anesth Analg* 1996;82:1091–3.

Grossman R. Magnesium sulphate for uterine inversion. *J Reprod Med* 1980;20:161–2.

Huntington JL, Irving FC, Kellog FS. Abdominal reposition in acute inversion of the puerperal uterus. *Am J Obstet Gynecol* 1928;15:34–40.

Kriplani A, Relan S, Kumar R, Mittal S, Buckshee K. Complete inversion of the uterus during Caesarean section: a case report. *Aust N Z Obstet Gynaecol* 1996;36:17–19.

Loeffler F. Postpartum haemorrhage and abnormalities of the third stage of labour. In: Chamberlain G, editor. *Turnbull's Obstetrics*. 2nd ed. Edinburgh: Churchill Livingstone; 1995. p. 729–34.

Manassiev N, Shaw G. Uterine inversion. *Modern Midwife* 1996;6(5):32–4.

Mohanty AK, Trehan AK. Puerperal uterine inversion: analysis of three cases managed by repositioning, and literature review. *J Obstet Gynecol* 1998;18:353–4.

Mwinyoglee J, Simelela N, Marivate M. Non-puerperal uterine inversions. A two case report and review of the literature. *Cent Afr J Med* 1997;43:268–72.

Obstetric emergencies

Ogueh O, Ayida G. Acute uterine inversion: a new technique of hydrostatic replacement. *Br J Obstet Gynaecol* 1997;104:951–2.

O'Sullivan J. Acute inversion of the uterus. *Br Med J* 1945;2:282–3.

Shah-Hosseini R, Evrard JR. Puerperal uterine inversion. *Obstet Gynecol* 1989;73:567–70.

Thomson AJ, Greer IA. Non-haemorrhagic obstetric shock. *Baillieres Best Pract Res Clin Obstet Gynaecol* 2000;14(1):19–41.

Watson P, Besch N, Bowes WA Jr. Management of acute and subacute puerperal inversion of the uterus. *Obstet Gynecol* 1980;55:12–16.

World Health Organization, UNFPA, UNICEG, World Bank. *Managing Complications in Pregnancy and Childbirth. A guide for midwives and doctors.* Geneva: WHO; 2001.

Algorithm 24.1 Retained placenta

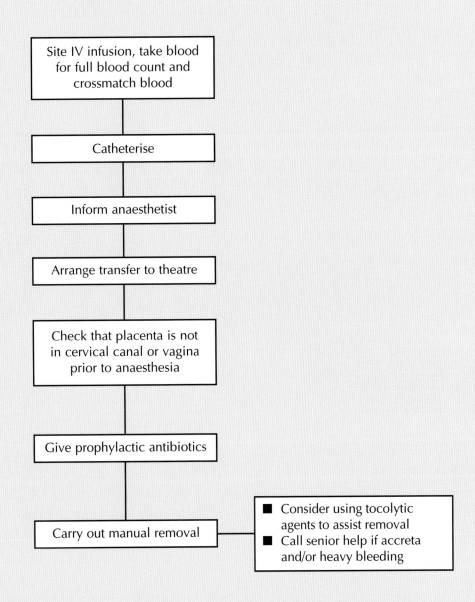

Site IV infusion, take blood for full blood count and crossmatch blood

Catheterise

Inform anaesthetist

Arrange transfer to theatre

Check that placenta is not in cervical canal or vagina prior to anaesthesia

Give prophylactic antibiotics

Carry out manual removal

- Consider using tocolytic agents to assist removal
- Call senior help if accreta and/or heavy bleeding

Chapter 24

Retained placenta

Objectives

On successfully completing this topic you will be able to:

- recognise risk factors for a retained placenta and morbidly adherent placenta
- provide adequate resuscitation and fluid management
- understand the technique of manual removal of the placenta
- discuss non-invasive treatments.

Introduction

Worldwide, postpartum haemorrhage accounts for the deaths of many thousands of women. Retained placenta features prominently within this group and in many cultures it is a dreaded complication of childbirth. Placenta accreta is now becoming more frequent and is correlated with the increasing incidence of caesarean sections in the UK.

Definitions, incidence and predisposing factors

Although 'retained placenta' has been observed to occur in at least 2% of deliveries, the diagnosis depends upon arbitrary time limits. Clearly, the shorter the time limit the more frequent the diagnosis and the more likely is 'obstetric intervention'. Much debate has focused on the relative benefits and risks of obstetric interference in the natural process of placental delivery.

It is widely agreed that women with a retained placenta are at a significantly increased risk of haemorrhage. In the UK, the risk ratio for major obstetric haemorrhage in women with a retained placenta was 5.15 (95% CI 3.4–7.9). This occurs predominantly within this first hour after birth. However, Combs and Laros found no increase in haemorrhage until the third stage exceeded 30 minutes. This has become the conventional cut-off point for the diagnosis of 'retained placenta'. Choosing a time limit on the basis of haemorrhage risk is supported by observations made in other studies. For example, Dombrowski et al., looking at retained placenta within a population of 45 852 women, found that the frequency of haemorrhage peaked by 40 minutes, regardless of gestational age.

A systematic review of the literature relating to injection of oxytocic agents into the umbilical vein for retained placenta defined a cut-off point of 15 minutes. Given the finding that 90% of placentas are spontaneously delivered at 14 minutes and the noninvasive nature of the 'medical' intervention that they were reviewing, this is reasonable.

The most extreme form of placental retention is placenta accreta, where the placenta is morbidly adherent to the uterus. Miller et al. reviewed hospital records of all cases of histologically confirmed accreta and found 62 (1/2510) among 155 670 deliveries.

Factors predisposing to retained placenta and placenta accreta

In a systematic review, which included the Hinchingbrooke trial, the need for manual removal of the placenta was found to be more likely with active management of labour than with expectant management (2.1% versus 1.5%) and was more likely with the longer-lasting uterotonic agent, ergometrine 500 micrograms and oxytocin 5 units/ml (Syntometrine®, Alliance) than with oxytocin (Syntocinon®, Alliance) alone (2.5% versus 1.6%). Oxytocin induces strong rhythmic uterine contractions, principally in the upper part of the uterus, whereas ergometrine, which has no physiologically produced counterpart, produces spasm of smooth muscle throughout the body and in the uterus affects primarily the lower segment and cervix. Syntometrine was developed for intramuscular use and begins to have an effect after about 2 minutes as the oxytocin starts to work; the ergometrine acts about 4–5 minutes later, causing the uterus and cervix to clamp down. These findings support the link between uterine constriction and placental retention (or entrapment).

A number of authors have undertaken multivariate risk factor analyses for 'retained placenta'. Among the common risk factors for retained placenta are:

- previous retained placenta
- multiparity
- induced and preterm labour
- small placenta
- history of previous instrumentation of the uterus (caesarean section, sharp or suction curettage)
- placenta praevia
- leiomyoma.

There appears to be a significant association with placental weight of less than 601 g.

The timing of placental delivery appears to relate closely to the gestation. Life-table analyses predicted that 90% of placentas would spontaneously deliver by 180 minutes at 20 weeks of gestation, by 21 minutes at 30 weeks and by 14 minutes at 40 weeks. Romero et al., noting the increased incidence of retained placenta in preterm pregnancies, speculated that the relatively larger size of a preterm placenta might require more uterine work and time.

There is a highly significant association between raised serum alphafetoprotein (AFP) and placenta accreta. Aberrant maternal–trophoblastic interaction in the placental bed is thought to be a key to the understanding of the pathogenesis of morbid placental adherence.

Placenta accreta is becoming more common and over the last 40 years the incidence has increased ten-fold. This phenomenon is due to the fact that lower segment caesarean section appears to increase the risk of subsequent placenta praevia and there is a well-documented association between placenta praevia and previous caesarean section with placenta accreta.

In a large cohort study, risk factors for placenta accreta were:

- placenta praevia (OR 54.2; 95% CI 17.8–165.5)
- abnormally elevated second-trimester AFP (> 2.5 MoM) (OR 8.3; 95% CI 1.8–39.3)
- raised serum beta-human chorionic gonadotrophin (OR 3.9; 95% CI 1.5–09.9)
- age 35 years and older (OR 3.2; 95% CI 1.1–09.4).

In another series, placenta accreta occurred in 55/590 (9.3%) of women with placenta praevia and in 7/155 080 (1/22 154) without placenta praevia.

Among women with placenta praevia, the risk of accreta ranged from 2% in women less than 35 years of age with no previous caesarean deliveries to almost 39% in women with two or more previous caesarean deliveries and an anterior central placenta praevia.

Management of retained placenta

Numerous traditional beliefs and practices exist related to delivering the placenta. There is an awareness of the risks of retained placenta and its link to haemorrhage is widely recognised. As a consequence, delivery of the placenta is considered of prime importance and many techniques have been devised for facilitating this. The majority of manoeuvres, described across cultures, relate to pulling on the placenta, squeezing the uterus and increasing intra-abdominal pressure by inducing vomiting. Inducing vomiting has been described in widely differing cultures across different continents.

Current conventional management of retained placenta is manual removal under anaesthesia. This therefore requires transfer to an operating theatre and a high level of expertise. In some countries with limited medical resources, transfer to theatre might take many hours or even days. In a survey of home deliveries, considerable delay in referral resulted in nearly one-third of women being admitted in shock, constituting 68% of emergency admissions.

Resuscitation

The potential for massive haemorrhage associated with retained placenta should never be underestimated.

Routine practice should be followed with regard to assessment of any woman with potential or actual haemorrhage, involving adequate intravenous access and appropriate fluid replacement. Blood should be made available (see Chapters 10 and 17).

Non-operative intervention

There has been considerable interest in finding a non-invasive treatment for retained placenta.

Intra-umbilical vein injections

In one trial, 37 women with retained placenta were randomised to have intra-umbilical vein injection of prostaglandin F_2, oxytocin or physiological saline or to immediate manual removal of the placenta. Spontaneous separation of the placenta occurred in all ten women after injection of prostaglandin and in six of ten that received oxytocin. In the UK, Gazvani *et al.* found a similar clinically important benefit from giving intra-umbilical oxytocin, compared to saline.

Carroli and Berger reviewed those studies that have examined the use of intra-umbilical oxytocic agents. Injection of saline solution with oxytocin after 15 minutes of placental retention was associated with a significant reduction in the need for manual removal of placenta (117/234, 50%, versus 129/220, 59%). Pipingas *et al.* suggested that the most likely explanation for the observed beneficial effects of volume infused oxytocin would be a direct action on the myometrium underlying the unseparated placenta.

Tocolytic agents

Glyceryl trinitrate (GTN) has come to the attention of obstetricians as a potent tocolytic agent. GTN is a nitric oxide donor and a potent endogenous smooth-muscle relaxant in vasculature, gut, genitourinary tract and the uterus. This may be useful for aiding fetal delivery. It has been used successfully for urgent tocolysis in cases of difficulties with delivery at caesarean section to provide tocolysis for external cephalic version. It has been used in the management of inverted uterus.

GTN has also been tried for the third-stage complications. Sublingual GTN has a rapid onset of action and has been used in the acute cardiac setting in place of the intravenous formulations. Sublingual GTN using a spray is an easy way of administering the drug and has been used in women requiring vaginal delivery of retained placenta, at an initial dose of 800 micrograms. Rapid uterine relaxation was obtained with no observed adverse effects. Sublingual GTN has a quicker effect if administered by spray than by tablet.

Intravenous GTN has also been used successfully, in doses ranging from 50 micrograms to 250 micrograms for placental extraction, with minimal adverse effects. The onset of action is within 1 minute and uterine contractility is restored by 5 minutes. However, it requires dilution, a time-consuming process with the possibility of error.

Manual removal of the retained placenta

- Bearing in mind the time expended after the delivery of the baby, procedures to deliver the placenta should be considered once half an hour has elapsed, or sooner if there is significant active bleeding.

- Transfer to theatre.

- Anaesthesia (see below).

- Consider appropriate antibiotic cover.

- Full aseptic precautions. Non-permeable gowns and/or gauntlet (up to elbow) gloves are useful, as fundal site placentas require the operator's arm to be inserted high into the uterus.

- Surgical technique:
  - If the umbilical cord is still attached it can be traced to the placenta. Often, due to enthusiastic traction on the cord during attempts to deliver the placenta, it gets snapped off and is not visible.
  - Uterotonic agents may help the operator access the uterine cavity.
  - The edge of the placenta needs to be identified and feels like a ridge which if followed will lead to the smooth membranous surface.
  - It is essential to keep one hand on the maternal abdomen to feel the uterus throughout the procedure, to avoid using increased force, which can cause an iatrogenic rupture or trauma.
  - The temptation to claw at the placenta must be resisted; this is best achieved by keeping all the fingers together like a spade to initiate separation in the correct plane. Blind grabbing of tissue can lead not only to piecemeal removal but the possibility of retained lobes with recurrence or uncontrolled postpartum haemorrhage.
  - Once the placenta has been sheared off and is in the operator's palm, manual compression, together with uterotonic agents, will ensure uterine contractility. A Syntocinon drip needs to be continued for at least 4 hours after the procedure.

Should a manual removal be unsuccessful or piecemeal, or should haemorrhage not abate, the possibility of placenta accreta should be considered. Futile or forceful attempts to remove a clearly stuck placenta should be resisted and the safest option if early diagnosis is made is to tie off the umbilical cord close to the placenta and adopt a wait and see approach. Managing a placenta accreta requires senior input, Doppler imaging to confirm and the possibility of methotrexate or uterine artery embolisation to be considered.

Placenta accreta/increta and percreta

These conditions of abnormal placental adherence or invasion of the myometrium are often associated with major haemorrhage.

An index of suspicion should provoke attempts to make the diagnosis antenatally. There are a number of options available but at present it appears that colour flow Doppler ultrasonography has the highest specificity and sensitivity and is therefore the greatest use in diagnosis. Other techniques include MRI scanning. Choice will depend on availability and local expertise.

In cases where an antenatal diagnosis of placenta praevia/accreta may have been made, a planned caesarean hysterectomy may be required. This may be performed in a routine theatre setting. Some centres have made provision for planning preoperative radiological intervention in the form of iliac artery catheterisation prior to starting the caesarean section. This will allow much easier control of haemorrhage, should it be necessary, by inflation of the balloon catheters at an appropriate site to reduce the uterine blood flow. This needs to be performed in a well-stocked theatre setting with access to facilities for monitoring and rapid transfusion and will require careful planning to allow optimal care during these occasional but life-threatening emergencies.

Placenta praevia/accreta

A traditional lower segment caesarean section can be carried out in the majority of cases of placenta praevia, even if anterior. The placenta does not need to be cut through but can usually be swept off the uterine wall and the baby delivered.

Troublesome bleeding can be controlled by a hydrostatic balloon or uterine packing with the tail brought out through the cervix and the lower segment packed last. The hydrostatic balloon can also be used in cases of placenta accreta where there is pressure to conserve the uterus.

In many cases of caesarean section with a morbidly adherent placenta, it may be necessary to proceed to hysterectomy.

An HDU setting for postoperative care for these women is mandatory, as the blood loss can be massive. There have been a few case reports on the management of morbidly adherent placenta using methotrexate. Alternatively, tying off the umbilical cord flush with the placenta to allow it to dry up has been used. Limited experience has suggested that methotrexate is particularly useful in the treatment of placenta percreta with bladder invasion due to the rapid resolution of the vascular invasion of the bladder.

In addition to possible anaesthetic complications, manual removal of placenta itself carries further risks of haemorrhage and trauma. A significant association between manual removal of the placenta and postpartum endometritis has also been shown. It is also possible that separation of mother and baby immediately after birth will affect bonding and breastfeeding.

Anaesthesia for manual removal of placenta

General anaesthesia will usually be considered if there is significant bleeding or cardiovascular instability, as it ensures control of airway and breathing, leaving the anaesthetist free to concentrate on fluid replacement and cardiovascular support. Maintenance of anaesthesia with inhalational agents has been used to produce uterine relaxation but this effect requires effective drug levels. Thus, endotracheal intubation is required, followed by another 2–4 minutes to achieve the depth of anaesthesia necessary for endometrial relaxation. There is concern that this form of anaesthesia will delay recovery of uterine contractility and also delay awakening from anaesthesia. There are thus complexities to the use of general anaesthesia.

Regional anaesthesia (spinal or epidural) avoids the risks associated with intubation in pregnant women provided there is cardiovascular stability.

Anaesthetic management should ensure the provision of cervico-uterine relaxation, which can be achieved with tocolytic drugs (see above).

Audit

■ All women with retained placenta should have an experienced/senior doctor present.

■ Time from birth of the baby to delivery of placenta should be less than 90 minutes.

■ Postnatal haemoglobin should be checked prior to discharge.

■ Prophylactic antibiotics should be given.

■ A large blood sample should be taken.

■ Peripheral lines × 2 should be inserted.

■ Blood pressure, pulse and urine output should be monitored.

Suggested further reading

Altabef KM, Spencer JT, Zinberg S. Intravenous nitroglycerin for uterine relaxation of an inverted uterus. *Am J Obstet Gynecol* 1992;166:1237–8.

Chan ASH, Rolbin SH. Alternating nitroglycerin and syntocinon to facilitate uterine exporation and removal of an adherent placenta. *Can J Anaesth* 1995;42:335–7.

Combs CA, Laros RKJ. Prolonged third stage of labor: morbidity and risk factors. *Obstet Gynecol* 1991;77:863–7.

Dombrowski MP, Bottoms SF, Saleh AAA, Hurd WW, Romero R. Third stage of labor: analysis of duration and clinical practice. *Am J Obstet Gynecol* 1995;172:1279–84.

Gazvani MR, Luckas MJM, Drakeley AJ, Emery SJ, Alfirevic Z, Walkinshaw SA. Intraumbilical oxytocin for the management of retained placenta: a randomised controlled trial. *Obstet Gynecol* 1998;91:203–7.

Hung TH, Shau WY, Hsieh CC, Chiu T, Hsu J, Hsieh T. Risk factors for placenta accreta. *Obstet Gynecol* 1999;93:545–50.

Inch S. Management of the third stage of labour. Another cascade of interventions? *Midwifery* 1985;1:114–22.

Jacques SM, Qureshi F, Trent VS, Ramirez NC. Placenta accreta: mild cases diagnosed by placental examination. *Int J Gynecol Pathol* 1996;15:28–33.

Khong TY, Khong TK. Delayed postpartum hemorrhage: a morphologic study of causes and their relation to other pregnancy disorders. *Obstet Gynecol* 1993;82:17–22.

McDonald S, Prendiville WJ, Elbourne D. Prophylactic syntometrine versus oxytocin for delivery of the placenta. *Cochrane Database Syst Rev* 2000;(2):CD000201 [update in *Cochrane Database Syst Rev* 2004;(1):CD000201].

Maine D, Rosenfield A, Wallis M, Kimball A, Kwast B, Papiernik E, *et al. Prevention of Maternal Deaths in Developing Countries.* New York: Centre for Population of Family Health; 1999.

Miller DA, Chollet JA, Goodwin TM. Clinical risk factors for placenta previa–placenta accreta. *Am J Obstet Gynecol* 1997;177:210–14.

Prendiville WJ, Elbourne D, McDonald S. Active versus expectant management of the third stage of labour. *Cochrane Database Syst Rev* 2000;(2):CD000007 [update in *Cochrane Database Syst Rev* 2000; (3):CD000007].

Sawhney H, Gopalan S. Home deliveries and third stage complications. *Aust N Z J Obstet Gynaecol* 1994;34:531–4.

Sorbe B. Active pharmacologic management of the third stage of labor. A comparison of oxytocin and ergometrine. *Obstet Gynecol* 1978;52(6):694–7.

Algorithm 25.1 Face presentation

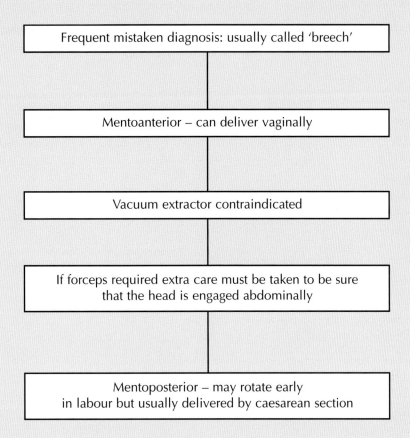

Frequent mistaken diagnosis: usually called 'breech'

Mentoanterior – can deliver vaginally

Vacuum extractor contraindicated

If forceps required extra care must be taken to be sure that the head is engaged abdominally

Mentoposterior – may rotate early in labour but usually delivered by caesarean section

Chapter 25

Face presentation

Objectives

On successfully completing this topic you will be able to:

- recognise and manage face presentation
- appreciate the importance of correct definition of presentation and position of the part.

Incidence

Face presentation occurs in approximately 1/500 to 1/1000 deliveries.

Aetiology

- Multiparity
- Prematurity
- Multiple pregnancy
- Loops of cord around neck
- Neck tumours
- Uterine abnormalities
- Cephalopelvic disproportion
- Fetal macrosomia.

Diagnosis

Primary face presentation might be detected on a late ultrasound scan. The majority of face presentations are secondary and arise in labour.

Abdominal examination

A large amount of head is palpable on the same side as the back without a cephalic prominence on the same side as the limbs.

Vaginal examination

In early labour the presenting part will be high.

Landmarks are the mouth, jaws, nose, malar and orbital ridges.

The presence of alveolar margins distinguishes the mouth from the anus.

The mouth and the maxillae form the corners of a triangle, while the anus is on a straight line between the ischial tuberosities.

Avoid damaging the eyes by trauma or antiseptics.

Management

- Make a diagnosis.
- Check for cord presentation or prolapse.
- Continuously monitor fetal heart rate.
- Examine regularly to check that progress is adequate.
- Give oxytocin if progress is not satisfactory.
- Do not use scalp electrodes or perform fetal blood sampling.
- If the position is mentoanterior, vaginal delivery should be possible.
- Perform an episiotomy.
- If the fetus is persistently presenting mentoposteriorly, deliver by caesarean section.

Background

Labour in face presentation

In early labour, minor deflexion attitudes are common, especially with occipitoposterior positions and multiparity. In such cases, uterine contractions often cause increased flexion. Occasionally, extension will increase, producing successively a brow presentation and finally the fully extended face. Most face presentations are thus secondary, becoming evident only in established labour.

Diagnosis is notoriously difficult. In approximately 50% of cases the diagnosis is not made until delivery is imminent.

Descent is usually followed by internal rotation, with the chin passing anteriorly. It must be remembered that the biparietal diameter is 7 cm behind the advancing face, so that, even when the face is distending the vulva, the biparietal diameter has only just entered the pelvis. Descent is thus always less advanced than vaginal examination would suggest, even when one allows for the gross oedema that is usually present. The value of abdominal examination in such cases cannot be overstressed. Anterior rotation having occurred, the neck comes to lie behind the symphysis pubis and the head is born by flexion, causing considerable perineal distension in the process. The shoulders and body are born in the usual way.

In cases of persisting mentoposterior position, the neck is too short to span the 12 cm of the anterior aspect of the sacrum. Additionally, the neck would have to be extended to pass under the symphysis but it is already maximally extended. Delivery is impossible unless, as can happen with a very small fetus or one that is macerated, the shoulders can enter the pelvis at the same time as the head. With satisfactory uterine action and a mentoanterior position, spontaneous delivery or easy 'lift out' (forceps only) assisted delivery will ensue in 60–90% of cases. Even with mentoposterior positions, anterior rotation will occur in the second stage in 45–65% of cases, so that persistent mentoposterior position or mentotransverse arrest is encountered in only 10% of face presentations.

Mentoposterior position

Persistent mentoposteriorly presenting fetuses are usually delivered by caesarean section to reduce fetal and maternal morbidity. Vaginal manipulation, including forceps delivery and the Thorn's manoeuvre to convert the fetal head to the occipitoanterior position, were reported to be highly morbid.

Historically, vaginal manipulation of persistent mentoposterior position has been contra-indicated because of the high risk of fetal injury. In a report by Newman *et al.*, intrapartum bimanual conversion of mentoposterior to occipitoanterior position was performed while using ritodrine. Eleven women involved were orthodox Jews who refused caesarean section delivery. In the ten cases where ritodrine was administered, the manoeuvre was successful and vaginal delivery was achieved. A ritodrine bolus was administered, with concurrent upward transvaginal pressure, and the fetal head was disengaged. Bimanual fetal head flexion was then attempted using ultrasound guidance and transabdominal palpation of the occiput with gentle flexion towards the maternal pubis. Once the occipitoanterior presentation was achieved, oxytocin infusion was started. The one failure in this report was the author's initial case, in which ritodrine was not employed. Maternal and neonatal outcomes were good in all cases.

After birth, oedema and bruising of a child's face may persist for some days and may make feeding difficult.

Suggested further reading

Benedetti TJ, Lowensohn RI, Truscott AM. Face presentation at term. *Obstet Gynecol* 1980;55:199–202.

Bhal PS, Davies NJ, Chung T. A population study of face and brow presentation. *J Obstet Gynecol* 1998;18:231:5.

Cruikshank DP, Cruikshank JE. Face and brow presentation: A review. *Clin Obstet Gynecol* 1981;24:333–51.

Cruikshank DP, White CA. Obstetric malpresentations: 20 years experience. *Am J Obstet Gynecol* 1973;116:1097–104.

Daw E. Management of the hyperextended fetal head. *Am J Obstet Gynecol* 1976;124:113–15.

Duff P. Diagnosis and management of face presentation. *Obstet Gynecol* 1981;57:105–11.

Mostar S, Akaltin E, Babunca C. Deflexion attitudes: median vertex, persistent brow and face presentations. *Obstet Gynecol* 1966;28:49–56.

Newman M, Beller U, Lavie O, Aboulafia Y, Rabinowtiz R, Diamant Y. Intrapartum bimanual tocolytic-assisted reversal of face presentation: preliminary report. *Obstet Gynecol* 1994;84:146–52.

Posner LB, Rubin EJ, Posner AC. Face and brow presentations: a continuing study. *Obstet Gynecol* 1963;21:745–9.

Schwartz Z, Dgani R, Lancet M, Kessler I. Face presentation. *Aust N Z J Obstet Gynaecol* 1986;26:172–6.

Algorithm 26.1 **Ruptured uterus**

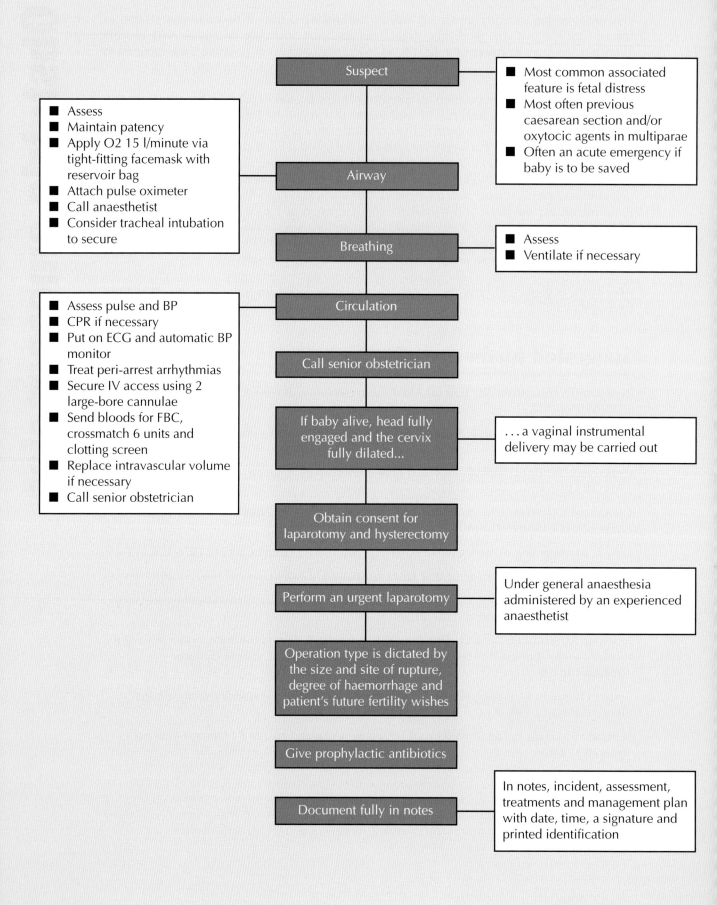

Suspect
- Most common associated feature is fetal distress
- Most often previous caesarean section and/or oxytocic agents in multiparae
- Often an acute emergency if baby is to be saved

Airway
- Assess
- Maintain patency
- Apply O2 15 l/minute via tight-fitting facemask with reservoir bag
- Attach pulse oximeter
- Call anaesthetist
- Consider tracheal intubation to secure

Breathing
- Assess
- Ventilate if necessary

Circulation
- Assess pulse and BP
- CPR if necessary
- Put on ECG and automatic BP monitor
- Treat peri-arrest arrhythmias
- Secure IV access using 2 large-bore cannulae
- Send bloods for FBC, crossmatch 6 units and clotting screen
- Replace intravascular volume if necessary
- Call senior obstetrician

Call senior obstetrician

If baby alive, head fully engaged and the cervix fully dilated...
...a vaginal instrumental delivery may be carried out

Obtain consent for laparotomy and hysterectomy

Perform an urgent laparotomy
Under general anaesthesia administered by an experienced anaesthetist

Operation type is dictated by the size and site of rupture, degree of haemorrhage and patient's future fertility wishes

Give prophylactic antibiotics

Document fully in notes
In notes, incident, assessment, treatments and management plan with date, time, a signature and printed identification

Chapter 26

Ruptured uterus

Introduction

Complete rupture of the uterus can be a life-threatening emergency. Fortunately, however, the condition is rare in modern obstetrics, despite the increase in caesarean section rates and serious sequelae are even more rare.

Incidence and predisposing factors

Federkow *et al.* reported their experience over 20 years in a major Canadian teaching hospital and referral centre. From 1966 to 1985, there were 15 cases of uterine rupture encountered in 52 854 deliveries: an overall incidence of 0.3/1000 deliveries. There was no change in the incidence over time. Of the 15 women who suffered a uterine rupture, only seven had previously had a caesarean section. In the other eight women, there was a suggestion that uterine trauma could have previously occurred in association with dilatation and curettage, hyteroscopy or forceps delivery. A bicornuate uterus, a precipitous delivery and use of oxytocin could explain the rupture in the other three women. Four of the ruptures were incidentally found at caesarean section. The rupture site was repaired in 11 and four women underwent a hysterectomy. In this series, none of the babies died.

A similar incidence has been reported by Gardeil *et al.* In their series of 65 488 deliveries between 1982 and 1991, there were also 15 cases of uterine rupture. They found no case of rupture in 21 998 primigravidae. However, 13 cases occurred to multigravidae with a previous caesarean section scar (1/304, equivalent to 0.3%). Although they had no maternal deaths, five women required a hysterectomy and there were five perinatal deaths, three of which were attributable to the rupture. A total of 13 women had received an oxytocic agent. The authors concluded that compared with earlier reports from Dublin (e.g. Flannelly), the incidence of uterine rupture is low, owing to an decrease in the number of ruptures associated with trauma or obstetric manipulation. However, their review highlighted the risk of uterine rupture when an oxytocic agent is administered to a multigravid woman with a previous caesarean scar. Sweeten *et al.* summarised the risk factors for spontaneous rupture of the unscarred uterus:

■ grand multiparity

■ undiagnosed cephalopelvic disproportion or malpresentation

■ oxytocin administration

- macrosomic fetus

- placenta percreta

- prior instrumentation of uterus

- version

- uterine abnormalities (e.g. rudimentary horn).

Data from Scotland (1985–1998), reported by Smith *et al.*, included the outcomes of 35 854 women with one previous caesarean delivery who gave birth to a singleton term infant by a means other than planned repeat caesarean section. The overall proportion of vaginal birth was 74.2% and of uterine rupture was 0.35%. The risk of intrapartum uterine rupture was higher among women who had not previously given birth vaginally and those whose labour was induced with prostaglandin. Although use of oxytocin and prostaglandin agents is often implicated in routine rupture, case–control comparisons do not show definitive pattern of uterine hyperstimulation. It would appear that their use is therefore not precluded in multigravidae or women who have had previous caesarean sections. To date, there have been no randomised controlled trials with reported data that compare outcomes in mothers and babies who planned a repeat elective caesarean section with outcomes in women who planned a vaginal birth where a previous birth had been caesarean.

Perinatal outcome

Leung *et al.* undertook a retrospective review of 106 cases of uterine rupture. They found that a higher incidence of perinatal mortality and morbidity was associated with complete fetal extrusion and that significant neonatal morbidity occurred when more than 18 minutes elapsed between the onset of prolonged decelerations and delivery. In terms of diagnosing uterine rupture, Farmer *et al.* noted that bleeding and pain were, somewhat surprisingly, unlikely findings (occurring in only 3.4% and 7.6% cases, respectively). The most common manifestation of scar separation was a prolonged fetal heart rate deceleration (70.3%).

CESDI data

In the 1995 CESDI report of intrapartum deaths, there were 12 cases of ruptured uterus. The two clinical features that stood out were:

- delay in making the diagnosis – fetal distress was invariably present but no action was taken

- the use of prostaglandins to induce labour.

In some cases, multiple doses of dinoprostone were used in a non-ripe cervix that had not been tested in a previous labour (previous caesarean section). It was not unusual to find a somewhat superficial indication for induction.

Following the publication of the fourth CESDI report (1997), a focus group was set up to review the cases of ruptured uterus. The findings of this group were reported in the fifth CESDI report (1998). Forty-two cases of ruptured uterus were found. It was estimated that these occurred within the context of a 2-year period when there were 1.3 million births. If 10% of women in antenatal clinics had experienced a previous caesarean section, 130 000 previous caesareans would have been included, of whom approximately half would have been offered a trial of labour. Given that the risk of uterine rupture with a lower segment scar is 0.1%, perhaps a total of 650 uterine ruptures would have occurred. If that were the case, then the fetal mortality for uterine rupture would be 7%. However, if the risk of rupture is higher (0.5%), then the risk of mortality is correspondingly smaller (1.4%).

Of the 42 cases, 75% were considered to have had significantly substandard care (CESDI grade III: 'different care would reasonably be expected to alter the outcome'), which can be compared with the figures for all intrapartum deaths (52%).

Risk factors

■ Obesity (46% BMI greater than 30 compared with 14% of the female population in this age group).

■ Uterine scar (30/42). Of the 12 women without a scar, only one was nulliparous.

■ Antenatal issues: absence of a recorded plan (five cases), failure to involve seniors (four cases), inappropriate decision about induction (four cases).

■ Labour issues: nine hysterectomies, no maternal deaths; three preterm.

■ Induction (60%) and augmentation (25%): all 12 women without scars had oxytocics. 23/30 of women with previous caesarean section had oxytocics. Prostaglandins: 85% greater than 1 mg; oxytocin: 80% used for slow progress at or near full dilatation.

■ 50% of ruptures occurred at or close to full dilatation.

■ Presence of warning signs: scar pain and tenderness (21 cases), vaginal bleeding (five cases), poor progress in labour (ten cases), fetal heart rate abnormality for longer than 1 hour (17 cases). In 18 cases, the diagnosis was first made at laparotomy. Delay in transfer to theatre (five cases).

■ Failure to involve senior staff was common.

■ Eight cases with poor records; nine where CTG unavailable; 14 no partogram.

CESDI (1997) recommendations for practice

Women with a uterine scar require:

■ antenatal management including plans for delivery and induction involving a documented discussion with senior obstetrician (ideally a consultant but at least SpR4 or higher)

■ attentive intrapartum fetal and maternal surveillance in a setting where caesarean section can be performed in 30 minutes

■ involvement of an experienced obstetrician in intrapartum decisions

■ no more than one dose of prostaglandin unless great vigilance is exercised

■ information about relevant symptoms to be reported to those caring for them in labour.

CEMD data

In the 2000–2002 CEMD report, maternal mortality statistics genital tract trauma accounted for one death, compared with two in 1997–1999 and five in 1994–1996.

National Institute for Health and Clinical Excellence recommendation

The NICE induction of labour guideline recommends that the induction should not occur on antenatal wards.

Hospital units need to provide:

■ local guidelines regarding the augmentation of labour

▓ local guidelines regarding the setting and standards of intrapartum fetal and maternal surveillance in women with a uterine scar.

Whenever uterine rupture occurs, it should be the subject of a departmental case review.

Training issues:

▓ All involved in intrapartum care of women must be aware of the factors that may lead to uterine rupture. In particular, they must recognise that women with a uterine scar are 'high risk' and should be managed appropriately.

▓ All involved in intrapartum care of women should undergo training in the use and interpretation of CTG.

Areas for future research:

▓ further evaluation of the risks of prostaglandin, especially repeated doses, in women with a uterine scar

▓ a national prospective study of all women labouring with a scarred uterus (SENTINEL audit)

▓ a review of all uterine ruptures.

Findings at the time of laparotomy

Lower uterine segment dehiscence is the most common current finding for rupture of the lower segment. The rupture of the lower segment may extend anteriorly into the back of the bladder or laterally towards the region of the uterine artery, or even into the broad ligament plexus of veins, causing extensive haemorrhage and damage. Posterior rupture of the uterus is uncommon and would be seen in relation to previous uterine surgery or intrauterine manipulation.

Management

Three options exist in terms of managing uterine rupture.

Total hysterectomy

Two experienced obstetricians should be present. There should be concern about the ureters (and there may be value in obtaining a postnatal renal ultrasound or intravenous urogram to check).

Subtotal hysterectomy

The choice of subtotal hysterectomy may be dictated by the individual's situation. For example, will the risks to the bladder and ureter be grave? The choice of subtotal hysterectomy in this situation would be preferable. Giwa-Osagie *et al.* reported a series of emergency obstetric hysterectomies in 61 women, of whom 37 had a ruptured uterus. The lowest mortality (4%) followed subtotal hysterectomy in booked women, while the highest mortality (50%) followed total hysterectomy in unbooked women.

Simple repair

The choice of simple uterine repair would depend on the size of the injury and on the wishes of the mother. In one series of 23 cases of ruptured uterus, hysterectomy was undertaken in 15 (65%) cases and repair in the other eight. Five successful further pregnancies were reported without repeat rupture (all delivered by caesarean section). In another Middle Eastern series of 11 cases of uterine rupture, eight had simple repair, all of whom became pregnant later and delivered by caesarean section.

26

Obstetric emergencies

Summary

- Constant vigilance, antenatal, as well as intrapartum.

- Listen to the woman.

- Anticipate complications.

- Monitor carefully.

- Respond quickly.

- Follow CESDI recommendations.

Suggested further reading

Al Sakka M, Hamsho A, Khan L. Rupture of the pregnant uterus: a 21 year review. *Int J Gynecol Obstet* 1998;63:105–8.

Enkin M. Labour and delivery following previous caesarean section. In: Chalmers I, Enkin M, Keirse MJNC, editors. *Effective Care in Pregnancy and Childbirth.* Oxford: Oxford University Press; 1989. p. 1196–215.

Fedorkow DM, Nimrod CA, Taylor PJ. Ruptured uterus in pregnancy: a Canadian hospital's experience. *CMAJ* 1987;137:27–9.

Flannelly GM, Turner MJ, Rassmussen MJ. Rupture of the uterus in Dublin; an update. *J Obstet Gynaecol* 1993;13:440–3.

Giwa-Osagie OF, Uguru V, Akinla O. Mortality and morbidity of emergency obstetric hysterectomy. *Obstet Gynaecol* 1983 4:94–6.

Leung AS, Farmer RM, Leung EK, Medearis AL, Paul RH. Risk factors associated with uterine rupture during trial of labor after cesarean delivery: a case control study. *Am J Obstet Gynecol* 1993;168:1358–63.

Leung AS, Leung EK, Paul RH. Uterine rupture after previous cesarean delivery: maternal and fetal consequences. *Am J Obstet Gynecol* 1993;169:945–50.

Neale R. Intrapartum stillbirths and deaths in infancy: the first CESDI report. In: Studd JWW, editor. *Progress in Obstetrics and Gynaecology Volume 11.* Edinburgh: Churchill Livingstone; 1996. p. 193–211.

Phelan JP, Korst LM, Settles DK. Uterine activity patterns in uterine rupture: a case–control study. *Obstet Gynecol* 1998;92:394–7.

Smith GC, Pell JP, Pasupathy D, Dobbie R. Factors predisposing to perinatal death related to uterine rupture during attempted vaginal birth after caesarean section: retrospective cohort study. *BMJ* 2004;329:375.

Soltan MH, Khashoggi T, Adelusi B. Pregnancy following rupture of the pregnant uterus. *Int J Gynecol Obstet* 1996;52:37–42.

Sweeten KM, Graves WK, Athanassiou A. Spontaneous rupture of the unscarred uterus. *Am J Obstet Gynecol* 1995;172:1851–6.

Vause S, Macintosh M. Evidence based case report: use of prostaglandins to induce labour in women with a caesarean section scar. *BMJ* 1999;318:1056–8.

Algorithm 27.1 Breech and external cephalic version

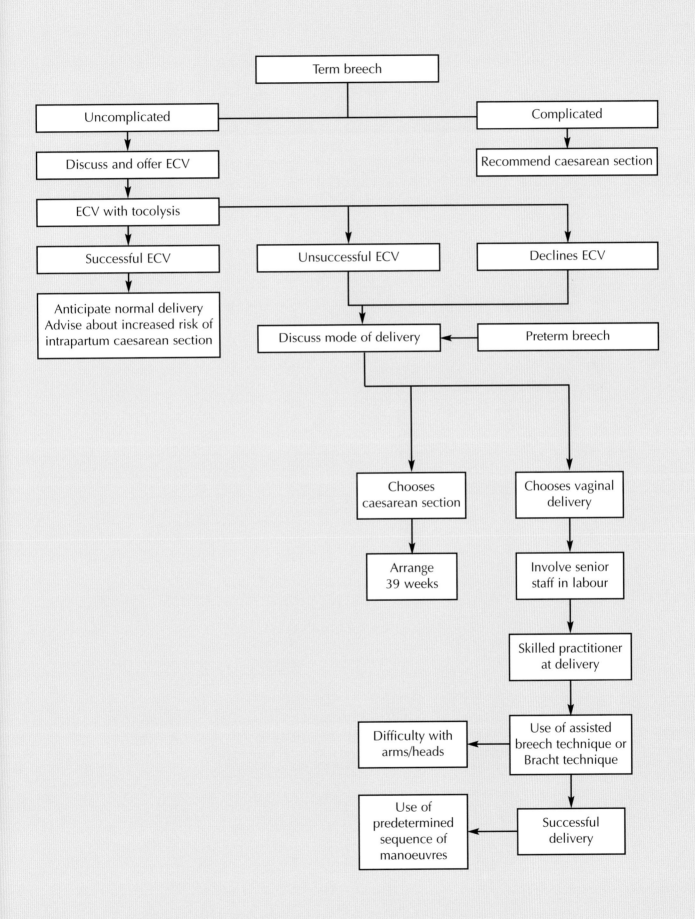

Term breech

Uncomplicated

Complicated

Discuss and offer ECV

Recommend caesarean section

ECV with tocolysis

Successful ECV

Unsuccessful ECV

Declines ECV

Anticipate normal delivery
Advise about increased risk of
intrapartum caesarean section

Discuss mode of delivery

Preterm breech

Chooses
caesarean section

Chooses vaginal
delivery

Arrange
39 weeks

Involve senior
staff in labour

Skilled practitioner
at delivery

Difficulty with
arms/heads

Use of assisted
breech technique or
Bracht technique

Use of
predetermined
sequence of
manoeuvres

Successful
delivery

27

Obstetric emergencies

Chapter 27

Breech delivery and external cephalic version

Objectives

On successfully completing this topic you will be able to:

- discuss the risks and benefits of external cephalic version
- understand the techniques of external cephalic version
- discuss the risks and benefits of vaginal breech delivery
- understand the techniques of vaginal breech birth.

Breech presentation

The incidence of breech presentation is about 20% at 28 weeks. Most fetuses turn spontaneously, so the incidence at term is 3–4%. It can be a consequence of fetal or uterine abnormality or can occur by chance. It has been widely recognised that there is higher perinatal mortality and morbidity with breech presentation, principally owing to prematurity, congenital malformation and birth asphyxia or trauma. Breech presentation, whatever the mode of delivery, is a signal for potential fetal handicap and this should inform antenatal, intrapartum and neonatal management. Caesarean section for breech presentation has been suggested as a way of reducing the associated fetal problems and in many countries in northern Europe and North America caesarean section has become the most common mode of delivery in this situation.

External cephalic version

External cephalic version (ECV) (the manipulative transabdominal conversion of the breech to cephalic presentation) has been practised since the time of Hippocrates and through the European Middle Ages to modern times though without much supporting evidence. In the late 1970s and 1980s, the procedure fell into disrepute following reports of increased perinatal mortality but subsequent trials and the decline in the choice of vaginal breech birth has led to its wide reintroduction. It has been an RCOG audit standard for some time to offer ECV to women with a diagnosed breech presentation at term.

Efficacy

ECV at term has been subjected to rigorous scientific appraisal in a number of randomised controlled trials. There is significant reduction in the risk of caesarean section in women where there is an intention to undertake ECV (OR 0.52, 95% CI 0.4–0.7) with no increased risk to the baby.

The perceived reduction in success rates in primigravid women has led to an examination of ECV before term. A systematic review of three older studies involving 900 women shows no reduction in caesarean section rate (RR 1.1, 95% CI 0.78–1.54). A more recent large pilot trial suggested a reduction in noncephalic births and caesarean section, although it did not reach statistical significance. A pragmatic trial to address this question is in progress.

ECV can be carried out in early labour with success but no randomised trials exist and studies are too small to assess safety.

ECV has been introduced successfully into practice in the UK. Although the success rate (conversion to cephalic presentation) found is less than that quoted in trials (e.g. over 80% in Africa), others have found similar success rates. Generalisation of these results in the UK would result in a significant reduction in the numbers of caesarean sections. With case selection, it is possible to achieve higher success rates and operators improve with experience. Among published US studies, an overall success rate of 65% was found.

Reversion to breech occurs after successful ECV, with between 3% and 7% being reported for term ECV. Rates of over 20% have been reported for preterm ECV.

Factors affecting success

Parity is the main factor that affects success with nulliparous success rates around one in three and multiparous success rates around two in three or greater. Amniotic fluid volume may affect success, though there is no consensus on whether there should be an absolute cut-off for attempting the procedure. Maternal weight and height affect success and fetal weight (both macrosomia and small for gestation) may be a factor. Even within the 'term' period, gestation may matter, and the degree of engagement of the fetal breech has an effect. Attempts to produce a predictive algorithm have not been helpful.

Techniques to improve success

Tocolysis and anaesthesia have been advocated to improve success rates. A Cochrane review showed a reduction in ECV failures with beta-agonist tocolysis (RR 0.74, 95% CI 0.64–0.87) and a reduction in caesarean section rate (RR 0.85, 95% CI 0.72–0.99). One further trial since this review confirms this efficacy. Others have used selective betamimetic treatment after failure of ECV without tocolysis demonstrating reduction in caesarean section rates with this approach (RR 0.33, 95% CI 0.14–0.8). Sublingual nitroglycerine was not found to be effective in the systematic review and in one subsequent large study. A trial comparing betamimetic with nitroglycerine tocolysis showed better success rates with betamimetic. One trial of fetal acoustic stimulation has shown fewer failures but this requires further study. Amnio-infusion has been advocated but there is no evidence of efficacy. Some groups have used epidural and spinal analgesia. Overall, there was no reduction in failure or caesarean section rates but there was heterogeneity of results, with the epidural studies suggesting benefit.

Alternative methods of producing cephalic version

Various postural methods such as knee–elbow, knee–chest, Indian and Zilgrie positions have been advocated. Review of clinical trials shows no increase in the rate of cephalic births.

The technique of moxibustion involves the use of burning herbs at acupoint BL 67 beside the outer corner of the fifth toenail. Although an early trial suggested an increase in cephalic presentations, a subsequent larger and better-conducted study has shown no benefit.

Complications of ECV

Systematic reviews of safety have been carried out. Transient fetal heart rate abnormalities occur in 5.7%, with persisting abnormal CTG in approximately 1/300. Placental abruption was rare, occurring in 1/1000 cases. A detailed examination of perinatal deaths in series of ECV suggests a perinatal mortality of 1.6/1000. This is not different from the perinatal mortality of pregnancies between 37 and 40 weeks.

There is a growing body of evidence that the caesarean section rate for women who have successful ECV is around twice that of cephalic-presenting pregnancies and that the vaginal operative delivery rate may also be increased. The data are sufficiently consistent that women undergoing ECV should be informed of this.

Women's views

Most women would choose ECV to allow vaginal delivery. However, some surveys have suggested that a substantial minority of eligible women would decline ECV, opting for caesarean section. In part, this may be a failure of education and uptake can be increased by well-constructed information packages.

Performance of ECV

There are no studies comparing different methods of performing ECV. Training is largely 'hands-on', although Burr et al. developed a model that has some promise.

Preparation

- Inform the woman fully of the risks, national and local success rates and about the procedure itself.
- Perform a CTG, which should be normal.
- Ultrasound examination should be carried out by a practitioner with appropriate training. The examination should determine:
  - fetal position
  - position of the legs
  - liquor volume
  - head flexion
  - it is useful to carry out an abdominal circumference measurement to exclude both small for gestation and macrosomia
  - written or informed and documented verbal consent should be obtained.
- Although serious complications are rare, the practitioner should ensure that there is immediate access to an obstetric operating theatre.
- Tocolysis, if preferred, should be given at this stage. Ritodrine hydrochloride is no longer available in the UK. Terbutaline 250 micrograms should be given by subcutaneous injection. The woman should be warned of the adverse effects and there should be no contraindications to betamimetic drugs.

Procedure

- Lay the woman flat and either on her side, with the fetal back upwards or tilted using a wedge. Some practitioners also tilt the bed, placing the woman partly head down.
- Disengagement of the fetal breech can be achieved by a number of methods, depending at present on personal preference. Most practitioners use the palmar surfaces of the fingers of both hands to gradually pull up the breech (Figure 27.1). Others use a modification of Paulik's grip to push up the breech. In some instances, an assistant may push the breech from below, if a woman or circumstances demand a more aggressive attempt at ECV.
- Some use talc or various oils. There is no evidence that the use of these influences success or comfort rates.

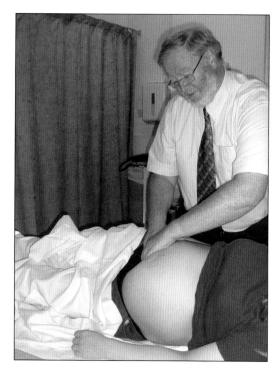 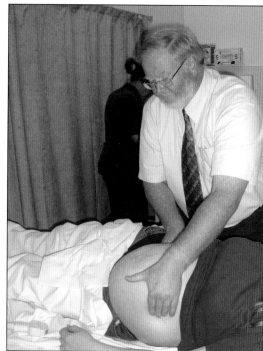

Figure 27.1 Disimpaction of the fetal breech   Figure 27.2 Flexion of the fetal head

■ Once disengaged, the breech is slowly pulled or pushed upwards and laterally to allow fetal flexion. Some practitioners rely totally on this manoeuvre, allowing the fetus to perform a forward somersault in its own time while maintaining the breech free and to the side. Others use one hand to grasp the free breech and the other to gently flex the fetal head by pressure on the occiput or nape of the neck (Figure 27.2). The hands follow the baby as he or she rotates.

■ The procedure should not be lengthy and there should be constant feedback from the woman on how uncomfortable she is. The fetal heart can be either auscultated or observed by scan if more than 2–3 minutes are needed. A maximum of three attempts can be made if the woman permits. Usually, forward somersault is the best direction but, if a third attempt is to be undertaken, a backward somersault approach can be considered. The fetal heart should be observed or auscultated between attempts.

Post-procedure

■ Whether successful or not, a repeat CTG should be performed.

■ If the woman is rhesus negative, then blood for Kleihauer estimation should be taken and 500 units of Rh immunoglobulin given.

■ If successful then spontaneous labour is awaited, and advice given on bleeding and reduced fetal movements.

■ If unsuccessful, then the reasons for this should be discussed. Arrangements can then be made either for a further attempt on another day, or for a discussion on the mode of delivery.

Vaginal breech delivery

Although the use of caesarean section as a primary choice of delivery mode for breech present-ation has been increasing in the developed world, the publication of the Term Breech Trial demonstrated clear fetal and neonatal advantages for elective caesarean section. Most subsequent large population studies have confirmed this advantage and Dutch data have shown that the alteration in practice to a higher caesarean section rate resulted in the predicted reduction in perinatal mortality. There are maternal disadvantages to a policy of caesarean section. In the UK setting, the vast majority of women balancing risks to themselves and their child choose to avoid risk to their child. In some healthcare settings, the maternal risks and culture may result in a higher proportion of women choosing vaginal breech birth at term.

There is more controversy as to whether caesarean section confers the same advantage in the preterm breech or where the second twin is breech and, at present, a policy of elective caesarean section for these indications is not justified.

As a consequence of these issues and of breech presentations being diagnosed for the first time in labour, vaginal breech birth will still occur and skill in delivering the breech will be needed.

Many of the manoeuvres used during an assisted breech delivery or Bracht manoeuvre should be used to deliver the breech at caesarean section and this, as well as formal manikin training, should be used to teach and maintain skills.

Conduct of labour

Where vaginal breech birth is being considered, ultrasound examination should be carried out to try to establish the type of breech presentation, the degree of flexion of the fetal head and the estiamted weight. If the presentation is footling (at term), if the head is hyperextended or if the estimated weight is more than 4000 g, then the woman should be advised to deliver by caesarean section and must be made aware of the additional risks should she decide to continue with planned vaginal birth.

At present, available data on complications of vaginal breech birth have derived from a hospital setting. There are a number of midwifery practitioners with experience of vaginal breech birth, using different techniques, but at present there is no published large case series data that can be used to incorporate these techniques into practice. This section will outline the conduct of a breech birth within a consultant led obstetric service.

Procedure

- On admission, senior midwifery, obstetric and anaesthetic staff should be alerted and the conduct of the labour should be supervised by the most experienced obstetrician available.

- One-to-one midwifery care with an experienced midwife should be put in place.

- If spontaneous labour, then issues of maternal and fetal surveillance should follow the same guidance as for any labour.

- Analgesia, as requested by the woman in consultation with her midwife, should be provided. There is no evidence that epidural analgesia is of specific benefit for breech labour and delivery.

- Labour can be accelerated using the normal doses of oxytocin where there is good evidence of poor uterine activity as a cause for poor progress in the first stage of labour. Evidence for and against augmentation is not robust and the decision to augment is best made at specialist level.

- Where continuous electronic fetal monitoring is used and is non-reassuring, fetal buttock sampling can be carried out but discussion at specialist level should occur if this is being considered.

- As soon as the second stage is diagnosed, a practitioner experienced in vaginal breech birth should be immediately available. The anaesthetic resident on call should be available on the delivery suite and the obstetric operating theatre free.

Conduct of the delivery

There are no recent data comparing safety or efficacy of the various techniques used in breech birth. Therefore, debates on whether classical techniques are superior to Bracht manoeuvres or whether forceps are superior to Mauriceau-Smellie-Viet techniques are simply personal debates. The last detailed comparison of Bracht techniques versus classical techniques was done in 1953 and actually recommended the Bracht technique. A study in 1991 showed no difference in neonatal outcomes comparing classical and Bracht techniques. The techniques used by midwifery practitioners are essentially derived from Bracht.

In all techniques, the avoidance of traction is the key.

Assisted breech delivery

■ Delay active pushing until the breech is distending the introitus (anus delivering).

■ Place the woman in lithotomy and perform episiotomy.

■ Initially 'hands-off'. The author, when teaching, places the stool at a distance from the maternal or manikin buttock that does not allow the operator to reach the breech. The only exception to a 'hands-off' approach is where the fetal back appears to be rotating from sacroanterior; if this occurs then it should be corrected.

■ Allow maternal effort to expel the breech to the level of the umbilicus. The back will arch towards the maternal symphysis. There is no evidence that pulling a loop of cord down at this point is of any benefit and handling of the cord produces arterial spasm and is not necessary.

■ If flexed, the legs will deliver spontaneously. If extended, it is legitimate to simply flex the hip by placing two fingers behind the thigh. No traction or handling of the rest of the baby is required.

■ Further expulsive efforts will continue to arch the fetal back. If the arms are flexed then they may deliver spontaneously. If not, they can be hooked down from the elbow. If this is not sufficient, two fingers can be passed over the shoulder to push the humerus across the chest, in a manoeuvre not dissimilar to that used in shoulder dystocia. At this point an assistant should be supporting the fetal body.

■ If the arms are extended or are behind the fetal neck, then Lovset's manoeuvre should be employed. The fetus is grasped by a femoral–pelvic grip (Figure 27.3) with the thumbs parallel along the spine. There is gentle downwards traction and the body is lifted towards the maternal symphysis. The baby is rotated through 180 degrees, bringing the posterior arm under the symphysis, where it can be hooked out by flexion of the elbow. The grip is maintained and the baby rotated back through 180 degrees to free the other arm.

■ Support the baby – do not allow it to 'hang', as this promotes head extension. Allow descent of the head within the pelvis and await the appearance of the nape of the neck. Allowing the baby to hang can promote head extension and gentle support can be provided at this stage.

■ Delivery of the head can be achieved using Wrigley's forceps or a pair of Piper forceps if you are lucky enough still to have a pair (Figure 27.4) or by the technique known as Mauriceau-Smellie-Viet. In both, an assistant is needed. Here, the baby is draped over one arm, with two fingers placed alongside the nose. The other hand is placed just under the occiput with the middle or index finger placed along the occiput (Figure 27.5). Both hands are used to promote flexion and delivery of the head.

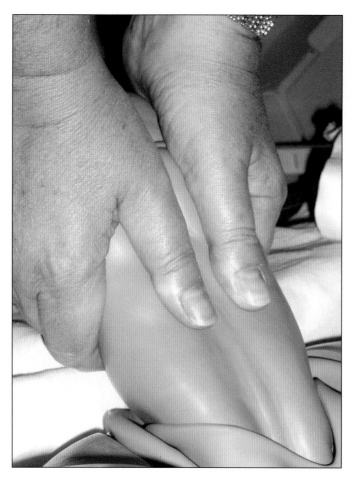

Figure 27.3 The pelvic grasp for Lovset's manoeuvre

Delivery using the Bracht technique

■ Delay active pushing until the presenting breech is distending the introitus.

■ Place the woman in lithotomy and perform episiotomy.

■ Allow delivery to the umbilicus.

■ Grasp the baby with the thumbs pressing the baby's thigh against its stomach and the rest of the hands over the sacral and loin area (Figure 27.6). While the woman is pushing, gently rotate or lift the baby around the maternal symphysis, maintaining upwards movement but without traction.

■ The legs will then deliver and, as the upwards rotation continues, the arms will follow.

■ Most practitioners of this technique also advise an assistant providing gentle but persistent pressure on the maternal abdomen to push the head downwards.

■ Where the arms do not follow then, though a range of manoeuvres are described by practitioners of the Bracht technique, it seems simplest to revert to the manoeuvres described above.

■ With continued upwards rotation the head may deliver spontaneously, not unlike the descriptions of the Burns-Marshall technique (Figure 27.7). If the head does not deliver then either forceps or the Mauriceau-Smellie-Viet procedure can be used.

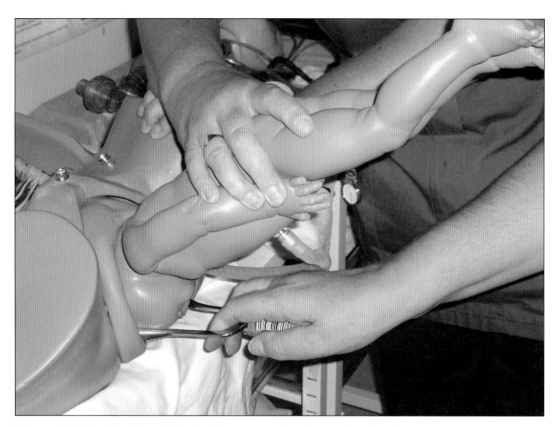

Figure 27.4 Application of Wrigley's forceps to the aftercoming head

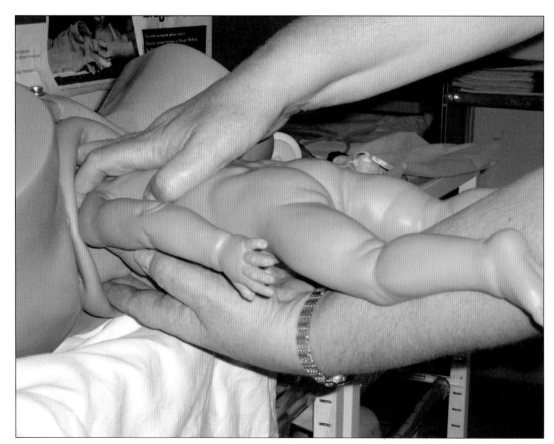

Figure 27.5 Mauriceau-Smellie-Viet manoeuvre

Failure to deliver

The great fear of vaginal breech delivery is head entrapment or nuchal arms that significantly delay delivery. Most experienced obstetricians will have dealt with each of these but experience is decreasing. Like any rare, unpredictable obstetric emergency, clinicians should have a plan or drill that they follow. There is no literature, other than case reports or small series to guide practice.

Nuchal arms

- Recognise nuchal arms by the fact that the shoulder is extended and the elbow flexed.

- Try Lovset's manoeuvre.

- If this fails, grasp the fetal feet. Rotate (swing) the fetus towards the hand of the posterior nuchal arm and above the level of the maternal symphysis. This may result in delivery of the posterior arm but, if not, it allows room for the occiput to slip below the elbow. A hand can be placed over the shoulder and behind the humerus to allow pressure on the humerus with delivery in front of the face.

- If the other arm does not deliver after this, then the procedure can be repeated.

- If this fails then time is important. It may be possible with the back anterior to insert a hand to grab the elbow of one arm and exert sufficient pressure to correct the shoulder extension, allowing reuse of Lovset's manoeuvre. If this fails then it is legitimate, in the author's opinion, to force the arm across the face to deliver. Humeral or clavicular fractures are very likely but will not cause long-term harm; perinatal hypoxia does.

Head entrapment

Intriguingly few recent texts mention how to deal with this when it occurs, merely providing advice on how to avoid it.

- Ensure adequate midwifery and anaesthetic support; prepare for immediate caesarean section; if available call for symphysiotomy equipment.

- Try to perform Mauriceau-Smellie-Viet manoeuvre if it is felt the head has entered the pelvis. Suprapubic pressure may also be worth considering, as in shoulder dystocia.

- Rotate the fetal body to a lateral position. Apply suprapubic pressure to flex head. Apply traction then rotation back to sacroanterior and deliver by forceps.

- Check that the cervix is still fully dilated, especially if preterm. If not, then incise at 4 and 8 o'clock.

- McRoberts' position.

- Attempt mid-cavity forceps if good analgesia is available.

- Perform symphysiotomy if you have adequate training; if not, then you should now be in a position to carry out caesarean section in the room if the baby is still alive. The baby needs to be pushed from below. The use of the ventouse has been described to assist.

Breech extraction

Breech extraction is most commonly used for the delivery of the second twin, though the technique is needed for delivery of an abnormal lie at caesarean section.

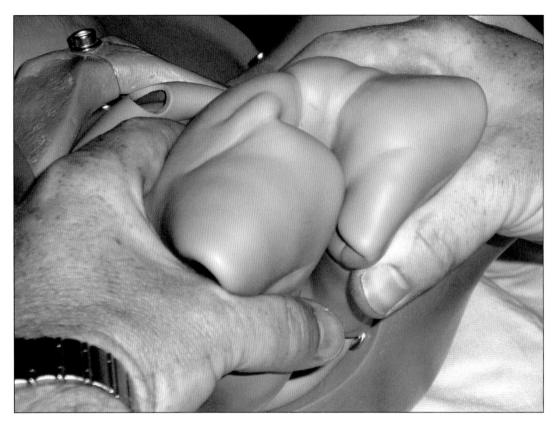

Figure 27.6 Initial placement of hands for Bracht technique

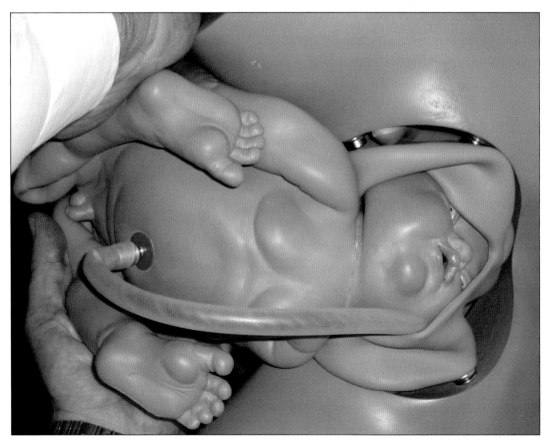

Figure 27.7 Delivery of the head by Bracht technique

Current evidence suggests that internal version and breech extraction of the second twin is superior to external version, with no differences in neonatal outcome and less likelihood of failure and caesarean section. There are few data on whether primary caesarean section for the abnormally presenting second twin confers any advantage for the infant.

There is no evidence that any single method of breech extraction or combination is superior to another.

Conduct of breech extraction

- The presence of a practitioner competent in the procedure is necessary; if there is not one present, then attempt ECV.

- Perform continuous monitoring of the fetal heart rate.

- Immediate access to obstetric theatre should be available.

- Ultrasound examination by a competent practitioner should be available.

- Good analgesia or anaesthesia is essential. Tocolysis may be necessary and should be available.

- One or preferably both feet are grasped through the membranes and gentle continuous traction started towards the introitus. This can be practised at caesarean section for abnormal lie.

- Either with the other hand or another operator, guide and stabilise the fetal head into the midline. Maintain a degree of pressure towards the pelvic inlet with this hand.

- Membrane rupture is left as late at possible. It should not occur until the feet are below the ischial spines and the lie is clearly longitudinal. Many prefer to wait until the foot is at or beyond the introitus.

- Once the fetus is delivered to the umbilicus, either assisted breech or Bracht techniques can be used.

- It is useful to maintain some pressure on the fetal head to guide it into the pelvis during these procedures.

Medico-legal issues

Medico-legal issues are increasingly rare for the singleton breech in the UK, as most breech presentations who decline or fail version choose caesarean section. However, if proper delivery techniques are not employed at caesarean section, trauma can result and this can lead to medico-legal issues.

Where vaginal breech delivery is to occur at any gestation, consultant or specialist input at every point in the decision process is vital. Although the literature is not supportive of absolute rules on oxytocin, continuous electronic monitoring, fetal buttock sampling and epidural analgesia, these are regarded by some practitioners as unacceptable practice. If these are being considered, the decision and discussions should be taking place at the most senior level.

For UK-trained practitioners, competence is now an issue. Even consultant or specialist-level staff may have little experience or confidence at conducting a vaginal breech birth and they should ensure the availability of other colleagues if necessary.

Although virtually all literature to date states that breech extraction of the second twin is superior to all other options, there is a perception among some that it is less safe. With decreasing skills, if there is insufficient time to allow an appropriately trained practitioner to be present, ECV or caesarean section may be a better risk management option.

Audit

■ The RCOG recommendations for audit are that 'all women with an uncomplicated breech presentation at term should be offered ECV'.

■ Maintain statistics on ECV success rates; annual comparison with predicted success rates.

■ All practitioners should maintain a record of competence or training in vaginal breech delivery.

■ The rate of caesarean section for the second twin should be monitored.

Summary

■ Offer and encourage ECV at term.

■ There is no simple algorithm for predicting ECV success.

■ Tocolysis with a betamimetic drug appears to increase ECV success rates.

■ Where vaginal breech birth is chosen, ensure early involvement of consultant staff in labour.

■ Assisted breech delivery or Bracht manoeuvre may be equally effective.

■ Ensure that drill for nuchal arms and entrapped head is in place.

■ Maintain competencies through practice at caesarean delivery for breech and through regular manikin training.

■ Audit uptake and success rates of ECV.

Suggested further reading

Chan LY, Leung TY, Fok WY, Chan LW, Lau TK. Prediction of successful vaginal delivery in women undergoing external cephalic version at term for breech presentation. *Eur J Obstet Gynecol Reprod Biol* 2004;116,39–42.

Chan LY, Tang JL, Tsoi KF, Fok WY, Chan LW, Lau TK. Intrapartum caesarean delivery after successful external cephalic version: a meta-analysis. *Obstet Gynecol* 2004;104:155–60.

Chauhan SP, Roberts WE, McLaren RA, Roach H, Morrison JC, Martin JN. Delivery of the nonvertex second twin: breech extraction versus external cephalic version. *Am J Obstet Gynecol* 1995;173:1015–20.

Cheng M, Hannah M. Breech delivery at term: a critical review of the literature. *Obstet Gynecol* 1993;82:605–18.

Collaris RJ, Guid Oei S. External cephalic version: a safe procedure? A systematic review of version-related risks. *Acta Obstet Gynecol Scand* 2004;83:511–18.

Edelstone DI. Breech presentation. In: Kean LH, Baker PN, Edelstone DI, editors. *Best Practice Labour Ward Management.* London: WB Saunders; 2000. p. 142–65.

Hannah ME, Hannah WJ, Hewson SA, Hodnett ED, Saigal S, Willan AR, for the TBT Group planned caesarean section versus planned vaginal birth for breech presentation at term: a randomised multicentre trial. *Lancet* 2000;356:1375–83.

Hofmeyr GJ. External cephalic version for breech presentation before term. *Cochrane Database Syst Rev* 2000;(2):CD000084.

Hofmeyr GJ, Gyte G. Interventions to help external cephalic version for breech presentation at term. *Cochrane Database Syst Rev* 2004;(1):CD000184.

Hofmeyr GJ, Kulier R. External cephalic version for breech presentation at term. *Cochrane Database Syst Rev* 2002;(2):CD000184.

Impey L, Pandit M. Tocolysis for repeat external cephalic version in breech presentation at term: a randomised, double-blinded, placebo-controlled trial. *BJOG* 2005;112:627–31.

Mukhopadhyay S, Arulkumaran S. Breech delivery. *Best Pract Res Clin Obstet Gynaecol* 2002;16:31–42.

Rabinovici J, Barkai G, Reichman B, Serr DM, Mashiach S. Internal podalic version with unruptured membranes for the second twin in transverse lie. *Obstet Gynecol* 1988;71:428–30.

Yogev Y, Horowitz E, Ben-Haroush A, Chen R, Kaplan B. Changing attitudes toward mode of delivery and external cephalic version in breech presentations. *Int J Gynecol Obstet* 2002;79:221–4.

Zhang J, Bowes WA, Fortney JA. Efficacy of external cephalic version: a review. *Obstet Gynecol* 1993;82:306–12.

27

Obstetric emergencies

Algorithm 28.1 **Prerequisites for instrumental vaginal delivery**

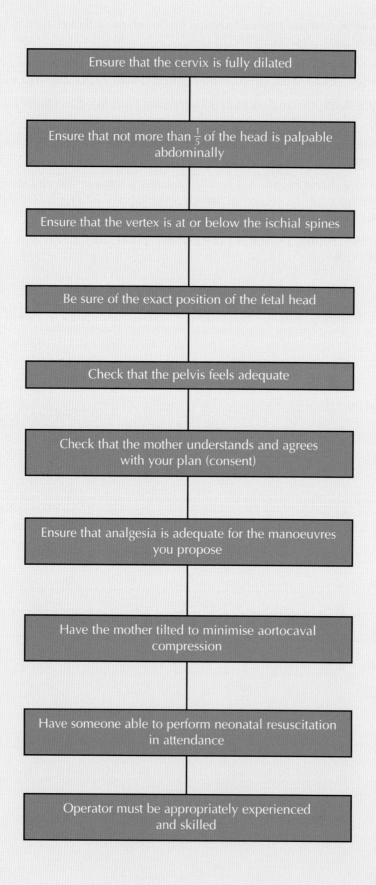

Ensure that the cervix is fully dilated

Ensure that not more than $\frac{1}{5}$ of the head is palpable abdominally

Ensure that the vertex is at or below the ischial spines

Be sure of the exact position of the fetal head

Check that the pelvis feels adequate

Check that the mother understands and agrees with your plan (consent)

Ensure that analgesia is adequate for the manoeuvres you propose

Have the mother tilted to minimise aortocaval compression

Have someone able to perform neonatal resuscitation in attendance

Operator must be appropriately experienced and skilled

Algorithm 28.2 **Rules for safety when conducting ventouse delivery**

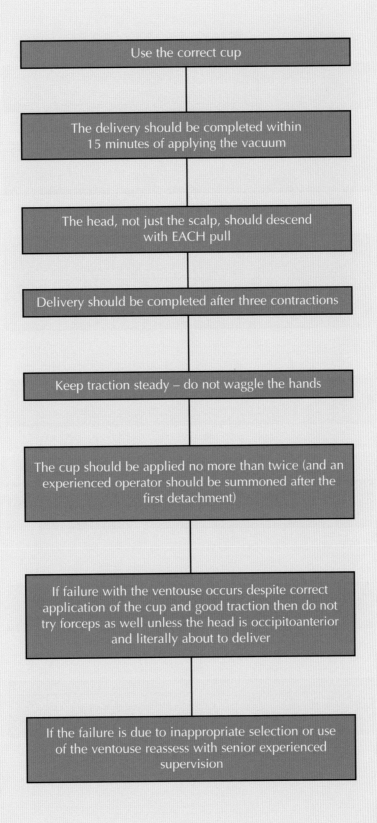

Use the correct cup

The delivery should be completed within 15 minutes of applying the vacuum

The head, not just the scalp, should descend with EACH pull

Delivery should be completed after three contractions

Keep traction steady – do not waggle the hands

The cup should be applied no more than twice (and an experienced operator should be summoned after the first detachment)

If failure with the ventouse occurs despite correct application of the cup and good traction then do not try forceps as well unless the head is occipitoanterior and literally about to deliver

If the failure is due to inappropriate selection or use of the ventouse reassess with senior experienced supervision

Algorithm 28.3 **Rules for safety when conducting forceps delivery**

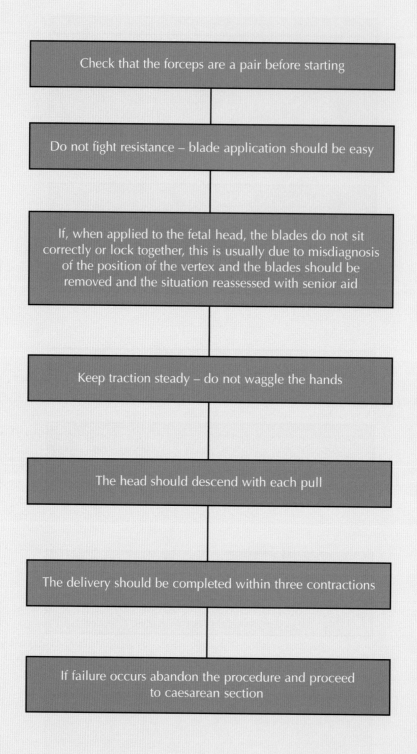

Check that the forceps are a pair before starting

Do not fight resistance – blade application should be easy

If, when applied to the fetal head, the blades do not sit correctly or lock together, this is usually due to misdiagnosis of the position of the vertex and the blades should be removed and the situation reassessed with senior aid

Keep traction steady – do not waggle the hands

The head should descend with each pull

The delivery should be completed within three contractions

If failure occurs abandon the procedure and proceed to caesarean section

Chapter 28

Ventouse and forceps delivery

Objectives

On successfully completing this topic you will be able to:

■ decide when an instrumental delivery is appropriate

■ decide which instrument is most appropriate in a specific circumstance

■ appreciate the techniques required for vacuum and forceps delivery

■ recognise and appreciate the causes of failure to deliver with the instrument selected

■ know what to do when the instrumental delivery has failed.

Introduction

Instrumental vaginal deliveries expedite the delivery of a baby who is believed to be at risk of compromise or when the mother is unable to push it out herself. Worldwide, assisted vaginal delivery remains an integral part of the obstetrician's duties. Rates vary from 1.5% of deliveries (Czech Republic) to 15% (Australia and Canada) and from 9% to 13% regionally in the UK. These varying rates reflect not only different clinical practices but also different attitudes. Low operative vaginal delivery rates may reflect high caesarean section rates, including those performed at full dilatation because of a reluctance to perform instrumental deliveries. Although instrumental vaginal delivery can be hazardous and should be undertaken with care, the difficulty of caesarean section at full dilatation should not be underestimated; it can be extremely difficult and is associated with high maternal morbidity.

Women who labour are, by definition, aiming for vaginal delivery and therefore efforts should be focused on helping them to achieve this normally and safely. Various techniques may help in achieving high spontaneous vaginal delivery rates, such as the use of a partogram, companionship in labour, delaying pushing in women who have had epidural anaesthesia, upright posture and active management of the second stage of labour using oxytocin in nulliparae with epidurals.

Indications for operative vaginal delivery

■ Delay in the second stage of labour.

■ Fetal compromise in the second stage of labour.

■ Maternal conditions which require either a short second stage or avoidance of Valsalva.

Prerequisites for operative vaginal delivery

Clinical examination should include both abdominal palpation and vaginal examination:

- the fetal head should not be palpable abdominally
- the cervix should be fully dilated
- the vertex (bone, not caput) should be at or below the ischial spines
- the exact position of the fetal head should be established
- the pelvis should feel adequate.

Informed consent is needed: check that the mother understands and agrees with your plan.

Adequate analgesia is needed but this will vary according to the type of delivery proposed, as discussed below.

Make sure the woman is tilted to minimise aortocaval compression during the procedure (this is best achieved by placing a wedge underneath her right hip).

Someone should be in attendance who is capable of performing neonatal resuscitation.

The operator must be appropriately experienced and skilled.

Safety issues and choice of instrument

When an assisted vaginal delivery is contemplated, careful clinical assessment is vital in order to confirm whether it is appropriate to proceed and to select the most suitable instrument. The different types of ventouse and forceps instruments both have their advantages and disadvantages. Promoting one type over another is inappropriate, as the instrument most suited for the situation at hand, with which the operator is experienced and skilled, is what matters to each individual mother and baby. The advantage of the ventouse cup over forceps relates to them being associated with significantly less maternal trauma and requiring less analgesia but they are more likely to cause fetal cephalohaematoma and retinal haemorrhage. In addition, ventouse deliveries are significantly more likely to fail than forceps deliveries. Using a combination of instruments is associated with increased complications. It is best to choose one likely to achieve success.

Different types of ventouse and forceps instruments are available to deal with lift out and rotational deliveries but the rotational deliveries require particular skills, especially when using forceps. Kjelland forceps have been known to be associated with traumatic deliveries for a long time but, in skilled hands, the overall rates of morbidity are low and can avoid the trauma associated with caesarean section at full dilatation. Whichever instrument is selected, the operator must be experienced and skilled in its use (or be supervised directly by someone who is). In all cases, as mentioned above, the exact position of the baby's head must be established before proceeding. It is universally acknowledged that the tendency to put a ventouse on a baby because the position is not clear is totally unacceptable and dangerous. One study demonstrated that 17 of 64 (27%) fetal head positions diagnosed clinically on digital vaginal examination were incorrect when checked with ultrasound and continued vigilance, training and supervision in this area is urgently needed.

Conditions where ventouse should be preferred to forceps

■ Urgent delivery required with no previous analgesia when a low lift out, easy delivery is anticipated.

■ Low lift out delivery, especially if there has been no prior analgesia.

■ Rotational delivery, if operator has inadequate experience with Kjelland forceps.

■ Operator or maternal preference, when either instrument would be suitable.

Conditions where forceps should be preferred to ventouse

■ Face presentation.

■ Aftercoming head of the breech.

■ Marked active bleeding from a fetal blood-sampling site.

■ Gestation of less than 34 weeks (between 34 and 36 weeks the ventouse is 'relatively' contraindicated).

■ Large amount of caput.

■ Mother who is unable or unwilling to push.

■ Operator or maternal preference when either instrument would be suitable.

Ventouse

There are a number of soft cups in common use which are smoothly applied to the contour of the baby's head and do not develop a 'chignon'. The vacuum achieved is particularly poor when soft cups are applied to moderate or severe caput (as adhesion to folds of oedematous skin is poor). In addition, they have limited manoeuvrability and cannot be correctly placed when the head is deflexed. Consequently, soft cups have a poorer success rate than metal cups but are less likely to be associated with scalp trauma. Being soft, they are easy to apply and unlikely to injure the mother. As they are cleaned and sterilised as one item, they present no problems with assembly or leakage.

The metal cups most widely used are the 'Bird-modification' cups. These have a central traction chain and a separate vacuum pipe. The anterior cups come in 4-, 5- and 6-cm sizes. The posterior cup is 5 cm in diameter and has either the standard chain or the new cord for traction. The posterior cup is designed to be inserted higher up in the vagina than the anterior cups, to allow correct placement when the head is deflexed.

It has been shown that successful delivery is most likely with the ventouse when the cup is applied over the flexion point, which lies in the midline just in front of the posterior fontanelle. A cup is ideally positioned when it covers the posterior fontanelle with the sagittal suture pointing to the centre of the cup. A well-placed cup will result in a well-flexed head (Figure 28.1), while failure to put the cup far enough back will result in deflexion.

Safe delivery with the ventouse

To minimise the chances of any fetal damage the basic rules for delivery with the ventouse should be followed. Overall, the risks of perinatal trauma using the vacuum extractor correlate with the duration of application, the station of the fetal head at the commencement of the delivery, the degree of difficulty of the delivery and the condition of the baby at the time of commencement of the procedure. When contemplating using the ventouse, in addition to the factors mentioned above, it is particularly important that there are good uterine contractions and

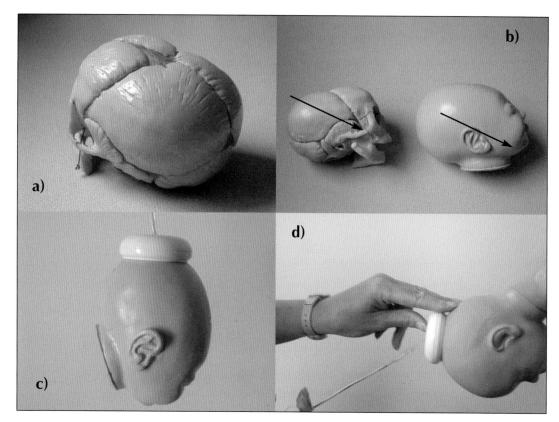

Figure 28.1 Ventouse; a) note how far back to the posterior fontanelle is; b) note the axis through the flexion point, which results in the smallest presenting diameter; c) the ventouse cup applied over the flexion point; d) traction (along the pelvic axis) and the three-finger grip of the ventouse cup with the second hand

that the mother is fully cooperative and able and willing to push. It is the author's opinion that the increasing tendency to perform operative deliveries in theatre as 'trials' (which are conducted under dense regional blockade with associated significant compromise to maternal efforts) are increasing the likelihood of failures with these instruments.

Basic rules for safe use of the ventouse

1. The delivery should be completed within 15 minutes of application of the vacuum (15 minutes is given as the maximum time allowed for application but the average time from insertion of the cup to delivery in over 400 deliveries was 6 minutes).

2. The head, not just the scalp, should descend with each pull.

3. Delivery should be complete within three pulls (if the head is crowning a fourth pull is allowed).

4. Keep the hands steady during traction – do not waggle, as this increases scalp trauma.

5. The cup should be reapplied no more than twice (and after one detachment an experienced operator should be summoned).

6. If failure with the ventouse occurs despite good cup placement and good traction, do not try the forceps as well.

Method

There is no need to catheterise the woman (unless there is another indication, such as epidural anaesthesia). No additional anaesthesia is required (perineal infiltration will suffice if an episiotomy is needed). Lithotomy is the most common position used (and should be used with lateral tilt) but delivery may be possible in dorsal, lateral or squatting positions.

Examine the woman carefully. Estimate the size of the baby by abdominal examination and ensure that the head is fully engaged (none of the head should be palpable). Confirm vertex presentation, position and the amount of caput through vaginal examination. Describe the attitude of the presenting part as 'flexed' or 'deflexed' (any situation where the anterior fontanelle can be felt easily) and take note of any asynctisim.

The appropriate cup should be chosen.

■ The **silicone rubber cup** can be used with any well-flexed vertex presentation, as long as the mother is cooperative, the baby is average-sized and there is minimal caput (i.e. by pressing firmly all details of the cranium should be felt, the skin will not be deep and will feel only slightly spongy). This cup is rarely suitable for occipitolateral positions, as the asynclitism associated with them tends to make placement of this cup over the posterior fontanelle difficult.

■ The **anterior metal cup** should be chosen if the baby is big, if the second stage is prolonged and if there is a moderate degree or more of caput (the skin may feel deep, may be folded and will definitely be spongy). It may also be used if the head is only slightly deflexed or slightly rotated, provided correct cup placement can be achieved. The 6-cm cup is preferable to the 5-cm cup because it allows greater traction without increasing the risk of scalp trauma. Only where the vagina is narrow should the 5-cm cup be used. The small 4-cm cup is reserved for use with the second twin, particularly if the cervix is no longer fully dilated.

■ The most valuable **posterior metal cup**, as its name indicates, is used for occipito-posterior positions, but also for occipito-lateral positions. It is particularly useful in situations with significant asynclitism and/or deflexion.

Once the correct cup has been chosen and connected to its pump as required (electric or hand) a check should be made for leakages prior to commencing the delivery. Common problems include suction bottles not tightly screwed in or tubing loosely attached to the metal cups (not locked with the small plastic ring). The metal cups should have a meshed bottom plate, which functions to maintain a clear space between the scalp and the cup so that an effective vacuum can be applied.

Silicone rubber cup

The silicone rubber cup is used in the following manner: it is folded and gently inserted into the vagina with one hand from above downwards, while the other hand parts the labia. A gentle twist may help it to unfold into place in the vagina and thereafter it is essentially not manoeuvrable, being larger in diameter than the metal cup and having a relatively inflexible handle.

Take the pressure up to $0.2\,kg/cm^2$, check that no maternal tissue is caught under the cup and then continue directly to $0.8\,kg/cm^2$, beginning traction with the next contraction after this pressure has been achieved. Where gentle to moderate traction is required it is reasonable to take the pressure to $0.6\,kg/cm^2$ and in those rare situations where deliveries are undertaken between 34 and 36 weeks it may suffice to stop at $0.4\,kg/cm^2$.

Traction should be along the pelvic axis for the duration of the contraction. One hand should rest on the bell of the cup (Figure 28.1) while the other applies traction. Malmstrom said 'Vacuum extraction is a matter of cooperation between the traction hand and the backward-pressing hand'. The hand on the cup detects any early detachment and also indicates whether the head moves downwards with each pull. The fingers on the head can promote flexion and can help to guide the head under the arch of the pubis by using the space in front of the sacrum. As the head crowns, the angle of traction changes through an arc of over 90 degrees but the fetal head should guide the hands, not the other way around: raising the hands too early causes extension of the fetal head, increasing the diameter of the presenting part. This, in turn, increases the risk of trauma to the perineum and can cause cup detachment.

At this point, if necessary, an episiotomy can be cut but if the perineum is stretching as normal, it is simply supported with the hand that was on the bell. Occasionally, an edge of the cup might lift off at the introitus (this is more likely to happen if there is caput present or if the hands have been raised too early). If this occurs, you must be careful not to catch maternal tissue under the cup as it reattaches, and thus this should be rechecked before final delivery of the head.

Anterior metal cup

The metal cup is lightly lubricated and then inserted sideways into the vagina. To orientate the cup, make sure the chain and vacuum pipe lie centrally over the posterior fontanelle. Check that no maternal tissue is included at low pressure then traction can commence once a negative pressure of $0.8\,kg/cm^2$ has been achieved. Otherwise, the controlled two-handed manner of delivery is similar to that described for the soft cup above, classically using the 'three-finger grip' for the fingers on the cup and head (Figure 28.1). This not only helps to confirm that the fetal head and not just the scalp is descending but also the fingers apply a force which opposes the lifting tendency of the upper edge of the rigid cup when pulling downwards earlier in the delivery and which oppose the lifting tendency of the lower edge when pulling upwards at the end of the delivery.

Posterior metal cup

When confronted with a deflexed head in an occipitoposterior position, the 'OP' cup should be used. It is applied as far back on the head as possible, again aiming to lie in the midline over the posterior fontanelle. To allow good placement of the cup, it sometimes helps to try to flex the head, with two fingers of the left hand pressing on the sinciput, while the right hand inserts the cup behind the head. Once correctly placed, the vacuum can be started and taken directly to the required level (because the cup lies parallel to the vagina it is unlikely to catch any maternal tissue).

The first pull will be in the direction required to flex the head and with this flexion the presenting diameter immediately becomes smaller. Thereafter, traction should be along the pelvic axis. The delivery may be completed simply by a standard spontaneous rotation with maternal effort and gentle assistance. It is important not to try to twist the cup to rotate the baby as this can increase scalp injuries.

Difficulty is sometimes encountered once the head flexes, as the suction pipe can tend to kink, making it more likely to detach. If the cup detaches at this point (after flexion and rotation) it may be simplest to change to an anterior cup or, if speed is essential, to perform a lift-out forceps.

Avoiding failure with the ventouse

Failure rates reported in the literature vary enormously but studies report rates from 6% to as much as 20–30%. There is increasing concern that failure rates are rising and with the evidence that caesarean sections in second stage are associated with significant morbidity attention to technique is vital. The following factors contribute to ventouse failure:

■ **inadequate initial assessment of the case: the head is too high**
  A classic mistake is to assume that because caput can be felt below the ischial spines the head must be engaged – always palpate the abdomen carefully.

■ **misdiagnosis of the position and attitude of the head**
Attention to simple detail will minimise the occurrence of this problem.

■ **incorrect instrument selected**
Failures with the silicone rubber cup will be common if it is used inappropriately when there is deflexion of the head, excess caput, a big baby, a prolonged second stage of labour or an uncooperative mother.

■ **either anterior or lateral placements of the cup will increase the failure rate**
Anterior placements are also more likely to be associated with fetal injury. In this respect, preterm infants are more vulnerable (even greater care should be taken to check position before application in these cases). If the cup placement is found to be incorrect, it may be appropriate to begin again with correct placement: mid-line over the posterior fontanelle or change to forceps.

■ **failures due to traction in the wrong direction**
These may be amenable simply to a change in angle of traction.

■ **excessive caput**
Rarely, even with the metal cups, adequate traction is not possible because of excessive caput and forceps may be more appropriate.

■ **poor maternal effort**
There is no doubt that maternal effort can contribute substantially to the success of the delivery. Adequate encouragement and instruction should be given to the mother.

■ **the incidence of cephalopelvic disproportion (true failure) is low**.

Special indications for ventouse delivery

The use of the ventouse in the first stage of labour has lost favour since two maternal deaths were reported on and reviewed in a recent Confidential Enquiry. If it is ever to be contemplated, all other prerequisites for ventouse delivery should be fulfilled. Use before full dilatation should be reserved for acute fetal distress (e.g. abruption), where a straightforward normal delivery would have been expected within the next half hour. Nevertheless, this is a potentially dangerous practice and should only be undertaken by an experienced operator.

In the hands of an experienced operator the ventouse can also be used to expedite delivery complicated by a prolapsed cord at full dilatation and for delivery of the second twin with fetal distress, (thereby avoiding a caesarean section).

Forceps

There are over 700 different makes of forceps. Most authors subscribe to a classification system that divides forceps into classic and specialised subtypes. Classic subtypes that are traction in design include Simpson, Anderson and Neville-Barnes forceps, while specialised forceps include Kjelland (for rotation) and Piper (for the aftercoming head of the breech). Variations in cephalic curvature, fenestration and design of shank allow selection to be made on the basis of individual circumstances. There have been no randomised controlled trials comparing different types of forceps and it is recognised that the choice is often subjective. One RCT was identified; in this study decreased facial marking was found when soft blade pads were used.

Safe delivery with forceps

It is important that the practitioner is comfortable with and skilled in the use of the instrument selected and that adequate supervision is available as required. To minimise morbidity the prerequisites for any instrumental delivery should be followed and particular points of safety for forceps delivery should be respected.

Basic rules for safe use of the forceps

■ Check the forceps are a pair before starting. This is done by locking them together and checking that they produce a symmetrical neat fit. It is also useful to check the maximum diameter between the two blades (a pair that is not true will have maximum diameter as little as 7 cm or 7.5 cm. The maximum diameter should be at least 9 cm).

■ If there is resistance when trying to apply the blades or if, when applied to the fetal head, the blades do not sit correctly or lock together, this is usually due to misdiagnosis of the position of the vertex and the blades should be removed and the situation reassessed with senior aid.

■ The head should descend with each pull.

■ Traction should be steady and the hands should not waggle, as this risks fetal injury.

■ The delivery should be completed within three contractions.

■ If failure occurs, abandon the procedure and proceed to caesarean section.

Method of delivery with traction forceps

The woman is placed in lithotomy and tilted by means of a wedge under the right hip.

An in–out catheterisation is required to empty the bladder prior to forceps delivery. Checks that the forceps are a pair.

The blades should be applied in turn when the uterus is relaxed between contractions with one hand guiding the blade in (while following in from the line of the contralateral femur) while the other protects the maternal soft tissues. If the blades do not insert easily then they should be removed and the situation reassessed with senior aid: there is no place for forcing the blades.

Once applied the blades should lock together easily (no force should be needed to achieve this) and their position should be checked relative to the fetal landmarks (Figure 28.2)

Traction during a contraction attempts to follow the pelvic curve by using Pajot's manoeuvre, which involves two separate components: the dominant hand applies traction while the other hand gently presses downwards on the shank of the forceps (Figure 28.3). The strength of the left hand is crucial to successful and safe delivery: too strong a left hand increases perineal trauma and too weak a left hand means the traction is transmitted too anteriorly – i.e. up against the bladder – causing inefficiency, possible failure and possible bladder trauma. This latter effect is also produced if the direction of traction is too vertical.

The timing of the episiotomy should be when the perineum has thinned out and once the operator is totally confident the delivery is going to be completed successfully.

As the head crowns, the hands will need to rise up but, as for ventouse delivery, they should follow the head, not lead it, to minimise perineal trauma.

Special indications for forceps delivery

Rotation

Rotational delivery for occipitotransverse or occipitoposterior positions can be effected following manual rotation or using a suitable ventouse cup as described above. However, Kjelland forceps still have an important place in operative obstetrics for rotational deliveries but they do require special expertise.

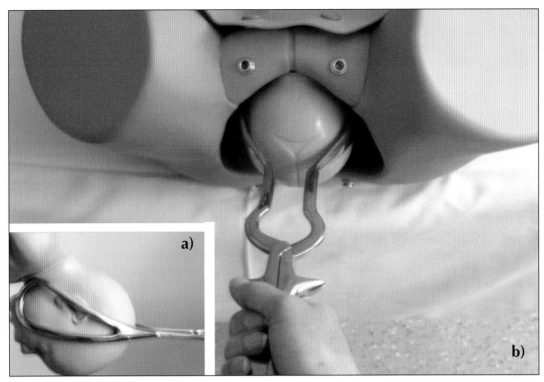

Figure 28.2 Forceps: a) correct forceps application; b) the forceps blades should lock adjacent to the lamboidal sutures and equi-distant from them on each side – always check the bony landmarks after forceps application and before traction

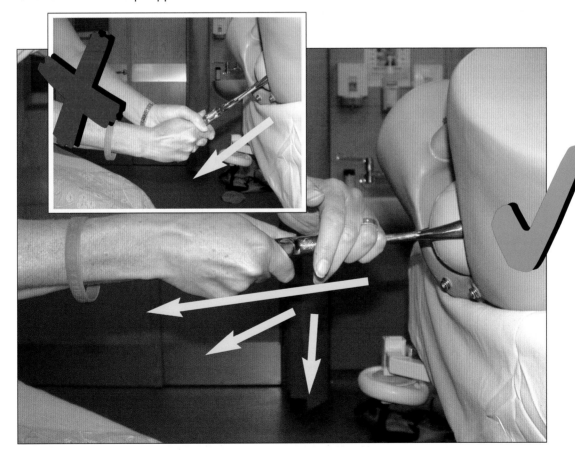

Figure 28.3 Direction of traction: dominant hand applies traction along the axis of the forceps blades while the second hand applies downward pressure on the shank of the blades; this produces a resultant direction of traction in line with the pelvic axis (Pajot's manoeuvre)

Be especially careful in the abdominal palpation to identify which side of the mother the baby's back is lying, as this will define which direction (clockwise or anticlockwise) that the baby's head should be rotated. When occiput and fetal back are on the same side direction of rotation is obvious but when they lie on opposite sides (sometimes seen with occipitoposterior positions) the occiput should be rotated towards the fetal back to avoid traction on the fetal neck (e.g. left occipitoposterior and fetal back on maternal right then rotation should occur clockwise ie the long way round).

Check that the blades are a pair. The blades are applied ensuring that the nipple on the shank is facing towards the occiput.

Blade application is achieved during uterine relaxation between contractions:

■ with occipitoposterior positions the blades are applied directly

■ with occipitotransverse positions the blade destined to lie anteriorly is applied first and usually wandered over from the lateral position across the brow. It should not be inserted far enough such that it ends up wandering over the face. Particular attention to this point should be made in training and supervising this technique. The posterior blade is then applied directly and negotiating the coccyx is usually the technically demanding part of this step.

Once the blades are applied they should be gently approximated and the lock engaged but rather than clasping the handles together as is done with other types of forceps (which compresses the Kjelland blades) they should be held with the thumb between the handles which serves to fix the blades together without squashing them (Figure 28.4). Their position relative to the fetal landmarks should be confirmed.

Once locked together, the handles are very likely to lie slightly removed from each other (enabled by the sliding lock on Kjelland) due to asynclitism. This is normal and attempts should not be made to force them to correct, as this should occur naturally as rotation is completed and asynclitism resolved.

Rotation should be attempted between contractions when the uterus is relaxed and the force required should be minimal. This is a feeling technique, it should never be forced and is usually achieved by lowering the hands and angling the forceps to encourage flexion of the head at the same time as rotation.

If a contraction develops during rotation, further movement should cease until it relaxes again but keep gentle hold of the handles of the forceps otherwise they tend to drift.

Once rotation is complete it is imperative that the fetal head is palpated to check its position and to confirm it is now occipitoanterior. The blades can slip round the fetal head and traction must not be applied until the operator is confident that this has not occurred.

Traction then proceeds as for a normal forceps delivery but taking care to maintain the safe Kjelland grip.

Face presentation

Face presentation is covered in Chapter 25, but it is noteworthy to reiterate that it is essential to judge the station of the head prior to embarking on a forceps assisted mentoanterior delivery. The head in these circumstances is always higher than one thinks and not only is careful abdominal palpation crucial but a careful vaginal examination is mandatory. If vaginal examination reveals a hollow sacrum then the head is not fully engaged and vaginal delivery is not appropriate.

The aftercoming head of the breech

The Piper forceps were designed for this manoeuvre but any traction forceps can be used. The breech delivery is covered in Chapter 27 and, as mentioned, forceps may not be needed but, if required, their principle of application and direction of traction is similar to that described above.

Obstetric emergencies

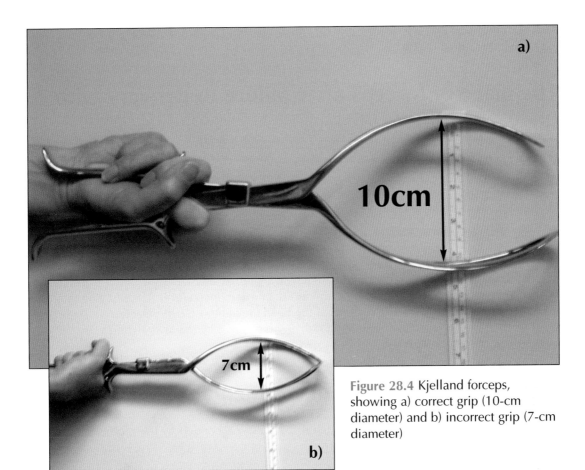

Figure 28.4 Kjelland forceps, showing a) correct grip (10-cm diameter) and b) incorrect grip (7-cm diameter)

The important safety points here are:

■ Forceps are not appropriate for delivery of the head of a breech that has not entered the pelvis. The nape of the neck/base of occiput must be seen before the baby's body is lifted up.

■ When conducting forceps delivery for the aftercoming head of the breech, an assistant is needed and coordination between operator and assistant must be maintained, as one is in control of the baby's body, the other the baby's head.

■ The baby should be lifted into the horizontal position but, as the arms tend to fall into the way, interfering with the forceps application, the assistant is advised to wrap the baby, including its arms, into a towel to keep things clear.

■ Hyperextension of the neck should be avoided at all times and the operator should keep strict control of the elevation of the baby provided by the assistant.

■ An episiotomy is required for delivery in this circumstance and, if not already cut when the breech distended the perineum, it should be cut after the application of the forceps.

The place of trial-of-instrumental delivery

If there is uncertainty about whether an instrumental delivery is appropriate because the operator is uncertain about the position or degree of engagement of the head good analgesia should be achieved to allow adequate examination. If uncertainty remains, someone of greater experience should be called to assess and assist prior to attempting delivery. There is no place for a 'try-it-and-see' approach in these situations and the suggestion that 'the indications for the use of the vacuum extractor as an alternative to forceps delivery include uncertainty with regard to the position of the sagittal suture and situations where the fetal head is assumed to be too high for application of forceps' is quite clearly both untrue and dangerous.

Any trial-of-instrument in theatre must be sanctioned and/or supervised by a consultant or experienced registrar.

The place of forceps after failure to delivery with the ventouse

There is no place for an attempt at forceps delivery if:

■ the position of the fetal head was correctly diagnosed

■ the cup was applied correctly

■ adequate traction was applied and there was no descent with the ventouse.

If these were not the case and there was a misdiagnosis, misapplication of a cup or traction was inadequate (due to caput, leaking equipment, no maternal assistance) it may be justified to change to forceps. This decision should be made at an experienced level. The situation may also arise that after good descent and rotation of the head the ventouse cup detaches: in such cases what might have been a difficult Kjelland delivery has now become a straightforward 'lift-out' anterior-cup or forceps delivery.

Following on from any instrumental delivery

■ If the baby is delivered in good condition it should be handed to the mother as soon as possible to encourage skin-skin contact.

■ After delivery, perineal damage should be assessed carefully with particular attention given to check for anal sphincter and anal mucosa integrity.

■ After repairing any tear or episiotomy, the swabs and instruments should be counted.

■ A vaginal and rectal examination should be performed at the end of the procedure to confirm restoration of anatomy, exclude any stray sutures having entered the rectum, and confirm no swabs have been retained.

■ Every aspect of the delivery should be documented.

■ Examine the baby's head, when you get a chance, to confirm the positioning of the instrument used relative to where you thought it was, and where it should have been. This is important in self-audit of your technique and in teaching and feedback for trainees.

Supervising an instrumental delivery

The supervising obstetrician must make a full clinical assessment, otherwise they have no way of knowing whether the operative delivery is appropriate or the instrument selected is suitable for the task.

During traction, the supervisor needs to be confident descent is occurring with each traction and, if in doubt, they should feel for themselves to confirm this fact. Leaving the trainee to pull for three contractions before assessing the situation leaves an almost impossible decision of whether and how to continue and risks inappropriate excessive attempts at delivery.

After delivery, a careful examination of the extent of perineal trauma should be conducted together. This is not only important in identifying third- or fourth-degree tears (which are often under-diagnosed clinically) but can provide useful feedback on instrument technique: tears or episiotomies which have extended may have been due to lifting the hands too early on crowning, or too strong a left hand with forceps deliveries.

Audit standards

The following should be audited routinely:

- rate of operative vaginal delivery
- rate of failed operative vaginal delivery
- rate of sequential instrument use
- rate of third and fourth degree tears
- rate of neonatal morbidity trauma and admissions for intensive care
- standard of documentation.

Suggested further reading

Akmal S, Kametas N, Tsoi E, Hargreaves C, Nicolaides KH. Comparison of transvaginal digital examination with intrapartum sonography to determine fetal head position before instrumental delivery. *Ultrasound Obstet Gynecol* 2003;21:437–40.

Attilakos G, Sibanda T, Winter C, Johnson N, Draycott T. A randomised controlled trial of a new handheld vacuum extraction device. *BJOG* 2005;112:1510–15.

Bird GC. The importance of flexion in vacuum extractor delivery. *Br J Obstet Gynaecol* 1976;83:194–200.

Johanson RB, Menon V. Soft versus rigid vacuum extractor cups for assisted vaginal delivery. *Cochrane Database Syst Rev* 2004;(2).

Johanson RB, Menon V. Vacuum extraction versus forceps for assisted vaginal delivery. *Cochrane Database Syst Rev* 2004:(2).

Lewis G, editor. *Why Mothers Die 2000–2002. Sixth Report on Confidential Enquiries into Maternal Deaths in the United Kingdom.* London: RCOG Press; 2004.

Murphy DJ, Liebling RE, Patel R, Verity L, Swingler R. Cohort study of operative delivery in the second stage of labour and standard of obstetric care. *BJOG* 2003;110:610–15.

Murphy DJ, Liebling RE, Verity L, Swingler R, Patel R. Early maternal and neonaatal morbidity associated with operative delivery in second stage of labour: a cohort study. *Lancet* 2001;358:1203–8.

O'Mahony F, Settatree R, Platt C, Johnson R. Review of singleton fetal and neonatal deaths associated with cranial trauma and cephalic delivery during a national intrapartum-related confidential enquiry. *BJOG* 2005;112:619–26.

Patel RR, Murphy DJ. Forceps delivery in modern obstetric practice. *BMJ* 2004;328:1302–5.

Roodt A, Nikodem VC. Pushing/bearing down methods used during the second stage of labour. *Cochrane Database Syst Rev* 2002;(1):CD003513 [DOI: 10.1002/14651858.CD003513].

Royal College of Obstetricians and Gynaecologists. *Operative Vaginal Delivery.* Guideline No. 26. London: RCOG; 2005.

Saunders NJ, Spiby H, Gilbert L, Fraser RB, Hall JM, Mutton PM, *et al.* Oxytocin infusion during second stage of labour in primiparous women using epidural analgesia: a randomized double-blind placebo-controlled trial. *BMJ* 1989;299:1423–6.

Towner D, Castro MA, Eby-Wilkens E, Gilbert WM. Effect of mode of delivery in nulliparous women on neonatal intracranial injury. *N Engl J Med* 1999;341:1709–14.

Vacca A. The place of the vacuum extractor in modern obstetric practice. *Fetal Medicine Review* 1990;2:103–22.

Algorithm 29.1 **Twin pregnancy**

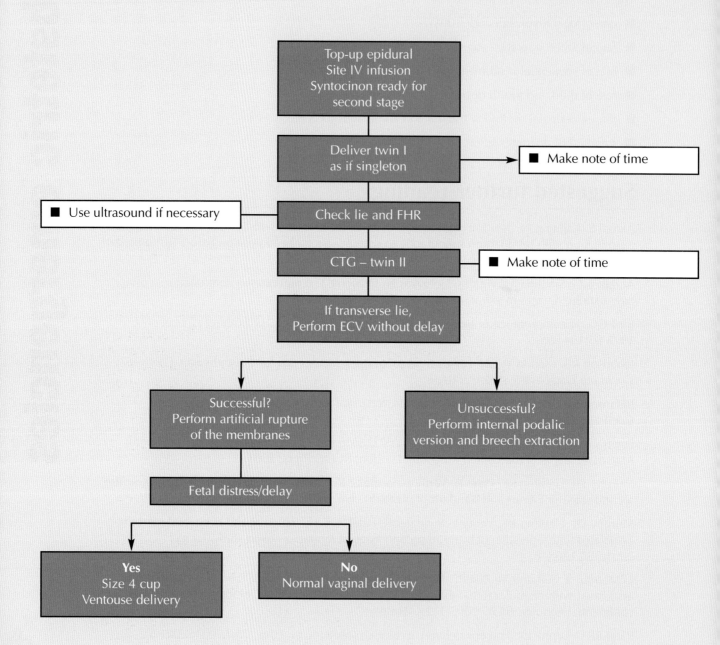

Chapter 29

Twin pregnancy

Objectives

On successfully completing this topic you will be able to:

■ assess the suitability for vaginal delivery

■ safely manage vaginal twin delivery.

Introduction

Dizygous twinning rates vary enormously depending on age, parity, racial background and assisted conception techniques. The incidence of twin pregnancies continues to increase with the success of assisted reproduction techniques giving a multiple birth rate of 15/1000 maternities in the UK in 2002. Monozygous twinning rates are relatively constant with incidence of 3.5/1000 births. Overall perinatal mortality and morbidity are higher in multiple gestations than in singletons. Premature delivery and the complications of prematurity are the main contributors to adverse outcomes. Other factors contributing to the risk are intrauterine growth restriction, congenital anomalies, malpresentation, cord prolapse and premature separation of the placenta.

The use of routine antenatal ultrasound assessment has facilitated the diagnosis of multiple gestations. Women who have attended for antenatal care should have had the chorionicity of the pregnancy determined and have undergone serial growth scans.

Currently, the evidence in the literature surrounding twin delivery is limited. A meta-analysis of the management of twin delivery did not find significant differences in outcome in terms of mortality or neonatal morbidity when comparing policies of planned vaginal delivery against planned caesarean section. A cohort study of 2890 twin pairs delivered after 36 weeks of gestation found that there were no deaths in those twins delivered by caesarean section but nine second-twin deaths in those delivered vaginally. An international multi-centred randomised controlled trial (the Twin Birth Study) is planned to study 2400 women randomly delivered by caesarean section and planned vaginal birth. This should answer many questions about twin delivery.

Vaginal delivery of twins, if judiciously managed, is generally considered to be safe. Until the results of the Twin Birth Study are available, this policy should continue to be adopted. However, some aspects of twin delivery remain controversial.

Presentation

Twin 1 vertex

Assess the suitability for vaginal delivery. As it is difficult to predict the eventual presentation of the second twin at the time of delivery, the situation should be favourable for breech delivery.

If the second twin is non-vertex, vaginal delivery is considered safe. Caesarean delivery of a non-vertex-presenting second twin is associated with increased maternal febrile morbidity and no improvement in the neonatal outcome when compared with vaginal delivery. The second twin presenting by the breech is best delivered by assisted breech delivery or breech extraction.

Twin 1 non-vertex

The incidence of locked twins is very low at 1/645. In the wake of the Term Breech Trial, vaginal delivery when twin 1 is non-vertex will need careful discussion with senior staff and parents. The Canadian Perinatal view is that the Term Breech Trial was a singleton study and the results should not be extrapolated to twins. In a large multicentre retrospective study of breech first births, no increased risk attributable to vaginal delivery was found. However, current opinion favours planned caesarean section when the first twin presents as a non-vertex – either breech or transverse.

Inter-twin delivery interval

The ideal time interval between the delivery of the first and second twin is not agreed. In one report, umbilical cord arterial and venous pH and base excess were shown to deteriorate with increasing twin-to-twin delivery interval. There were no second twins with an umbilical pH less than 7.00 when delivered within 15 minutes of twin 1. If the inter-twin delivery interval was greater than 30 minutes, 27% had an umbilical artery pH of less than 7.00. Among those with an inter-twin delivery interval of greater than 30 minutes, 73% had evidence of fetal distress that required operative intervention.

Studies have previously suggested that no specific time interval needs to be set providing there is continuous electronic fetal heart rate monitoring of twin 2 and it is reassuring.

ECV versus internal podalic version

Confusion still exists over whether ECV or internal podalic version and breech extraction should be performed. Many investigators report success with attempt at ECV in the first instance. However, other authors have reported lower success rates with ECV or increased maternal complication rates. Nevertheless, given that ECV is less invasive, it should seem reasonable to consider this in the first place. The experience of the operator is probably the most important factor.

Higher multiples

Even though the incidence of triplets is rising, most obstetricians have relatively little experience of delivering triplets and even less of delivering them vaginally. Although a study from the Netherlands reported improved outcome for triplets with vaginal delivery, when compared with caesarean section, the unit was particularly experienced at this type of delivery. For most obstetricians the safer option would almost certainly be caesarean section.

Previous caesarean section

Although there is little evidence, what there is suggests that a trial of labour is a safe option in the absence of a contraindication to vaginal birth. Scar dehiscence rates have been reported to be 0–3%.

Preterm/very-low-birthweight twins

There seems to be little difference in outcome between vaginal and caesarean delivery in very-low-birthweight gestations and little difference in terms of perinatal outcome.

> **Indications for caesarean section**
> - Conjoined twins
> - Monoamniotic twins
> - Placenta praevia
> - Certain congenital anomalies
> - Possible interlocking twins

Intrapartum management of vaginal twin delivery

Management of stage 1

- Admit to delivery suite.
- Intravenous line.
- Blood tests – full blood count, group and save serum.
- Continuous cardiotocograph on a twin monitor
  - fetal heart rate abnormalities twin 1 take fetal blood sample
  - fetal heart rate abnormalities twin 2 perform caesarean section.

  If at any stage either twin cannot be monitored then caesarean section may be the only safe option. It is imperative that both twins are monitored and the trace should be scrutinised to ensure that this is the case.

- Ultrasound assessment should be performed by an appropriately trained practitioner to determine:
  - presentation of each fetus
  - liquor volume assessment
  - placental site
  - viability of each fetus
  - estimation of fetal weight if not recently performed
  - for ECV
  - may be used to guide the operator undertaking internal podalic version.
- The use of epidural analgesia may be justified for possible intrauterine manipulations required for the delivery of the second twin.
- Inform:
  - anaesthetist
  - paediatrician
  - neonatal unit.

Management of stage 2

- Provide appropriate analgesia.

■ Prepare oxytocin 10 iu in 1 litre Hartmann's solution if not already receiving oxytocin infusion.

■ Deliver twin 1 as if singleton.

■ Perform abdominal palpation to determine lie.

■ Confirm lie, presentation and fetal heart with ultrasound scan.

■ Monitor electronic fetal heart rate continuously.

■ If transverse lie, perform ECV or internal podalic version.

■ When lie longitudinal and presenting part in pelvis, perform amniotomy with contraction.

■ If no contractions within 5–10 minutes commence oxytocin infusion.

Management of stage 3

■ Give Syntometrine 1 ampoule (or Syntocinon 5 iu if Syntometrine contraindicated) with the delivery of the second twin.

■ Deliver the placenta.

■ Consider commencing oxytocin infusion (40 iu oxytocin in 1 litre Hartmann's solution), as there is a risk of uterine atony following delivery of multiple gestations.

Internal podalic version

A fetal foot is identified by recognising a heel through intact membranes. The foot is grasped and pulled gently and continuously lower into the birth canal. The membranes are ruptured as late as possible. This procedure is easiest when the transverse lie is with the back superior or posterior. If the back is inferior or if the limbs are not immediately palpable, ultrasound may help to identify to the operator where they may be found. This will minimise the risk of bringing down a fetal hand.

Communication and team working

In the delivery of twins and higher multiples, team working is essential to optimise the outcome for mother and babies. Obstetricians, midwives and paediatricians should be present at the delivery. An anaesthetist should be available on the delivery suite should it become necessary to perform a caesarean section urgently.

Suggested further reading

Adam C, Allen AC, Baskett TF. Twin delivery: influence of the presentation and method of delivery on the second twin. *Am J Obstet Gynecol* 1991;165:23–7.

Crowther CA. Caesarean delivery for the second twin. *Cochrane Database Syst Rev* 2000;(2):CD000047.

Feng TI, Swindle REJ, Huddleston JF. A lack of adverse effect of prolonged delivery interval between twins. *J Matern Fetal Investig* 1995;5:222–5.

Fishman A, Grubb DK, Kovacs BW. Vaginal delivery of the nonvertex second twin. *Am J Obstet Gynecol* 1993;168:861–4.

Gocke SE, Nageotte MP, Garite T, Towers CV, Dorchester W. Management of the nonvertex second twin: primary cesarean section, external version, or primary breech extraction. *Am J Obstet Gynecol* 1989; 161:111–14.

Hogle KL, Hutton EK, McBrien KA, Barratt JFR, Hannah M. Cesarean delivery for twins: A systematic review and meta-analysis. *Am J Obstet Gynecol* 2003;188:220–7.

Leung TY, Tam WH, Leung TN et al. Effect of twin to twin delivery interval on umbilical cord blood gas in the second twins. *BJOG* 2002;109:63–7.

Miller DA, Mullin P, Hou D, Paul RH. Vaginal birth after cesarean section in twin gestation. *Am J Obstet Gynecol* 1996;175:194–8.

Rabinovici J, Barkai G, Richman B, Serr DM, Mashiach S. Internal podalic version with unruptured membranes for the second twin in transverse lie. *Obstet Gynecol* 1988; 71:4280–300.

Rabinovici J, Barkai G, Reichman B, Serr DM, Mashiach S. Randomised management of the second nonvertex twin: vaginal delivery or caesarean section. *Am J Obstet Gynecol* 1987;156:52–6.

Rao A, Sairam S, Shehata H. Obstetric complications of twin pregnancies. *Best Pract Res Clin Obstet Gynaecol* 2004;18:557–76.

Smith GC, Pell JP, Dobbie R. Birth order, gestational age and risk of delivery related perinatal death in twins: retrospective cohort study. *BMJ* 2002;325:1004.

Spinillo A, Stronati M, Ometto A, Fazzi E, de Seta F, Lasci A. The influence of presentation and method of delivery on neonatal mortality and infant neurodevelopmental outcome in nondiscordant low-birthweight. *Eur J Obstet Gynecol Reprod Biol* 1992;47:189–94.

Tchabo JG, Tomai T. Selected intrapartum external cephalic version of the second twin. *Obstet Gynecol* 1992;79:421–3.

Wildschut HIJ, Van Roosmalen J, van Leeuwen E. Planned abdominal compared with planned vaginal birth in triplet pregnancies. *Br J Obstet Gynaecol* 1995;102:292–6.

Algorithm 30.1 Symphysiotomy

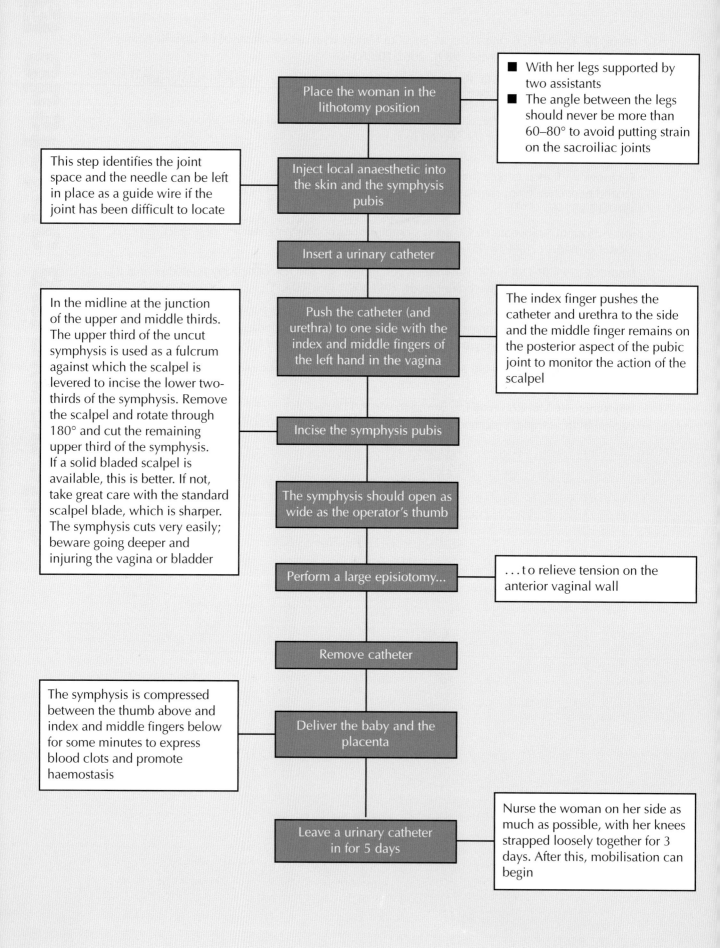

Place the woman in the lithotomy position
- With her legs supported by two assistants
- The angle between the legs should never be more than 60–80° to avoid putting strain on the sacroiliac joints

Inject local anaesthetic into the skin and the symphysis pubis
This step identifies the joint space and the needle can be left in place as a guide wire if the joint has been difficult to locate

Insert a urinary catheter

Push the catheter (and urethra) to one side with the index and middle fingers of the left hand in the vagina
The index finger pushes the catheter and urethra to the side and the middle finger remains on the posterior aspect of the pubic joint to monitor the action of the scalpel

Incise the symphysis pubis
In the midline at the junction of the upper and middle thirds. The upper third of the uncut symphysis is used as a fulcrum against which the scalpel is levered to incise the lower two-thirds of the symphysis. Remove the scalpel and rotate through 180° and cut the remaining upper third of the symphysis. If a solid bladed scalpel is available, this is better. If not, take great care with the standard scalpel blade, which is sharper. The symphysis cuts very easily; beware going deeper and injuring the vagina or bladder

The symphysis should open as wide as the operator's thumb

Perform a large episiotomy...
...to relieve tension on the anterior vaginal wall

Remove catheter

Deliver the baby and the placenta
The symphysis is compressed between the thumb above and index and middle fingers below for some minutes to express blood clots and promote haemostasis

Leave a urinary catheter in for 5 days
Nurse the woman on her side as much as possible, with her knees strapped loosely together for 3 days. After this, mobilisation can begin

Chapter 30

Symphysiotomy

Objectives

On successfully completing this topic you will be able to:

- discuss the indications for symphysiotomy
- understand and practise the technique.

Introduction

Symphysiotomy is a relatively common procedure in the developing world, where it is used in situations of cephalopelvic disproportion when caesarean section is not available. Symphysiotomy leaves no uterine scar and subsequent risk of ruptured uterus in future labours is not increased. Van Roosmalen illustrated the potential morbidity and mortality of caesarean sections carried out in developing country rural hospitals. Mortalities of up to 5% and an incidence of uterine scar rupture in subsequent pregnancies of up to 6.8% have been reported. Symphysiotomy has a low maternal mortality, with three deaths reported in a series of 1752 symphysiotomies. All three deaths were unrelated to the procedure.

Hartfield reviewed the cases of 138 women in whom symphysiotomy had been performed. Early and late complications were few and rarely serious if recommended guidelines were followed. He also reviewed published series of women followed up for 2 years or more after symphysiotomy and concluded that permanent major orthopaedic disability only occurs in 1–2% of cases.

Pape carried out a prospective review of 27 symphysiotomies performed between 1992 and 1994. Five women had paraurethral tears needing suturing, nine had oedema of the vulva or haematomas tracking from the symphysiotomy. All made a full recovery and severe pelvic pain was not a feature in any woman.

In 2001, the question of legal action against obstetricians in Ireland who carried out symphysiotomies was raised. Verkuyl made the point that many symphysiotomies were performed in Roman Catholic countries because contraception was illegal even for medical reasons and women were spared repeated operative deliveries.

Symphysiotomy is a useful technique that is occasionally required in UK practice. One report highlighted four cases where it has been used successful in this country.

Bjorkland published a comprehensive retrospective review of the literature based on papers published between 1900 and 1999; 5000 symphysiotomies and 1200 caesarean section operations were included and the results indicated that symphysiotomy is safe for the mother and life saving for the child. Severe complications are rare.

Indications

■ Trapped aftercoming head of breech due to cephalopelvic disproportion.

■ Severe cases of shoulder dystocia that do not resolve with routine manoeuvres.

■ In cases of cephalopelvic disproportion with a vertex presentation and a living fetus (in the developing world), when at least two-thirds of the fetal head has entered the pelvic brim. Note that the use of forceps is contraindicated.

■ In cases of cephalopelvic disproportion with a vertex presentation when caesarean section is declined by the mother.

Technique

1. Place the woman in the lithotomy position with her legs supported by two assistants. The angle between the legs should never be more than 60–80 degrees to avoid putting a strain on the sacroiliac joints and tearing of the urethra and bladder.

2. Inject local anaesthetic into the skin and symphysis pubis. This step identifies the joint space and the needle can be left in place as a guide wire if the joint has been difficult to locate.

3. Insert a firm urinary catheter. Apply antiseptic solution suprapubically.

4. Push the catheter (and urethra) aside with the index and middle fingers of the left hand in the vagina. The index finger pushes the catheter and urethra to the side and the middle finger remains on the posterior aspect of the pubic joint to monitor the action of the scalpel.

5. Incise the symphysis pubis in the midline at the junction of the upper and middle thirds. Use the upper third of the uncut symphysis as a fulcrum against which to lever the scalpel to incise the lower two-thirds of the symphysis. Cut down through the cartilage until the pressure of the scalpel blade is felt on the finger of the vagina.

    Remove the scalpel and rotate it through 180 degrees and the remaining upper third of the symphysis is cut. If a solid-bladed scalpel is available, this is better. If not, take great care with the standard scalpel blade, which is sharper. The symphysis cuts very easily; beware of going deeper and injuring the vagina or bladder.

6. The symphysis should open as wide as the operator's thumb.

7. After separating the cartilage remove the catheter to decrease urethral trauma.

8. Use a large episiotomy to relieve tension on the anterior vaginal wall.

9. After delivery of the baby and placenta, compress the symphysis between the thumb above and index and middle fingers below for some minutes, to express blood clots and promote haemostasis.

10. Re-catheterise and leave a urinary catheter in place for 5 days.

11. Apply elastic strapping across the front of the pelvis from one iliac crest to the other to stabilise the symphysis and reduce pain. The woman needs to be nursed on her side as much as possible, with her knees strapped loosely together for 3 days. After this, mobilisation can begin.

Summary

■ Symphysiotomy is a useful procedure that can be used in certain emergency situations.

■ It must only be performed by trained clinicians.

■ Prompt decision is required to avoid fetal morbidity.

■ Intrapartum and postpartum management are important to minimise maternal morbidity.

Obstetric emergencies

Suggested further reading

Björklund K. Minimally invasive surgery for obstructed labour: a review of symphysiotomy during the twentieth century (including 5000 cases). *BJOG* 2002;109:236–48.

Goodwin TM, Banks E, Millar L, Phelan J. Catastrophic shoulder dystocia and emergency symphysiotomy. *Am J Obstet Gynecol* 1997;177:463–4.

Hartfield VJ. Late effects of symphysiotomy. *Trop Doct* 1975;5:76–8.

Hartfield VJ. Subcutaneous symphysiotomy: time for a reappraisal? *Aust N Z J Obstet Gynaecol* 1973;13:147–52.

Menticoglou SM. Symphysiotomy for the trapped aftercoming parts of the breech: a review of the literature and a plea for its use. *Aust N Z J Obstet Gynaecol* 1990;30:1–9.

Pape GL. 27 Symphysiotomies. *Trop Doct* 1999;29:248–9.

Payne G. Ireland orders enquiry into barbaric obstetric practices. *BMJ* 2001;322:1200.

Spencer JA. Symphysiotomy for vaginal breech delivery: two case reports. *Br J Obstet Gynaecol* 1987;94:716–18.

Van Roosmalen J. Safe motherhood: cesarean section or symphysiotomy? *Am J Obstet Gynecol* 1990;163:1–4.

Van Roosmalen J. Symphysiotomy as an alternative to casarean section. *Int J Gynecol Obstet* 1987;25:451–8.

Verkuly DAA. Symphysiotomies are an important option in the developed world. *BMJ* 2001:323:809.

World Health Organization, UNFPA, UNICEG, World Bank. *Managing Complications in Pregnancy and Childbirth. A guide for midwives and doctors.* Geneva: WHO; 2001.

Wykes CB, Johnston TA, Paterson-Brown S, Johanson R. Symphysiotomy: a lifesaving procedure. *BJOG* 2003;110:219–21.

Greisen G. Three-year follow-up of eight patients delivered by symphysiotomy. *Int J Gynecol Obstet* 1985;23:203–5.

Algorithm 31.1 **Destructive operations**

Destructive operations are useful, although rare procedures in modern obstetric practice

In situations of fetal demise destructive operations should be considered as a first line to assist vaginal delivery rather than using the alternative abdominal approach

Obstetricians can be trained using manikins

Destructive operations can avoid unnecessary abdominal delivery and subsequent risks to the mother

Chapter 31

Destructive operations

Objectives

On successfully completing this topic you will be able to:

- understand the role of destructive operations
- understand the procedures involved in destructive operations.

Introduction

Destructive operations are fairly common in the developing world in cases of obstructed labour, where absent prenatal care and poor intrapartum care at peripheral hospitals have resulted in fetal demise. Reported incidences range between 0.094% and 0.98% of all deliveries. A destructive procedure is an alternative to abdominal delivery that may carry considerable risk to the mother.

With the use of prophylactic antibiotics and thromboprophylaxis, caesarean section has become safer and there is only a limited role in modern practice for destructive procedures in the developed world.

Destructive procedures

Destructive operations may be required where the fetus is dead and where a vaginal delivery is being attempted. It may be the appropriate method for delivery to minimise maternal risk or it may be the only route by which the mother wishes to be delivered. Whenever a destructive procedure is being considered it must only be performed with the mother's consent.

- Initially, basic resuscitation must be carried out quickly to avoid undue delay in delivering a dead fetus.

- Catheterise.

- Since urinary and genital tract infections are common, antibiotic prophylaxis should be used.

- General or regional anaesthesia combined with sedation is ideal for the procedure.

- The cervix should be fully dilated, although destructive surgery may be performed by an experienced operator when the cervix is dilated by 7 cm or more.

- The genital tract and rectum must be carefully examined after the procedure.

- A catheter should be left in place for at least 48 hours.

The three most common destructive procedures are:

- craniotomy
- perforation of the aftercoming head
- decapitation.

Craniotomy

Indications

Craniotomy is indicated for the delivery of a dead fetus in situations of cephalopelvic dispro-portion and hydrocephalus.

Method

- The fetal head should be no more than three-fifths above the pelvic brim, except in cases of hydrocephalus.
- Ask an assistant to steady the head from above the pubic symphysis.
- Perforate the skull via the fontanelle using a Simpson's perforator with the instrument at right angles to the surface of the skull, to minimise the risk of slipping. If a fontanelle cannot be palpated, the perforator should be inserted through the bone.
- Push the blades as far as their shoulders and separate first in one direction and then in another direction, at right angles to the first.
- Evacuate the brain and deliver the fetal head by a pull on the skull using vulsellum forceps and counter-traction. It may be gentler to attach the vulsellum to a 1-kg weight (for example, a 1-litre bag of fluid) using a bandage. This will allow a slower and possibly more 'normal' delivery.
- If the fetus is very large, reduction in the size of the shoulder girdle by cleidotomy may be required after delivery of the head. This can be achieved by cutting the clavicle at its midpoint using either scissors or scalpel.

Aftercoming head of the breech

The aftercoming head of a breech can be managed similarly by craniotomy, with perforation of the head through the base of the skull, beginning at the nape of the neck, aiming towards the vertex. If the head is deflexed, perforation of the occiput may be achieved in the region of the posterior fontanelle.

Where there is hydrocephalus and accompanying spina bifida, cerebrospinal fluid can either be withdrawn by exposing the spinal canal and passing a catheter into the canal and up into the cranium. The hydrocephalic head can be decompressed transabdominally under ultrasound control using a spinal needle.

Decapitation

Indications

Decapitation is indicated in cases of neglected, obstructed labour with shoulder presentation and a dead fetus. In an already emotionally fraught situation, the prospect of explaining the options to parents may be distressing for all. Nevertheless, in terms of minimising harm to the mother, a very early delivery remains optimal.

Method

■ If the fetus is small and the neck can easily be felt, it may be severed with stout scissors. However, for the larger fetus, and especially where the neck is not easily accessible, the Blond-Heidler decapitation tool is the safest instrument.

■ If possible, an arm is brought down and firmly pulled on by an assistant, which brings the neck lower to make it more accessible.

■ Thread the saw around the fetal neck and keep the handles attached to the ends of the saw close together. This prevents injury to the vagina and the neck is soon severed after a few firm strokes.

■ Deliver the trunk by traction on the arm, with the operator's hand protecting the vagina from laceration by spicules of bone.

■ Deliver the aftercoming head by grasping the stump with a heavy vulsellum and performing the Mauriceau-Smellie-Veit manoeuvre. It is easy to restore anatomic continuity with skin sutures to the neck.

■ The baby should be wrapped neatly before showing the parents.

Background

In the developing world, caesarean section carries significant risks. Potential problems include haemorrhage from uterine extension, generalised peritonitis and the risk of rupture of the scar in a subsequent pregnancy. Gogoi showed a much lower morbidity and mortality with craniotomy than with caesarean section in a group of 158 women who were grossly infected. Peritonitis occurred in 66% of women after caesarean section and was nil after destructive operations, The maternal mortality in the caesarean section group was 13/107 (12%) compared with 1/37 (2.7%) in the craniotomy group.

Marsden *et al.* described a series of four cases where the Blond-Heidler saw was used in the case of a dead baby in a transverse lie. They had no complications and suggested that in such situations this method of delivery is more appropriate than caesarean section, when a classical incision may often be required, which significantly increases the risk to the mother.

Reports from the developing world of maternal morbidity and mortality following destructive procedures illustrate that most problems encountered can be attributed to obstructed labour, which often necessitates their performance in the first place. It is often not easy to differentiate the complications of one from the other. Ekwempu reported on a series of 112 patients treated by embryotomy between 1974 and 1975. The only complications that he could attribute to the destructive procedure were seven cases of soft-tissue (mainly vaginal and perineal) laceration. The procedures themselves have been shown to be simple with little morbidity.

There are several reports from the developing world of postoperative vesicovaginal fistula. These are often attributed to pressure necrosis in obstructed labour. However, it has been suggested that they could be secondary to the use of sharp instruments or from bony spicules exposed during the procedure. This can be avoided by regular training using dummies and appropriate case selection.

Suggested further reading

Amo-Mensah S, Elkins T, Ghosh T, Greenway F, Waite V. Obstetric destructive procedures. *Int J Gynaecol Obstet* 1996;54:167–8.

Arora M, Rajaram P, Oumachigui A, Parveena P. Destructive operations in modern obstetrics in a developing country at tertiary level. *Br J Obstet Gynaecol* 1993;100:967–8.

Ekwempu CC. Embryotomy versus caesarean section. *Trop Doct* 1978;8:195–7.

Giwa-Osaigie O, Azzan B. Destructive operations. In: Studd J, editor. Progress in Obstetrics and Gynaecology Volume 6. Edinburgh: Churchill Livingstone; 1987. p. 211–21.

Gogoi M.P. Maternal mortality from Caesarean section in infected cases. *J Obstet Gynaecol Br Empire* 1971;78:373–6.

Gupta U, Chitra R. Destructive operations still have a place in developing countries. *Int J Gynaecol Obstet* 1993;44:15–19.

Hudson CN. Obstructed labour and its sequelae. In: Lawson JB, Harrison KA, Berström S, editors. *Maternity Care in Developing Countries.* London: RCOG Press; 2001. p. 201–14.

Konje JC, Obisesan KA, Ladipo OA. Obstructed labour in Ibadan. *Int J Gynaecol Obstet* 1992;39:17–21.

Lawson J. Embryotomy for obstructed labour. *Trop Doct* 1974;4:188–91.

Maharaj D, Moodley J. Symphysiotomy and fetal destructive operations. *Best Pract Res Clin Obstet Gynaecol* 2002;16:117–31.

Marsden DE, Chang AS, Shin KS. Decapitation and vaginal delivery for impacted transverse lie in late labour: reports of 4 cases. *Aust N Z J Obstet Gynacol* 1982;22:46–9.

Mitra KN, John MP. Decapitation by thread saw. *J Obstet Gynaecol India* 1950;1:65–73.

Moir C, Myerscough P. *Munro Kerr's Operative Obstetrics.* 8th ed. London: Ballière Tindall and Cassell; 1971. p. 191, 715.

Chapter 32

Perinatal psychiatric illness

Introduction

Mental health problems are common in the community at large, with an incidence of at least 20%. The most common mental health problems are mixed anxiety and depression. Women are at least twice as likely to suffer from these conditions as men and they are most prevalent amongst younger women with children under the age of 5 years. Serious mental illnesses such as schizophrenia and bipolar illness (manic depressive illness) are less common, with a prevalence of approximately 1% for each condition and are no more common in women than in men.

Mental health problems in pregnancy

The prevalence of psychiatric disorder of all severities during pregnancy is much as that at other times. Antenatal depression and anxiety is therefore common and no less common than it is after delivery, affecting 10–20% all women.

The incidence (new onset) of serious mental illness (schizophrenia, psychoses and bipolar illness), during pregnancy is markedly reduced compared with other times. However, serious mental illness does sometimes occur for the first time during pregnancy and poses particular management problems. A more frequent situation is that of a woman who already has a chronic serious mental illness and becomes pregnant. Approximately 2/1000 births are to women with chronic serious mental illness. Pregnancy is not protective against a relapse of these conditions, particularly if patients stop taking their medication. However, continuing medication may pose problems for management during labour and for the care of the newborn.

Mental health problems after delivery

In contrast, there is a dramatic increase in the incidence of serious affective illness following delivery. Women face a relative risk of 32 of developing a psychotic illness in the first 3 months following delivery. These illnesses are thought to belong to the bipolar group of illnesses. There is also an increased risk (relative risk 10) of developing a severe unipolar depressive illness. There is no increase in risk of developing schizophrenia. Women who have a previous history of bipolar illness, puerperal psychosis or severe postnatal depression have at least a 50% risk of recurrence of this condition following delivery, even if they have been well for many years. Fifty percent of puerperal psychoses will have presented by day 7, 75% by day 14 and all by 42 days. Women without a personal history but with a family history of bipolar illness, particularly if it is of postpartum onset, also face an elevated risk of developing a serious mental illness following delivery.

These serious postpartum mental illnesses, which become manifest in the early days following delivery, are life threatening. Women are acutely disturbed, very frightened and bewildered, and the illness poses a risk both to their physical health and safety. They require expert assessment and treatment and should be admitted to a mother and baby unit rather than to a general psychiatry ward.

Severe but nonpsychotic depressive illness tends to develop more gradually and present later in the first 12 weeks following delivery. While it benefits from specialist psychiatric care it can frequently be managed at home with the usual treatments for severe depressive illness, modified by whether or not the woman is breastfeeding.

The more common mild to moderate depressive illness often associated with marked features of anxiety, described as 'postnatal depression' or 'PND' is in fact no more common following childbirth than in women who have not given birth. These conditions usually present later in the postpartum year, after 3 months, and are best managed in primary care. For these conditions psychosocial treatments are often as effective as antidepressants.

Confidential Enquiries into Maternal Deaths

The last two reports of the CEMD reveal that 25% of maternal deaths (including late deaths) are caused by psychiatric disorder and 15% by suicide. Suicide is therefore the leading cause of maternal death in the UK. The most important findings for obstetricians and midwives are:

▓ Women who died from suicide were in the main older, more socially advantaged and better educated than in other causes of maternal death. Suicide is not associated with the same socioeconomic factors as other causes of maternal death.

▓ The majority were seriously mentally ill before they died. They had been well during pregnancy and developed either a puerperal psychosis or very severe depressive illness. Over 50% of these women had had a previous episode requiring inpatient psychiatric treatment, even though they had been well for some time before giving birth. This identifiable risk factor had, in the majority of cases, neither been identified at booking nor had the management of this risk been planned during pregnancy. Both psychiatric and maternity services had failed to take the opportunity to anticipate the risk following delivery. The rapid deterioration of a sudden onset illness appears to have taken all by surprise.

▓ There was little evidence of communication taking place between psychiatric and maternity teams and the lack of planning was reflected in the lack of information that was passed between involved professionals.

▓ The remainder of the psychiatric deaths, those not due to suicide, were due to women dying from physical illness that could either be directly attributable to their psychiatric disorder (in half the cases the consequences of alcohol or drug misuse) or because their life-threatening illness was missed or misattributed to psychiatric disorder. Obstetricians and midwives are reminded that serious physical illness can present as, complicate or co-exist with psychiatric disorder.

Implications for obstetric practice

The long-standing knowledge of the epidemiology and distinctive clinical features of perinatal psychiatric disorder, together with the findings of the CEMD, provide the evidence base for obstetric and midwifery practice and for the psychiatric care of pregnant and postpartum women.

▓ All women with serious mental illness and those taking psychotropic medication should discuss with their general practitioner, psychiatrist or obstetrician their plans for becoming pregnant, with regard to the risks to their mental health and to the risks to the developing fetus of their medication.

▓ All women should be asked in a systematic and sensitive way about their previous as well as current psychiatric history at booking in early pregnancy. These questions should be structured so that those with a previous or current history of serious mental illness can be identified. Those responsible for booking should receive training to enable them to distinguish between serious psychiatric disorder and common mental health problems.

■ Women with serious mental health problems currently or those with a past history of a serious psychiatric disorder should have a written management plan, shared between the woman, the general practitioner, obstetrician and psychiatrist, with regard to her peripartum management and the management of her risk in the early weeks following delivery.

■ Women with serious mental health problems complicating pregnancy and the early post-partum period should have access to a specialist psychiatrist in perinatal mental health, supported by a specialist multidisciplinary team.

However, despite many national recommendations (Perinatal Maternal Mental Health Services, recommendations for provision of services for childbearing women from the Royal College of Psychiatrists (CR88), Perinatal Mental Health Services, Women's Mental Health Strategy and Children and Young Peoples and the Maternity National Service Framework) specialist perinatal mental health teams have yet to be developed in the majority of maternity localities and there are insufficient mother and baby units in the UK to ensure equity of access for all. In addition, both the psychiatric and maternity professions have yet to fully acknowledge and implement the need for screening and proactive management of this high-risk group of women. Therefore, sadly, midwives and obstetricians will still be presented with women in late pregnancy and shortly after delivery with serious psychiatric disorder who have not been previously identified as well as those who develop illnesses at this time which could not have been anticipated.

Management of well 'at risk' women

The well 'at-risk' woman will have been well often for many years but will have a previous history of either puerperal psychosis or severe postnatal depression or a previous episode of bipolar illness. She may not have been in contact with psychiatric services for some time and will not be taking any medication. Ideally, she should have been detected at the booking clinic and should have been seen by a specialist psychiatrist during pregnancy. The risk of a recurrence of the condition and a management plan should have been drawn up during pregnancy. However, often this has not happened and the risk may be identified only in late pregnancy or on admission to the labour suite.

There are no particular management issues during labour. If no management plan is in place then the risk of recurrence of the puerperal psychosis or bipolar illness should be explained to the woman and her family. She should be seen by the psychiatrist serving the maternity hospital as soon as possible following delivery, preferably before she is discharged. The maximum risk of a recurrence of the condition is in the first 2 weeks following delivery so early contact is essential. The minimum requirement will be that the community midwife is alerted and that together with the psychiatric team the woman's mental health should be closely monitored over the first 6 weeks following delivery. Ideally, there should be a specialist perinatal mental health team involved but these are not available to all maternity services. The psychiatrist may consider using prophylactic medication such as lithium carbonate or an antipsychotic (small dose of atypical or newer atypical antipsychotic) if this is acceptable to the woman. In these circum-stances she should not breastfeed. The evidence for the prophylactic effect of antidepressants is less strong but many women may wish to consider it.

Management of women with chronic severe mental illness

Women with chronic severe mental illness are usually still under the care of psychiatric services. They may be suffering from either chronic schizophrenia and receiving antipsychotic medi-cation or from recurrent bipolar illness and receiving mood stabilisers, antidepressants or antipsychotic medication. Ideally, these women should not present unannounced. There should have been frequent communication and joint management during the pregnancy, consideration given to the choice of medication and the possibility of tapering medication prior to delivery if the woman's mental health permitted it. There should also be clear and written management plans for both the peripartum period and her care following delivery. However, sadly, this is sometimes not the case.

Women with bipolar illness may be taking lithium carbonate. The haemodynamics of later pregnancy and increased clearance of lithium may well have resulted in increasing oral doses of lithium in order to maintain a therapeutic lithium level (0.6–0.9 mmol/l) during pregnancy. During labour, this situation will alter and the woman will need a reduction of her dose of lithium and frequent monitoring of her serum lithium levels at least twice in 24 hours during labour and daily for the first 3–4 days following delivery to guard against increasing serum lithium levels and the possibility of lithium toxicity (levels higher than 1.5 mmol/l). Following delivery, the dosage of lithium carbonate will need to be reinstated at her usual prepregnancy dose. The neonatal paediatricians will need to be alerted.

Many women with bipolar disorder will be taking an anti-epileptic mood stabiliser as an alternative to lithium. The most common preparation in use for the management of bipolar illness is sodium valproate. Despite clear guidance from the National Institute for Health and Clinical Excellence guidelines on the management of epilepsy and the management of bipolar disorder that sodium valproate should not be used in pregnancy and in women of reproductive age unless there is no reasonable alternative, this situation still arises. The neonatal paediatrician should be alerted. Following delivery, the dose of the sodium valproate should be adjusted back to the prepregnancy dose and continued, because of the high risk of a relapse of the bipolar disorder following delivery. If the woman wishes to breastfeed, the sodium valproate or other antiepileptic mood stabilisers should be given in divided dosage and the infant monitored for drowsiness and rashes.

A variety of antipsychotic medication may be taken by women with chronic serious mental illness, including the older antipsychotics (such as trifluoperazine and haloperidol). These preparations have been in use for many years and do not appear to be associated either with an increased risk of major congenital abnormalities or any particular problems during pregnancy. Many women will be taking the newer or atypical antipsychotics (including olanzapine and risperidone). There are fewer data available on these newer drugs and there has been some concern expressed about the association of olanzapine with gestational diabetes. In an ideal world, these issues will have been discussed by the psychiatrist and obstetricians prior to delivery and consideration given to switching medication and the possibility of tapering before delivery. If this has not happened, the neonatal paediatricians will need to be alerted because of the possibility of withdrawal effects in the infant. Following delivery, the prepregnancy dose will need to be reinstated because of the risk of relapse postpartum. Breastfeeding is not advised in women who are taking atypical antipsychotics but can proceed with caution in those taking the older psychotics. However, they should be given in divided dosage.

Many women both those suffering from serious mental illness and milder mental illness are taking antidepressants during pregnancy. These may be the older tricyclic antidepressants (for example, imipramine, amitriptyline or dosulepin or the newer selective serotonin re-uptake inhibitors such as paroxetine or fluoxetine). There has been concern that these may be associated with an increased risk of ventricular septal defect and pulmonary hyperplasia with first-trimester exposure. There is more robust evidence that their use at term is associated with withdrawal effects in the neonate and in the case of SSRIs with the serotonin syndrome in the newborn. If time allows and the woman's mental health is stable, consideration should be given to tapering the dose of antidepressants prior to delivery. However, if this has not happened then the neonate should be observed for withdrawal symptoms. Following delivery, the medication should be continued. Breastfeeding should be avoided if the woman wishes to continue taking SSRIs in the early weeks. Tricyclic antidepressants can be continued when breastfeeding but should be given in divided dosage.

Labour ward crises

True psychiatric emergencies occurring in the labour ward are extremely uncommon. Women with chronic serious mental illness who are under the care of psychiatric teams should probably be accompanied during labour by a familiar mental healthcare professional, particularly if they are frightened, unable to fully comprehend what is happening to them or if they are symptomatic. Women who are well but at risk because of a previous history should be managed as other women are but attention paid following delivery to their need for close surveillance in the early postpartum period.

Occasionally, acute episodes of distress may occur in women either in early labour or in the minutes and hours following delivery. These acute episodes of distress will usually be understandable (if not proportional to) the contextual meaning of events or procedures in the light of previous experience. Examples would be: previous sexual abuse, previous experience of a traumatic delivery or loss of a baby, misattribution of sensations or procedures, to name but a few. Women will be more vulnerable to the possibility of this occurring if they have previous experience of panic attacks, if they cannot speak English or if they are frightened for a wide variety of reasons.

The overwhelming majority of these situations will respond to calm kindness and reassurance. However, some women will be suffering from panic attacks. These will usually be evident because of hyperventilation and are associated with feelings of imminent disaster, a fear of dying or suffocation, losing control or even imminent insanity. Panic attacks are the great imitators. The CEMD describes individual cases where women with cardiac and respiratory disease were mistaken for panic attacks but conversely panic attacks can be mistaken for pulmonary embolus and other physical emergencies. Swift differential diagnosis is therefore necessary. In many cases, encouragement to control hyperventilation would be sufficient, together with an explanation to the woman of what is happening to her. However, on other occasions it may be necessary to use a short acting benzodiazepine tranquilliser. Lorazepam 0.5–1.0 mg is best suited to use in labour because of its swift action and short duration.

Neonatal paediatrician

The neonatal paediatrician needs to be alerted in the following circumstances:

- **Lithium** – Infants born to mothers taking lithium during pregnancy are at increased risk of suffering from cardiac abnormalities. Ebstein's anomaly is rare (approximately 2/1000 exposed pregnancies) but other cardiac abnormalities are more common (up to 10% of all exposed pregnancies). Continuing use throughout pregnancy is associated with an increased risk of hypothyroidism, large-weight infants, nephrogenic diabetes insipidus and the floppy baby syndrome following delivery.

- **Sodium valproate** – Infants born to mothers taking sodium valproate are at increased risk of neural tube defects, fetal valproate syndrome and cardiac abnormalities following first trimester exposure. Continuing use throughout pregnancy is associated with an increased risk of neurodevelopmental and cognitive problems in later childhood.

- **Antipsychotic medication** – Infants born to mothers receiving antipsychotic medication may experience withdrawal symptoms, jitteriness and convulsions as well as short term and reversible extra pyramidal symptoms.

- **Antidepressants** – Infants born to mothers receiving tricyclic antidepressants at full therapeutic dosage may be at risk of withdrawal symptoms, neonatal jitteriness and convulsions as well as anticholinergic adverse effects.

- Infants born to mothers receiving **SSRI medication** may experience withdrawal effects, jitteriness, irritability, feeding difficulties and problems maintaining blood sugar and temperature.

Summary

Most perinatal psychiatric crises can be predicted and avoided by identification of potential psychiatric problems in early pregnancy, proactive management and collaborative perinatal management plans between psychiatry and obstetrics. However, occasionally crises and emergencies do arise during labour and more frequently in the early days following delivery. The effective management of these requires the rapid response of a specialist perinatal mental health team. The possibility of neonatal consequences of maternal psychiatric medication needs to be born in mind following delivery.

Suggested further reading

Dean C, Kendell RE. The symptomatology of puerperal illness. *Br J Psychiatry* 1981;139:128–33.

Kendell RE, Chalmers JC, Platz C. Epidemiology of puerperal psychoses. *Br J Psychiatry* 1987;34:662–73.

Lewis G, editor. *Why Mothers Die 1997–1999. The Fifth Report of the Confidential Enquiries into Maternal Deaths in the United Kingdom.* London: RCOG Press; 2001.

Lewis G, editor. *Why Mothers Die 2000–2002. The Sixth Report of the Confidential Enquiries into Maternal Deaths in the United Kingdom.* London: RCOG Press; 2004.

Chapter 33

Domestic violence

Objectives

On successfully completing this topic you will be able to:

■ appreciate the incidence of domestic violence

■ understand the implications for the woman and fetus during pregnancy and in the postnatal period

■ plan to identify cases and familiarise yourself with local support services.

Introduction

Domestic violence is a major public health issue, which threatens the health, emotional wellbeing and lives of women and their families.

Domestic violence is defined as the intentional abuse inflicted on one partner by another in an intimate relationship. The abuse can be physical, psychological or sexual. It can occur within the context of a heterosexual or homosexual relationship and need not occur in the home. Women are more likely to be victims in heterosexual relationships (90%). Domestic violence affects all social classes, all ethnic groups, occurs in any part of the world and affects all age groups.

Scale of the problem

■ One in three women experiences domestic violence at some point in their lives.

■ One in ten women will have experienced domestic violence in the past year.

■ Over one million domestic violence incidents are recorded by the police each year.

■ 30% of domestic violence starts in pregnancy.

■ 40% of women who are murdered are killed by a current or ex-partner.

■ Domestic violence is more common than violence in the street or a public house.

■ In the 2000–2002 Confidential Enquiries into Maternal Deaths, it was reported that 11 women were murdered by their partners during or soon after pregnancy.

What keeps women in violent relationships?

To outsiders it seems almost bizarre that anyone would stay within a violent relationship. However, women all too often do. The reasons for staying are often multiple:

■ Fear   If she leaves she or her family will experience more violence or possibly be killed.

■ Financial   Control of her resources by her abuser.

■ Family   Pressures to stay with the abuser.

■ Father   Wanting a father figure for her children.

■ Faith   That she places in a religious doctrine.

■ Forgiveness   Because the abuser is often contrite.

■ Fatigue   From living under high and constant stress and erosion of self-esteem.

Domestic violence and pregnancy

The incidence of domestic violence in pregnancy is reported as being 0.9–20.1%. Domestic violence often begins or escalates during pregnancy. In some cases, domestic violence commences in the puerperium. The risk of moderate-to-severe violence appears to be greatest in the postpartum period. Women suffering physical abuse are at increased risk for miscarriage, premature labour, placental abruption, low birthweight infants, fetal injury and intrauterine fetal death. Often, as a result of the violence, women are 15 times more likely to abuse alcohol, nine times more likely to abuse drugs, three times more likely to be clinically depressed and five times more likely to attempt suicide. These all obviously have implications for both the mother and fetus.

Classically, injuries toward the pregnant abdomen, genitals and breasts are seen in pregnancy. However, the injuries can be multiple affecting any part of the woman's body. Campbell reported that 9.5% of women reported sexual abuse and 13.9% were raped by their partners.

Recognising domestic violence in pregnancy

Women who are being abused often book late and may be poor attenders. Their partners may not give them enough money to get to the hospital. Alternatively, they may attend repeatedly with trivial symptoms and appear reluctant to be discharged home. If the partner accompanies the woman, he may be constantly present not allowing for private discussion. The woman may seem reluctant to speak in front of or contradict her partner.

Any signs of violence on the woman's body will be minimised. As with child abuse, the mechanism of injury often does not fit with the apparent injury. There may be untended injuries of different ages or the late presentation of injuries. A history of behavioural problems or abuse in the children may be indicative. Often the patient will give a history of psychiatric illness.

Diagnosing domestic violence

As domestic violence often begins or escalates during pregnancy, it is essential that we, as obstetricians and midwives, routinely ask women whether they are subject to violence. Violent pregnancies are high risk and violence is much more prevalent than most other complications of pregnancy, such as pre-eclampsia or gestational diabetes mellitus. Standard questions should therefore be included, in the same way as we would ask about medical disorders, smoking or alcohol use. Systematic multiple assessment protocols lead to increased detection and reporting of violence during pregnancy. RADAR was developed by the Massachusetts Medical Society as a tool to guide enquiry about domestic violence (Gerard 2000).

R	**Routinely enquire**
A	**Ask direct questions**
D	**Document your findings**
A	**Assess safety**
R	**Review options and choices**

Obstetric emergencies

Health professionals should be given appropriate training and education to improve awareness. Questions should be asked in a non-judgemental, respectful, supportive manner. Obstetricians and midwives should be aware of what help is available should a woman request help. Questions such as the following may allow the woman to disclose that she is subject to violence:

- I have noticed you have a number of bruises. Did someone hit you?

- You seemed frightened by your partner. Has he ever hurt you?

- You mention that your partner loses his temper with the children. Does he ever with you?

- How does your partner act when drinking or on drugs?

If routine questioning is to be introduced it is important that local guidelines are developed for referral to appropriate agencies. Other strategies such as questionnaires in the female toilets may help those women whose partners are constantly by their sides. Community midwives visiting women at home may have the privacy to discuss such sensitive issues. The provision of interpreters is essential (CEMD 2000–2002). It is not acceptable to rely on family members to act as interpreters as this does not allow free dialogue to occur. Documentation in the medical notes is important, even if the woman does not want to prosecute at the current time. Women often prosecute many years later and evidence of the pattern of domestic violence helps to secure a conviction.

Medico-legal issues

Following the Domestic Violence Crime and Victims Act 2004, a case against a perpetrator can now proceed if there is sufficient evidence even if the victim withdraws their statement. The case proceeds in 40% of cases where the victim retracts their complaint. If a victim is pregnant then healthcare workers including midwives and obstetricians will be approached for a statement if it is known that the victim was pregnant.

Communication and teamwork

Domestic violence is an area where multi-agency working is essential. No one agency is able to address all the issues of domestic violence. Working collaboratively will ensure appropriate help and support is given. Unit guidelines should incorporate referral pathways for multi-agency working.

Audit standard

All women should be seen on their own at least once during the antenatal period to enable the disclosure of such information.

Summary

- Domestic violence is a major health and social problem in pregnancy.

- Domestic violence represents a serious threat to the physical and emotional health of women and their children.

- All health professionals have an obligation to identify cases of domestic violence and provide support and help to the victims.

Useful contacts

Women's Aid Federation of England
PO Box 391, Bristol BS99 7WS
Tel: 0117 944 4411 (office)/0808 2000 247 (helpline)
Email: helpline@womensaid.org.uk
Website: www.womensaid.org.uk

Victim Support National Office
Cranmer House, 39 Brixton Road, London, SW9 6DZ
Tel: 020 7735 9166 (enquiries)
Email: contact@victimsupport.org.uk
Website: www.victimsupport.org.uk
Victim Support Line
Tel: 0845 30 30 900

Rape Crisis
PO Box 69, London, WC1X 9NJ
Tel: 020 7837 1600 (24-hour helpline)
Email: info@rapecrisis.co.uk
Website: www.rapecrisis.co.uk

Refuge
0808 2000 247 (24-hour national helpline)
Website: www.refuge.org.uk

Samaritans
Tel: 0845 7909 090
Website: www.samaritans.org.uk

Police – Domestic Violence Group
contact your local police station for details.

National Association of Citizens Advice Bureaux
Middleton House, 115–123 Pentonville Road, London, N1 9LZ
Tele: 020 7833 2181

Suggested further reading

Abbasi K. Obstetricians must ask about domestic violence. *BMJ* 1998;316:9.

Ballard TJ, Salzman LE, Gazmararian JA, Spitz AM, Lazorick S, Marks JS. Violence during pregnancy: mMeasurement issues. *Am J Public Health* 1998;88:274–6.

Bewley S, Friend J, Mezey G, editors. *Violence Against Women*. London: RCOG Press; 1997.

Campbell JC. Nursing assessment for risk of homicide with battered women. *Adv Nurs Sci* 1986;8:36–51.

Covington DL, Diehl SJ, Wright BD, Piner M. Assessing for violence during pregnancy using a systematic approach. *Matern Child Health J* 1997;1(2):129.

Gerard M. Domestic violence: how to Screen and Intervene. *Registered Nurse* 2000;62:52–6.

Gibson E, Klein S. *Murder 1957–1968*. Home Office Research Study No 3. London: HMSO; 1989.

Gielen AC, O'Campo PJ, Faden RR, Kass NE, Xue X. Interpersonal conflict and physical violence during the childbearing year. *Soc Sci Med* 1994;39:781–7.

Grunfeld A, MacKay K. Diagnosing domestic violence. *Canadian Journal of Diagnosis* 199714:61–9.

Heath I. Domestic violence and the general practitioner. *Matern Child Health* 199419:316–20.

Lewis G, editor. *Why Mothers Die 1997–1999. The Fifth Report of the Confidential Enquiries into Maternal Deaths in the United Kingdom.* London: RCOG Press; 2001.

Lewis G, editor. *Why Mothers Die 2000–2002. The Sixth Report of the Confidential Enquiries into Maternal Deaths in the United Kingdom.* London: RCOG Press; 2004.

Mezey GC, Bewley S. Domestic violence and pregnancy. *Br J Obstet Gynaecol* 1997;104:528–31.

Royal College of Midwives. *Domestic Abuse in Pregnancy.* Position Paper No. 19. London: RCM; 1997.

Stark E, Flitcraft A. *Women at Risk.* London: Sage; 1996.

Widding Hedin L. Postpartum, also a risk period for domestic violence. *Eur J Obstet Gynecol Reprod Biol* 2000;89:41–5.

Algorithm 34.1 Anaesthetic complications in obstetrics

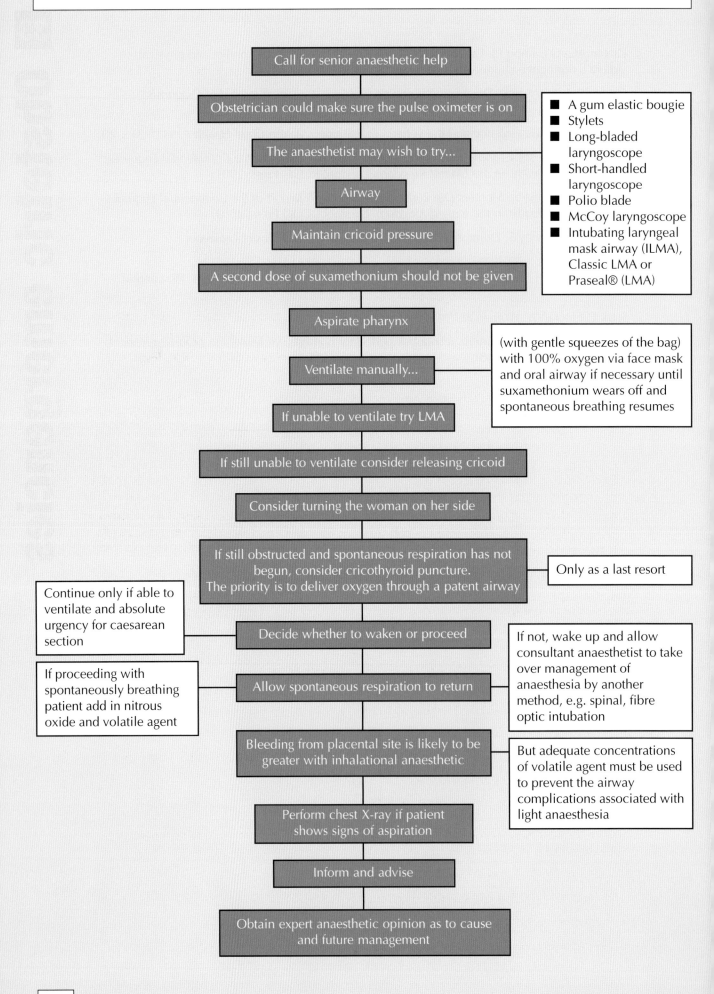

Call for senior anaesthetic help

Obstetrician could make sure the pulse oximeter is on

The anaesthetist may wish to try...

- A gum elastic bougie
- Stylets
- Long-bladed laryngoscope
- Short-handled laryngoscope
- Polio blade
- McCoy laryngoscope
- Intubating laryngeal mask airway (ILMA), Classic LMA or Praseal® (LMA)

Airway

Maintain cricoid pressure

A second dose of suxamethonium should not be given

Aspirate pharynx

Ventilate manually...

(with gentle squeezes of the bag) with 100% oxygen via face mask and oral airway if necessary until suxamethonium wears off and spontaneous breathing resumes

If unable to ventilate try LMA

If still unable to ventilate consider releasing cricoid

Consider turning the woman on her side

If still obstructed and spontaneous respiration has not begun, consider cricothyroid puncture. The priority is to deliver oxygen through a patent airway

Only as a last resort

Continue only if able to ventilate and absolute urgency for caesarean section

Decide whether to waken or proceed

If not, wake up and allow consultant anaesthetist to take over management of anaesthesia by another method, e.g. spinal, fibre optic intubation

If proceeding with spontaneously breathing patient add in nitrous oxide and volatile agent

Allow spontaneous respiration to return

Bleeding from placental site is likely to be greater with inhalational anaesthetic

But adequate concentrations of volatile agent must be used to prevent the airway complications associated with light anaesthesia

Perform chest X-ray if patient shows signs of aspiration

Inform and advise

Obtain expert anaesthetic opinion as to cause and future management

Chapter 34

Anaesthetic complications in obstetrics

Objectives

On successfully completing this topic you will:

■ be able to appreciate the risks posed to the pregnant women by anaesthetic drugs and techniques

■ have a working knowledge of anaesthetic emergency problems befalling the pregnant woman.

Introduction and incidence

The 2000–2002 Confidential Enquiries into Maternal Deaths in the United Kingdom reported seven deaths that were directly owing to the actions or omissions of anaesthetic services or staff. All deaths related to the administration of general anaesthesia; four of these deaths were related to anaesthesia for caesarean section.

The use of general anaesthesia has declined with the increasing use of regional anaesthesia but its continued use is estimated to carry a risk of death of 1/20 000 caesarean section operations.

The case reports concerning anaesthesia highlighted:

■ the need for the proper checking of anaesthetic machines

■ the danger of unrecognised oesophageal intubation and the importance of always using a capnograph to confirm tracheal placement

■ the contribution of isolated sites in delaying the provision of senior help and of blood products

■ the increased risks associated with obesity (body mass index greater than 30)

■ the need for staff to possess advanced life support skills

■ the need for staff to able to manage anaphylaxis.

There were a further 20 deaths to which anaesthesia in some way contributed. The report specifically highlights:

■ issues of timely and effective communication and consultation

■ failures to appreciate the severity of maternal illness

■ inadequate usage of invasive monitoring

■ substandard care in women who have sepsis, pre-eclampsia and haemorrhage.

Failed intubation

To learn about the management of the airway in a pregnant woman without mention of the potential and management of failed intubation would be wrong. Failed intubation is more likely in the pregnant than the nonpregnant woman and is more likely in the heavily pregnant woman. It occurs in any setting but will be most often seen when giving a general anaesthetic for caesarean section. It is potentially fatal and must be professionally managed.

Algorithm 34.1 applies to failed intubation at the time of general anaesthesia for caesarean section. Every anaesthetist will have a mentally rehearsed drill, which may vary slightly between individuals. The algorithm is suggested and described, not for the obstetrician to necessarily institute, as the drill should be guided by the anaesthetist, but so that the obstetrician is familiar with the drill, is able to offer help and is aware that they will be asked to take part in decision making.

Regional blocks (epidural and spinal anaesthesia)

Terminology

Spinal injection is into the intrathecal space and is sometimes called an intrathecal injection. It may also be called a subarachnoid injection. The epidural space is immediately peripheral to the dura, contains nerve roots, fat and blood vessels and extends from the foramen magnum to the sacral hiatus. See Figure 34.1.

An injection of local anaesthetic is often described as a 'block' because nerve conduction of painful impulses is blocked. A 'nerve block' refers to block of a single nerve and a 'regional block' refers to groups of nerves, as happens with a spinal or epidural injection.

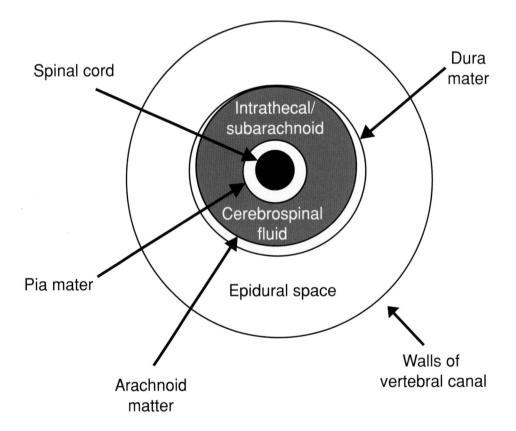

Figure 34.1 Anatomy of the spinal cord

Anatomy

The spinal cord, like the brain, is surrounded by three meninges:

■ the pia mater

■ the arachnoid mater

■ the dura mater.

The pia mater is a vascular membrane that closely invests the spinal cord.

The arachnoid mater lies between the pia mater and the dura mater. It is separated from the pia mater by a wide space, the subarachnoid space, which is filled with cerebrospinal fluid.

The arachnoid mater is continued along spinal nerve roots. The inner surface of the dura mater is in contact with the arachnoid mater. It is separated from the walls of the vertebral canal by the extradural (epidural) space. This contains loose areolar tissue and the internal vertebral venous plexus.

The dura mater extends along each nerve root as they cross the epidural space and exits via the transverse foramen and it becomes continuous with the connective tissue surrounding each nerve. Spinal nerves have communications with the sympathetic trunk.

Characteristics of spinal versus epidural anaesthesia

Epidural anaesthesia is conventionally used for analgesia for vaginal delivery and spinal anaesthesia is used for obstetric surgery. Conventionally, an 'epidural' refers to the placement of an epidural catheter in the epidural space so that drug can be repeatedly added to the space or continuously infused to give analgesia for the duration of labour, irrespective of how long that is. Occasionally, a spinal injection may be used as a method of analgesia for labour, for speed, and then an epidural catheter is used for the rest of the labour. This is called combined spinal/epidural analgesia (CSE). A 'spinal' refers to a one-off injection into the intrathecal space. The effect lasts for about 2 hours, which is long enough to carry out a caesarean section. Intrathecal infusions are not conventionally used in obstetric practice. Epidural incremental top-ups were formerly used for anaesthesia for caesarean section and may be indicated in certain patients where a slow onset of anaesthesia is desirable. For emergency sections or other operative procedures such as retained placenta, existing epidurals can be topped up or spinal analgesia given.

A single-shot spinal injection gives a dense, complete (no 'missed' – unanaesthetised – dermatomal segments) block of rapid onset. Its downside is that it causes marked vasodilatation (owing to the effect of local anaesthetic on lumbar sympathetic nerves) with consequent hypotension unless fluid loading, with or without vasopressors, is used. The height of the block is somewhat unpredictable and uncontrollable but is a function of dose.

The desired height of block for caesarean section is to the T4 level (sternal angle of Louis) but above this a spinal is described as 'high' and can cause cardiovascular and respiratory problems (see below).

Dosage

Calculation

A simple way to calculate local anaesthetic doses is to multiply by ten:

■ 0.5% bupivacaine contains 5 mg/ml; 10 ml therefore contains 50 mg

■ 0.5% means 0.5 g in 100 ml (equivalent to 500 mg in 100 millilitres; divide by 100 to get 5 mg in 1 ml)

Typical dose

A typical dose for a spinal for caesarean section (in the absence of pre-existing epidural) would be 2.2–2.7 ml of 0.5% hyperbaric (see below for explanation of this) bupivacaine. Opioids are commonly added to improve the quality of the block (for example, fentanyl) and to provide postoperative analgesia (for example, morphine or diamorphine).

A typical dose of bupivacaine immediately after siting an epidural for analgesia during the first stage of labour would be 10 ml of 0.25% or 0.5% bupivacaine (followed by top-ups or an infusion). Opioids are commonly added to the bupivacaine to improve the quality of the block (for example, fentanyl) and to minimise the local anaesthetic dose. Levobupivicaine and ropivicaine, two newer local anaesthetics, are both less cardiotoxic and therefore safer for labour epidural analgesia.

Complications

Complication can be grouped as follows:

■ Owing to the drugs used
Local anaesthetics and opioids are used both for spinal and epidural techniques. Local anaesthetic alone is still used occasionally. Opioids are used in combination but not alone.

■ Due to the technique.

Complications of local anaesthesia

■ Hypotension
   □ Defined as a greater than 20% fall in blood pressure.
   □ Occurs because of block of sympathetic nerves providing tone to the blood vessels; nausea may be a heralding sign.
   □ Likely to happen with both epidural and spinal blocks but more likely with a spinal block.
   □ Treat by checking airway and breathing, tilting the patient or displacing the uterus to the left, fluid loading – run in 1 litre Hartmann's immediately unless other reason not to do so.
   □ May require ephedrine in 3-mg increments intravenously approximately every 2 minutes until blood pressure recovers.
   □ Prophylactic infusions of vasopressors (phenylephrine or ephedrine) commonly used.

■ Motor block
   □ Dense motor blockade is required for operations under regional anaesthesia but is unwanted with labour epidural analgesia. Motor block depends on the dose of local anaesthetic used and the duration of labour.
   □ Labour is more likely to result in instrumental delivery if there is motor block (loss of power).
   □ Pressure sores are a potential complication of epidural analgesia as there is a prolonged period of relative immobility and a loss of sensation to discomfort.

■ Sensory block
   □ Full bladder unnoticed by patient and unopposed parasympathetic block predisposes to urinary retention.
   □ Can minimise motor and sensory block by reducing dose of local anaesthetic, at the price of complete analgesia or by supplementing local anaesthetic with opioids.

Toxic effects

The toxic dose of bupivacaine is 2 mg/kg nonpregnant weight in any 4-hour period and 3 mg/kg lignocaine (without adrenaline).

Toxicity can occur from any route of injection. It is dependent upon absorption and therefore is more likely from an area of high vascularity (e.g. interpleural space) or following direct intravascular injection (inadvertent).

It does not occur with spinal anaesthesia since only tiny doses of drug are used but can occur if an epidural catheter has migrated into a vein.

Toxicity is due to membrane stabilising properties and affects mainly the brain and heart.

Symptoms change with increasing plasma level:

- low dose: (affecting the nervous system) tingling or numbness of tongue and perioral area, dizziness, tinnitus, twitching, anxiety, confusion, convulsions.

- high dose: cardiovascular depression (can be cardiac arrest) and arrhythmias. Most likely rhythms are ventricular tachycardia (VT) and ventricular fibrillation (VF).

Management

- Stop administration of local anaesthetics.

- Call for help, cardiac arrest team, resident anaesthetist and obstetrician and resuscitation equipment and defibrillator.

- Displace the uterus and or tilt the patient to the left.

- Airway:
  - assess
  - open the airway and maintain patent
  - apply oxygen 15 litres/minute (hypoxia is more likely the cause of cardiovascular depression than direct effect)
  - put on pulse oximeter
  - consider intubation.

- Breathing:
  - assess
  - ventilate
  - protect airway.

- Circulation:
  - assess
  - cardiopulmonary resuscitation if necessary
  - tilt to left
  - put on ECG monitor
  - treat periarrest arrhythmias
  - treat hypotension with IV fluids and 3-mg bolus of ephedrine titrated against BP
  - use adrenaline as dictated by the cardiac arrest protocol
  - intravenous access, send bloods for urea and electrolytes, start intravenous infusion.

- Control seizures with diazepam 5–10 mg intravenously. If this fails to quickly control fits, make sure anaesthetist present, as thiopentone with intubation is required.

- Check fetal heart and consider timing and method of delivery. Deliver baby as matter of urgency. Inform paediatrician.

- Keep record chart to include pulse, blood pressure, respiratory rate, SpO_2, level of consciousness, fetal heart and treatments given.

- Consider transfer to intensive care unit.

- Document in notes, with time, date, a signature and printed identification and report to consultant obstetrician.

Cardiac arrest from local anaesthetic toxicity should be managed as any other but may need larger doses of adrenaline because larger capacitance of vasculature as it is vasodilated.

Local anaesthetic-induced VT and VF are often resistant to electrical defibrillation. Amiodarone 300 mg is the anti-arrhythmic drug of choice. Prolonged CPR may be required. There are some recent data suggesting that the use of intralipid (fat emulsion) may help to bind the bupiricaine and improve the outcome.

High spinal

If there is bradycardia, hypotension, tingling or weakness in the hands or complaint of difficulty in breathing or talking, suspect a high spinal block. Check the level of sharp sensation. If there is reduced sensation above the nipples then this is a high spinal block.

A high spinal block is a local anaesthetic block involving the spinal nerves above the level of T4. It may occur due to excessive (unpredictable) spread of a subarachnoid (spinal) injection of local anaesthetic (typically 2–3 ml of 0.5% bupivacaine) or following unintentional subarachnoid injection of an epidural dose of local anaesthetic, via a wrongly placed catheter or via migration of the catheter (typically 10 ml of 0.25% or 0.5% bupivacaine). Large volume epidural top-ups for caesarean section may produce a similar picture.

Symptoms depend upon the height of the block:

T1–T4   Bradycardia due to block of sympathetic cardiac nerves; severe hypotension due to effect of bradycardia superimposed on the effect of vasodilatation.

C6–C8   Hand paraesthesia and weakness, likely to be an effect on adequacy of breathing.

C3–C5   Diaphragmatic paralysis, with definite respiratory compromise.

Total spinal

Intracranial spread can also occur. It produces loss of consciousness due to the direct action of local anaesthesia on the brain. This is referred to as a 'total spinal'.

Hypotension with bradycardia occurs from the vasodilation caused by blockade of the sympathetic nervous system (T1–L2) and is exaggerated by the drug effects on the vasomotor centres in the brainstem. Hypoxia and respiratory arrest can occur because of phrenic nerve involvement and medullary depression.

Management of high and total spinal

- Turn off epidural infusion, if present.

- Call for help, cardiac arrest team, resident anaesthetist and obstetrician and resuscitation equipment and defibrillator.

- Displace the uterus and/or tilt the woman to the left.

- Airway:
  - [ ] assess
  - [ ] open and maintain patent
  - [ ] apply oxygen 15 litres/minute via tight-fitting facemask with reservoir bag
  - [ ] put on pulse oximeter.

- ◼ Breathing:
  - ☐ assess
  - ☐ ventilation assistance if necessary.
    The patient may complain of difficulty in breathing because of intercostal or diaphragmatic muscle paralysis. If this compromises her ventilation, she should be anaesthetised and intubated to assist ventilation until the effect of the local anaesthetic block wears off.
  - ☐ if patient is apnoeic, intubate
  - ☐ if patient is hypoxic, assist ventilation with facemask and self-inflating bag until anaesthetist arrives
  - ☐ protect airway by intubation if patient is unconscious.

- ◼ Circulation:
  - ☐ assess pulse rate and blood pressure
  - ☐ CPR
  - ☐ tilt to left
  - ☐ put on automatic blood pressure and ECG monitor
  - ☐ treat periarrest arrhythmias
  - ☐ IV access, send blood samples for full blood count, urea and electrolytes
  - ☐ treat hypotension with intravenous colloids and ephedrine, 3-mg increments titrated against blood pressure
  - ☐ treat bradycardia with atropine 0.6 mg intravenously.

- ◼ Check fetal heart and consider timing and method of delivery.

- ◼ Consider and exclude other causes of unconsciousness, e.g. hypoglycaemia, epilepsy, opioid drugs, intracranial lesion.

- ◼ Keep record chart of pulse, blood pressure, respiratory rate, SpO_2, fetal heart rate and treatments given.

- ◼ Document in notes with time, date, a signature and printed identification and inform consultant anaesthetist and obstetrician.

It is not always necessary to intubate a woman who says that she has difficulty breathing. Leave this decision to the anaesthetist unless the patient is apnoeic.

When using 'heavy', i.e. hyperbaric (heavier than cerebrospinal fluid) local anaesthetic as is used for spinals, the position of the woman affects where the local anaesthetic lies and can be used to influence the height of the block. A block that has not reached the required height can be brought higher by placing the woman in the head-down position. Similarly, a high spinal can be stopped from going higher by placing the woman head up. Gravity can be made to influence the height of the block for up to 20 minutes after the injection. A pillow under the shoulders and head virtually eliminates the spread of a spinal dose beyond the thoracic level.

Local anaesthetic toxicity and high or total spinal can cause cardiac arrest.

Unrecognised migration of an epidural catheter into the cerebrospinal fluid effectively results in a high or total spinal.

Complications of opioids

- ◼ Pruritus
- ◼ Urinary retention
- ◼ Late respiratory depression in absence of overdose, especially with long acting opioids.

Respiratory depression should be treated by ventilatory assistance and the use of naloxone in 0.1-mg increments intravenously, titrated against response. Any woman who has had spinal or epidural opioids must be closely monitored for late respiratory depression.

Anaphylaxis

All drugs can cause anaphylaxis.

Anaphylaxis is an exaggerated response to a substance to which an individual has become sensitised, in which histamine, serotonin and other vasoactive substances are released. This causes symptoms that can include pruritus, erythema, flushing, urticaria, angio-oedema, nausea, diarrhoea, vomiting, laryngeal oedema, bronchospasm, hypotension, cardiovascular collapse and death. Anaphylactic reactions usually begin within 5–10 minutes of exposure and the full reaction usually evolves within 30 minutes. Anaphylactic and anaphylactoid reactions are indistinguishable and managed in the same way. They have a different immunological mechanism.

In a patient with latex allergy, repeated vaginal examination with gloves containing latex and other exposure to latex can lead to anaphylaxis. Diagnosis is made on clinical grounds – suspect.

Management

- Stop administration of drug(s)/blood product likely to have caused anaphylaxis.
- Displace the uterus and/or tilt the woman to the left.
- Call for help, including anaesthetist and obstetrician and resuscitation equipment.
- Airway:
  - assess
  - open and maintain patent
  - apply oxygen 15 litres/minute via tight-fitting facemask with reservoir bag
  - consider tracheal intubation.
- Breathing:
  - assess
  - ventilate
  - protect airway.
- Circulation:
  - assess pulse, blood pressure
  - secure intravenous access with large-bore cannula
  - CPR
  - put on ECG and blood pressure monitor
  - treat periarrest arrhythmias.
- Give adrenaline/epinephrine either 0.5–1.0 mg (0.5–1.0 ml of 1:1000) intramuscularly every ten minutes until improvement in pulse and blood pressure or 50–100 micrograms (0.5–1.0 ml of 1:10 000) intravenously titrated against blood pressure if cardiovascular collapse. 0.5–1.0 mg (5–10 ml of 1:10 000) may be required intravenously in divided doses titrated against response. Give at a rate of 0.1 mg/minute and stop when a response has been obtained.
- Start intravascular volume expansion with crystalloid or synthetic colloid. Large volumes are often required.
- Give secondary therapy:
  - antihistamines: chlorpheniramine 10–20 mg by slow intravenous infusion
                        consider ranitidine 50 mg intravenously
  - corticosteroids: hydrocortisone 100–300 mg intravenously.
- Reassess airway, breathing and circulation.

■ Consider catecholamines if blood pressure still low:

☐ summon intensive care help and plan to insert arterial line and central venous line

☐ adrenaline (epinephrine) 0.05–0.10 micrograms/kg/minute (approximately 4–8 micrograms/minute)

☐ 5 mg adrenaline (epinephrine) in 500 ml saline gives 10 micrograms/ml

☐ noradrenaline (norepinephrine) 0.05–0.1 micrograms/kg/minute (approximately 4–8 micrograms/minute)

☐ 4 mg noradrenaline (norepinephrine) in 500 ml dextrose gives 8 micrograms/ml.

■ Perform arterial blood gases:

☐ consider bicarbonate for acidosis (0.5–1.0 mmol/kg intravenously)

☐ 0.5–1.0 mmol is equivalent to 0.5–1.0 ml of an 8.4% solution of sodium bicarbonate.

■ Consider bronchodilators if persistent bronchospasm; e.g., salbutamol 2.5 mg via oxygen-driven nebuliser or 250 micrograms intravenously slowly, or aminophylline 250 mg intravenously over 20 minutes.

■ Check fetal heart and continuously monitor by CTG and consider timing and method of delivery.

■ Keep a record chart to include pulse, BP, respiratory rate, SpO_2, fetal heart and treatments given.

■ Document fully in notes and inform consultant obstetrician.

■ Investigate: serial blood and urine samples looking for evidence of histamine release.

Complications due to the technique

■ Failure: complete, missed segment, unilateral block.

■ Headache.

■ Backache.

■ Neurological damage.

■ Migration of catheter causing relative intrathecal overdose.

■ Infection.

Failure

Failure is unlikely with a spinal block but when it occurs the block may need to be repeated.

An epidural block can fail to provide adequate analgesia if the catheter is not correctly in the epidural space. Even if it is in the epidural space, analgesia can be inadequate as a result of a unilateral block or 'missed segment' or if the block has not spread high enough. The segment that most commonly fails to be blocked is the L1 nerve root (groin).

The remedies for unilateral or unblocked segments are to reposition the patient and to give further local anaesthetic and/or opiates.

An epidural that is persistently providing inadequate analgesia usually needs to be resited.

Headache

A puncture of the dura can cause a post-dural puncture headache. The likelihood of headache is related to the size of the needle that punctured the dura and how many times it was punctured. During an epidural there is no intention to puncture the dura but this can occur accidentally. The incidence is 2–3% among staff in training. An epidural needle (Tuohy 16G or 18G) is larger than a spinal needle (24G or 25G). The incidence of headache following dural puncture with a Tuohy needle is 70%.

Post-dural puncture headache can occur following a spinal but it is less common due to the smaller needles used. The incidence is 1/150.

Style and orientation of the needle to the fibres of the dura has a bearing.

A low pressure headache occurs secondary to the leak of cerebrospinal fluid and traction on the meninges, which in turn causes traction on intracranial structures. A typical post-dural puncture headache is frontal and or occipital and worse on being in the upright position. It can come on immediately or be delayed.

Management:

■ The anaesthetic team should always be informed.

■ The definitive treatment is an epidural blood patch (20 ml of the woman's own blood injected under aseptic conditions into the epidural space). This may need to be repeated.

■ Conservative measures may be taken initially: simple analgesics, encourage oral fluids, consider intravenous fluids, encourage caffeine intake but, if the headache is severe, consider a blood patch early.

■ Consider differential diagnosis, which can include:
  □ migraine
  □ meningitis
  □ cerebral venous sinus thrombosis
  □ subarachnoid haemorrhage.

If any doubt exists, easy access to neuroimaging and neurology opinions should be sought.

Backache

There is no evidence for an increase in long-term backache in those who have had regional blocks. Local discomfort is reported at the area of needle entry.

Treat with simple analgesics and non-steroidal anti-inflammatory drugs if no contraindication. Consider referral to a physiotherapist for ultrasound therapy.

Women may present with severe backache postpartum, which may be due to an acute disc prolapse. This should be managed appropriately. A differential diagnosis in a woman who has received a regional blockage would include epidural haematoma or abscess.

Neurological damage

Neurological symptoms and signs in the postpartum period may be due to regional techniques or as a result of compression injuries during labour and delivery. Symptoms and signs suggestive of compression should be investigated urgently with an MRI scan to exclude surgically treatable pathology. The anaesthetic team will need to consult with a neurologist or a neurosurgeon and, depending on the findings, urgent spinal decompression may be required to avoid permanent neurological deficit.

Neuropraxia

Neuropraxia occurs due to the piercing of a nerve with a needle (intraneural injection). A report of pain at the time of injection would be suggestive (the injection should not have proceeded if pain was reported at the time).

Infection (epidural abscess or discitis)

These are serious neurological conditions and are extremely rare. They have potentially devastating complications. Signs and symptoms include severe backache, neurological deficit including bowel/bladder dysfunction and unexplained fever. Suspicion should lead to immediate investigation: CT scan or MRI and neurological consultation. Check the patient's temperature and send blood samples for white count. Seek neurological advice immediately.

Effects of complications on the fetus

Maternal compromise, such as hypoxia and cardiovascular instability, causes compromise to the fetus. Opioids may cross the placenta and the paediatrician should be informed that maternal opioids have been given.

Suggested further reading

Lewis G, editor. *Why Mothers Die 2000–2002. The Sixth Report of the Confidential Enquiries into Maternal Deaths in the United Kingdom.* London: RCOG Press; 2004.

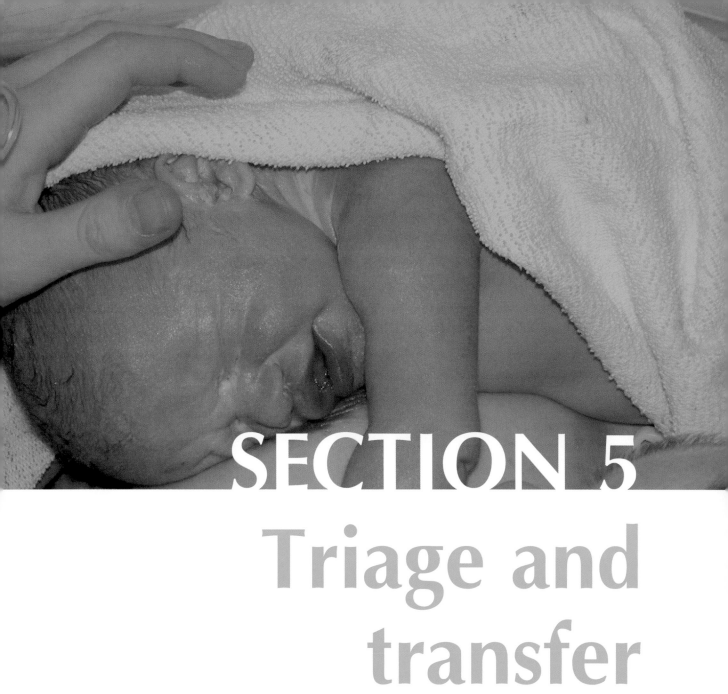

SECTION 5
Triage and transfer

Chapter 35

Triage

Objectives

On successfully completing this topic you will:

- understand the systematic approach advocated for prioritisation when casualties exceed resources available.

Introduction

The word 'triage' is derived form the French *trier*, to sort or to sift as through a sieve. The word was originally used to describe the process of selecting coffee beans. Triage was first described in modern times by Baron Dominique Jean Larrey, who was Napolean's Surgeon Marshal. He introduced a system of sorting casualties presenting to field dressing stations to ensure that soldiers with only minor wounds could be returned quickly to the battlefield with minimum treatment. In more recent times, triage has become a daily management tool within civilian accident and emergency departments.

The aims of triage, wherever it is done, are not only to deliver the right patient to the right place at the right time so that they receive the optimum treatment but also to 'do the most for the most', accepting that valuable medical resources should not be diverted to treating an irrecoverable condition. It can be deduced from this that triage principles should be applied whenever the number of casualties exceeds the skilled help immediately available.

Triage can be applied to acute medical and obstetric workloads. It can take place formally, as in the management of some major incidents, or informally and almost unnoticed as it often does in our day-to-day practice in resuscitation rooms or on delivery suites. Triage must reflect the changing state of the patient and is therefore a dynamic rather than a static process; regular reassessment of priorities across patients is vital.

The end point of the triage process is the allocation of a priority. This priority is then used in conjunction with other factors to determine optimum care. Most triage systems have four categories of patients. There has to be a method of assessment to determine the category (Figure 35.1).

The triage priorities given in Table 35.1 reflect the need for clinical intervention, not the severity of injury. For example, a shocked patient bleeding from a simple scalp wound may need urgent intervention (priority red) but the injury itself may be relatively minor. By prioritising such a patient in a high category, a simple manoeuvre (application of pressure dressing) may save the casualty's life. Similarly, a patient with a large burn to the extremities clearly has a severe, possibly life-threatening anatomical injury, certainly worse than the patient with the scalp laceration. However, their prognosis may not be altered by receiving their care within the first few hours rather than minutes.

335

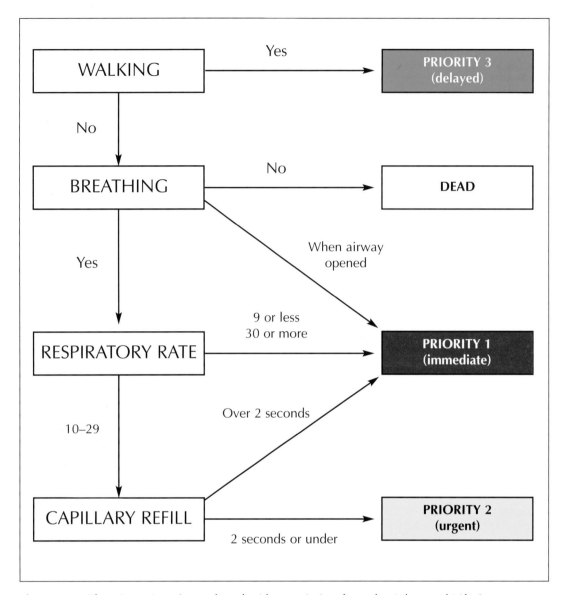

Figure 35.1 The triage sieve (reproduced with permission from the Advanced Life Support Group)

In the third-trimester pregnant woman, assessment of the fetus would immediately follow assessment of the mother.

If the 'P' system is in use then the use of the fourth category is very much a decision for the senior personnel involved. The decision must be based on an overall assessment of the situation: it must take into account both the patient load and the resources available. If the category is used, patients must be only considered to be within the category after assessment by senior medical personnel.

The principles of obstetric triage are the same, involving the ability to identify immediately life-threatening conditions and to deal with them in the correct order.

Table 35.1. Major incident triage categories (reproduced with permission from the Advanced Life Support Group)

Category	Description	Colour	Priority system	Treatment system
Immediate	Casualties who require immediate life saving treatment	Red	P 1	T 1
Urgent	Casualties who require treatment within 6 hours	Yellow	P 2	T 2
Delayed	Less serious cases who require treatment but not within a set time	Green	P 3	T 3
Expectant	Casualties who cannot survive treatment The degree of intervention required is such that in the circumstances their treatment would seriously compromise the provision of treatment for others	Blue		T 4
		Blue		T 4
Dead	Dead	White	Dead	Dead

Assessment of the mother

The priority category is determined by the identification of problems which are likely to kill and the order in which they are likely to kill: the ABCs. In the pregnant woman, triage category is determined firstly by threats to maternal life and then presence of life threats to the fetus.

- Think A B C.

- Assess before treating.

- Assess mobility then assess A B C.

- Is the patient walking?

- If so, the patient has a patent airway, is breathing and has sufficient circulating blood volume to allow locomotion. Move on.

- Is the patient talking?

- If so, the airway is open, the patient is breathing and there is sufficient circulating blood volume to allow oxygenation of the brain. Move on.

- Is the patient breathing but unconscious?

- If so, they have a potentially urgent airway problem.

- Is the patient not breathing?

- Open the airway.

- Is the patient still not breathing?

- Probably dead, especially in the trauma scenario.

- Assess fetal wellbeing and viability.

Scenario 1

You are the on-call SpR for obstetrics. You are on the labour ward reviewing a CTG when you hear a horn blaring followed by a loud crash and then splintering noises. A truck transporting an MRI scanner has crashed into the building, demolishing a wall. You run towards the affected room to find student midwife A covered in debris walking out in a dazed way bleeding from a scalp wound. As you enter the labour room, you find that the truck has gone through the window, the truck driver is still in his cab, which has stoved inwards and the windscreen has shattered. He is grasping the steering wheel and breathing very rapidly. He was not wearing a seat belt.

Mrs B is on the bed in established labour, her legs are in lithotomy as the SHO was about to perform a ventouse delivery for prolonged second stage. The CTG machine is still running: the fetal heart appears to be normal. Mrs B is panting and saying she needs to push. The SHO is on the floor groaning, with a large piece of masonry on his pelvis. Midwife C is lying on top of Mrs B, motionless with an obvious injury to the back of her head.

Mr B appears unscathed but grabs you on entry telling you that you must immediately deliver his baby.

Order of priority

■ Midwife C may have an airway problem, she may be unconscious or dead. Quickly assess her airway, breathing and the presence of circulation. If she is not breathing after checking her airway is not obstructed there is nothing further that can be done.

■ The truck driver has a breathing problem, there is likely to be a chest injury, which will need early assessment. He may be trapped in the cab and may also have a circulatory problem secondary to fractured long bones. He must have early attention.

■ The SHO is groaning and therefore does not have an airway or breathing problem. He is likely to have a significant circulatory problem.

■ Student midwife A has a circulation problem. Her confusion may be secondary to cerebral hypoxia/hypovolaemia, or due to concussion from a blow to the head.

■ Mrs B appears not to have an airway or breathing problem, the midwife has shielded her from injury although her fall onto Mrs B's abdomen may cause some trauma. There is no immediate urgency to deliver the baby.

■ Mr B does not require any immediate medical attention.

Scenario 2

You are the SpR arriving for your shift at 0800 hours on a Sunday morning on the labour ward. The midwife in charge tells you it has been a very busy night. The previous team has recently gone to theatre with a patient who had an anterior placenta praevia and was bleeding heavily; the consultant is with them. She goes through the labour ward board with you:

Room	Parity	VE	Epidural	Syntocinon	Comments
1	1+0	0730 5 cm	No	No	Gp B Streptococcus carrier
2	5+1	Del 0630	No	No	Retained placenta; cord snapped, PPH 600 ml and continues to trickle
3	0+0	0500 4 cm	Yes	Yes	38/40 induced for marked oedema and protein++++, poor urine output, BP 160/95
4	2+0				Term + 14 for induction
5	0+0	0730 9 cm	Yes	No	CTG late decelerations FBS pH 7.21 at 0730
6	2+1	0600 fully	No	No	
7	1+0		No	No	34 weeks c/o decreased FM and abd pain, previous SB at 38 weeks

Just as you finish report the support worker comes in with an urgent message from the midwife in room 7, who is unable to hear the fetal heart. The buzzer then goes off in room 1 where the midwife has recently given her patient intravenous penicillin, she is complaining of itching and is now very breathless.

Order of priority

Room 1 has a breathing problem that could become an airway problem, as she may be having an anaphylactic reaction and needs urgent attention.

Room 3 could be developing a breathing and airway problem; her blood pressure is inadequately controlled, she needs early review.

Room 2 has a circulation problem, ensure intravenous access and crossmatched; she will need to go to theatre for a manual removal of placenta as soon as possible.

Room 7 may have a circulatory problem as she has probably had an abruption. She will need intravenous access, crossmatch and clotting studies.

Room 5 has a fetal concern; the CTG should be reviewed and a decision made if further fetal blood sampling is necessary.

Room 6 should have delivered and will need review if there is delay in the second stage.

Room 4 is not a problem and induction should be deferred until there are sufficient staff to safely care for her.

As there are several major problems requiring attention, it will be necessary to divide the resources available; if there are an anaesthetist and an SHO also coming on duty they could be sent to rooms 1 and 3. Theatre should be made aware that there are other problems so that a speedy turnaround is possible and the consultant can be freed to help as soon as the bleeding is under control.

Summary

■ Triage is the key component whenever the number of casualties to treat exceeds the available resources.

■ More details on the process of triage are outside the scope of the manual and are covered in ALSG training courses such as Hospital MIMMS.

Suggested further reading

Advanced Life Support Group. Carley S, Mackway Jones K, editors. *Major Incident Medical Management and Support: The Practical Approach at the Scene.* Oxford: Blackwell Publishing; 2002.

Advanced Life Support Group. Carley S, Mackway Jones K, editors. *Major Incident Medical Management and Support: The Practical Approach in the Hospital.* Oxford: Blackwell Publishing; 2005.

Manchester Triage Group. *Emergency Triage.* Oxford: Blackwell Publishing; 2005.

Chapter 36

Transfer

Objectives

On successfully completing this topic you will:

■ have an overview of the principles of the safe transfer or retrieval of critically ill patients

■ understand the systematic 'ACCEPT' approach for managing such patients.

Introduction

The aim of a safe transfer policy is to ensure that maternal and neonatal care is streamlined and of the best standard. Transfer may be necessary for maternal or fetal reasons (specialised neonatal care or the availability of neonatal unit cots). Maternal transfer may be for an obstetric problem such as pre-eclampsia or for a problem not directly related to the pregnancy.

To achieve successful transfer or retrieval, the right patient has to be taken at the right time, by the right people, to the right place by the right form of transport and receive the right care throughout. The added complexity in obstetrics of dealing with 'two patients' demands a highly systematic approach that incorporates a high level of planning and preparation prior to the patient being moved. One such approach is the ACCEPT method developed by the Advanced Life Support Group.

The ACCEPT systematic approach to patient transfer

A   Assessment

C   Control

C   Communication

E   Evaluation

P   Preparation and packaging

T   Transportation

Following ACCEPT ensures that assessments and procedures are carried out in the right order. This method also correctly emphasises the preparation that is required before the patient is transported. The component parts of ACCEPT are outlined below.

Assessment

The clinician involved in the transportation may have been involved in the care given up to that point. However, the transporter may have been brought in especially for that purpose and will have no prior knowledge of the patient's clinical history. It is the responsibility of the person undertaking the transfer to appraise himself fully.

Control

Once assessment is complete, the transport organiser needs to take control of the situation. This requires:

■ identifying the clinical team leader

■ identifying the tasks to be carried out

■ allocating tasks to individuals or teams.

The lines of responsibility must be established urgently. In theory, ultimate responsibility is held jointly by the referring consultant clinician, the receiving consultant clinician and the transfer personnel at different stages of the transfer process. There should always be a named person with overall responsibility for organising the transfer.

Communication

Moving ill patients from one place to another requires cooperation and the involvement of several people. Therefore, key personnel need to be informed when transportation is being considered.

People who need to know about a transfer

The neonatologists in referring and receiving units should communicate directly. Who to involve in maternal care depends on whether the mother is being transferred for an obstetric problem or a non-obstetric problem. If the transfer is for a non-obstetric problem, obstetric care also has to be continued in the receiving unit and has to be transferred to an obstetric team at the receiving unit.

■ The consultant responsible for current maternal clinical care

■ The consultant responsible for current obstetric care if different from above

■ The consultant responsible for current neonatal clinical care

■ Special care unit staff in transferring hospital

■ The consultant responsible for the transfer of the patient (if different from above)

■ The consultant responsible for maternal intensive care if appropriate

■ The senior midwife in transferring unit

■ The patient's relatives

■ The consultant responsible for maternal clinical care in the receiving unit

■ The consultant responsible for obstetric care in the receiving unit

■ The consultant responsible for neonatal care in the receiving unit

■ Special care unit staff in the receiving unit

■ The senior midwife in the receiving unit

■ Ambulance control or special transportation controls (when appropriate)

■ If anaesthetists have been involved in the obstetric care they should communicate directly.

Communication may take a long time to complete if one person does it all. It is therefore advisable to share the tasks between corresponding teams, taking into account expertise and the local policies. Team to team communication is imperative. In all cases it is important that information is passed on clearly and unambiguously. This is particularly the case when talking to people over the telephone. It is useful to plan what to say before telephoning and to use the systematic summary shown below.

Key elements in any communication

- Who are you?
- What is needed (from the listener)?
- What are the relevant patient's details?
- What is the problem?
- What has been done to address the problem?
- What happened?

The second question can be repeated at the end to help summarise the situation. The response to all these questions should be documented in the patient's notes. The person in overall charge can then assimilate this information so that a proper evaluation of the patient's requirements for transportation can be made.

Evaluation

The dual aims of evaluation are to assess whether transfer is appropriate for the patient and, if so, what clinical urgency the patient has. While evaluation is a dynamic process which starts from first contact with the patient, it is only when the first phase of ACCEPT (that is, A C C) has been completed that enough information will have been gathered.

Is transfer appropriate for this patient?

Transfer may be indicated for maternal reasons or in the fetal interest. The need for neonatal intensive care may be reason for in utero transfer. If the woman herself requires transfer for delivery it is important that her condition is stabilised. Severe pre-eclampsia/eclampsia might be one reason for transfer either in the maternal or fetal interest.

The risks involved in transfer must be balanced against the risks of staying and the benefits of care that can only be given by the receiving unit.

Clinical urgency?

With the indication for transfer clear, the urgency must be evaluated. The degree of urgency for transfer and the severity of illness may be used to rank the woman's and fetus's transfer needs. This hierarchy also helps determine both the personnel required and the mode of transport.

Transfer categories

- Intensive
- Time-critical
- Ill – unstable
- Ill and stable
- Unwell
- Well

Preparation and packaging

Preparation and packaging both have the aim of ensuring that the patient transport proceeds with the minimum change in the level of care provided and with no deterioration in the patient's condition. The first stage (preparation) involves completion of patient stabilisation and preparation of transfer team personnel and equipment. The second stage (packaging) involves the final measures that need to be taken to ensure the security and safety of the patient during the transportation itself.

Patient preparation

To ensure best outcome for mother and fetus and to reduce the likelihood of complications during the journey, meticulous resuscitation and stabilisation should be carried out prior to transfer. This may involve carrying out procedures requested by the receiving hospital or unit (maternal or fetal). The standard airway, breathing and circulation (A B C) approach should be taken. Consideration should be given to securing a definitive airway in the patient with potential to fit. Hypovolaemic patients tolerate the inertial forces of transportation very poorly. Fetal wellbeing must be assessed to be certain that transfer is in the fetal interest before delivery. Steroids should be given if the woman is preterm.

All basic investigations should have been performed and the results clearly recorded in the accompanying notes or telephoned through as soon as available.

Inadequate resuscitation or missed illnesses and injuries will result in instability during transfer and will adversely affect outcome.

Equipment preparation

All equipment must be functioning.

Supplies of drugs and fluids should be more than adequate for the whole of the intended journey.

Particular care should be taken with supplies of oxygen, inotropes, sedative drugs and batteries for portable electronic equipment.

All lines and drains should be secured to the patient, the patient should be secured to the trolley and the trolley must be secured to the ambulance. The patient should be tilted to prevent aortocaval compression.

Specialist equipment may also be required for particular patients; for example, children and those patients with spinal injuries.

A member of the team should be allocated the task of ensuring that all of the patient's documents, including case notes, investigations reports and a transfer form, accompany the patient.

The transferring personnel should know exactly the location at which they are expected.

The team requires a telephone and contact names and numbers to enable direct communication with both the receiving and base unit. In addition, all personnel need appropriate clothing, food if the journey is long and enough money to enable them to get home if needed.

Personnel preparation

The number and nature of staff accompanying patients during transport will reflect their transfer category.

The sick, pre-eclamptic patient would normally be escorted by an anaesthetist and midwife.

All staff must practise within their areas of competence. For an intensive care transfer, the Intensive Care Society recommends that the accompanying physician 'should have received training in intensive care and transport medicine, had involvement in previous transfers and preferably have at least 2 years' experience in anaesthesia, intensive care medicine or other equivalent specialty'. In addition, they should be accompanied by another experienced doctor, nurse, paramedic or technician familiar with intensive care procedures and with all transport equipment.

Whatever category the patient, all personnel should be competent in the transfer procedure, and familiar with the equipment to be used as well as the details of the patient's clinical condition. The team should carry accident insurance with adequate provision for personal injury or death sustained during the transfer.

Packaging

Chest drains should be secured and unclamped with any underwater seal device replaced by an appropriate commercial drainage valve and bag system. If the patient has a simple pneumothorax, or is at risk of developing one, a chest drain should be inserted prophylactically.

Transportation

Mode of transport

The choice of transport needs to take into account several factors:

- nature of illness
- urgency of transfer
- mobilisation time
- geographical factors
- weather
- traffic conditions
- cost.

Road ambulances are by far the most common means used in the UK. They have a low overall cost, rapid mobilisation time and are less affected by weather conditions. They also give rise to less physiological disturbance.

Air transfer may be used for journeys over 50 miles or 2 hours in duration, or if road access is difficult. The speed of the journey itself has to be balanced against organisational delays and also the need for inter-vehicle transfer at the beginning and end of the journey.

Care during transport

Tilt should be maintained during transfer.

Physiological problems that occur during transportation may arise as a result of the effects of the transport environment on the deranged physiology of the patient. Careful preparation can minimise the deleterious effects of inertial forces, such as tipping, acceleration and deceleration, as well as changes in temperature and barometric pressure.

The standard of care and the level of monitoring carried out prior to transfer need to be continued as far as possible during the transfer. Monitoring will include oxygen saturation, ECG and direct arterial pressure monitoring in all patients. End-tidal CO_2 monitoring should be used in all patients who are intubated.

Fetal monitoring may be appropriate.

The patient should be well covered and kept warm during the transfer. Road speed decisions depend both on clinical urgency and the availability of limited resources such as oxygen.

With adequate preparation, the transportation phase is usually incident free. However, untoward events do occur. Should this be the case, the patient needs to be reassessed using the A B C approach. Appropriate corrective measures should then be instituted. This may require a stop at the first available place. Following any untoward events, communications with the receiving unit are important. This should follow the systematic summary described previously.

Handover

At the end of the transfer, direct contact with the receiving teams must be established, so that a succinct, systematic summary of the patient can then be provided. This should be accompanied by a written record of the patient's history, vital signs, therapy and significant clinical events during transfer. All the other documents that have been taken with the patient should also be handed over. While this is going on, the rest of the transferring team can help in moving the patient from the ambulance trolley to the receiving unit's bed. The team can then retrieve all equipment and personnel and make their way back to their home unit.

Summary

- The safe transfer and retrieval of a patient requires a systematic approach.
- By following the ACCEPT method important activities will be carried out at the appropriate time.
- Specific training is available for staff undertaking transfers on of the Safe Transfer and Retrieval Course (STaR) delivered by ALSG.

Suggested further reading

Advanced Life Support Group. *Safe Transfer and Retrieval: The Practical Approach.* Oxford: Blackwell Publishing; 2006.

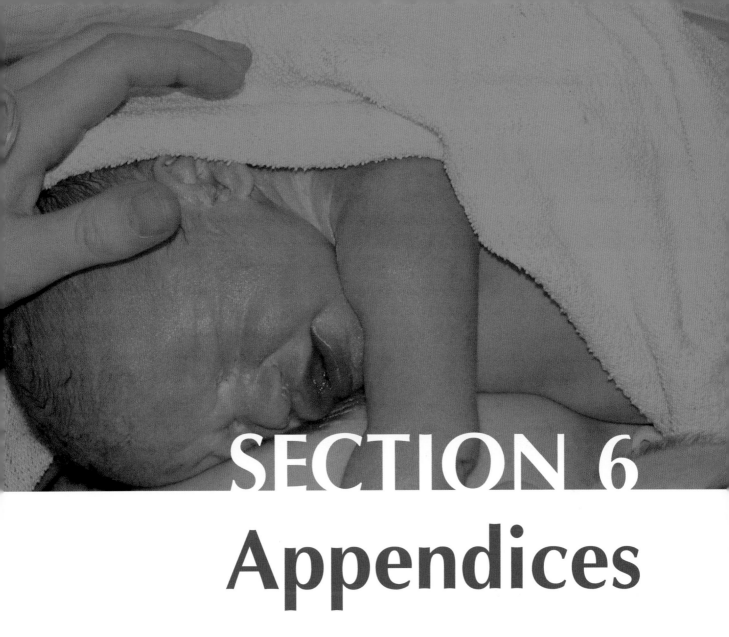

SECTION 6
Appendices

Appendix A

Perineal and anal sphincter trauma

Introduction

Perineal trauma resulting from childbirth remains a common problem that is associated with considerable maternal morbidity and may have a devastating effect on family life and sexual relationships. More than 85% of women sustain perineal trauma after childbirth and up to two-thirds need suturing.

Recognised anal sphincter rupture is reported in about 2.5% of vaginal deliveries in centres that practise mediolateral episiotomy and about 11% in centres that practise midline episiotomy. However, 33% of women sustain 'occult' anal sphincter injury (i.e. defects in the anal sphincter detected by anal endosonography) during vaginal delivery. The most plausible explanation for an 'occult' injury is either lack of recognition or misclassification as a second degree tear. As a result of inconsistency in classification and under-reporting it is difficult to establish the true global incidence of perineal trauma.

Definition of perineal trauma

Perineal trauma may occur spontaneously during vaginal birth or as a result of a surgical incision (episiotomy) that is intentionally made to facilitate delivery. It is also possible to have both an episiotomy and a spontaneous tear (e.g. extension of an episiotomy). Anterior perineal trauma is defined as injury to the labia, anterior vagina, urethra or clitoris. Posterior perineal trauma is defined as any injury to the posterior vaginal wall, perineal muscles or anal sphincters.

The following classification of spontaneous perineal trauma described by Sultan has now been accepted by the Royal College of Obstetricians and Gynaecologists and also internationally by the International Consultation on Incontinence.

First degree	Injury to vaginal or perineal skin only.
Second degree	Injury to perineal muscles but not involving the anal sphincter.
Third degree	Anal sphincter muscles torn. Further subdivided into: 3a: < 50% thickness of external sphincter torn. 3b: > 50% thickness of external sphincter torn. 3c: internal sphincter also torn.
Fourth degree	A third-degree tear with disruption of the anal epithelium.

An isolated rectal tear without involvement of the anal sphincter is rare and should not be included in the above classification.

Episiotomy

Episiotomy is a surgical incision made with scissors or a scalpel in the perineum to increase the diameter of the vulval outlet and facilitate delivery. The two main types of episiotomy incision are midline and mediolateral. A midline episiotomy is an incision from the midpoint of the posterior fourchette directed vertically towards the anus, in contrast to a mediolateral (posterolateral) episiotomy, whereby a similar incision is made but directed directly away from the anal sphincter and rectum at an angle of 40–60 degrees from the midline. However, in practice this angle is not always achieved.

Episiotomy is still being performed routinely in many parts of the world in the belief that it protects the pelvic floor. However, evidence from randomised controlled trials suggests that routine episiotomy does not prevent severe posterior perineal tears. There is currently an absence of clear, evidence-based clinical indications for the use of episiotomy. However, it is reasonable to suggest that an episiotomy should be performed to accelerate vaginal delivery:

- in cases of fetal distress

- to facilitate delivery during shoulder dystocia

- to minimise severe perineal trauma during an instrumental delivery (particularly forceps)

- to aid vaginal delivery when the perineum appears thick and inelastic

- when prolonged 'bearing down' may be detrimental to the mother's health (e.g. severe hypertension or cardiac disease).

These indications are not absolute and therefore clinical discretion is recommended.

Assessment of perineal trauma

- The perineum must be examined thoroughly following the birth, with good exposure and lighting.

- The assessment should include a rectal examination to exclude anal sphincter injury (Figure A.1). This is of considerable importance, as 'buttonhole' injuries of the rectum (Figure A.2) can occur in isolation even with an intact perineum.

- The anal sphincter should be palpated with the index finger in the rectum and the thumb on the perineum or over the posterior fourchette while performing a pill-rolling motion. In the absence of an epidural, the woman could be asked to contract her anal sphincter to accentuate any anal sphincter disruption.

- It is essential that, prior to examination or suturing, the procedure is explained to the woman and her partner and consent obtained.

Repair of first-degree tears

First-degree tears must be sutured if there is excessive bleeding or there is any uncertainty regarding alignment of the traumatised tissue which may affect the healing process.

If the tear is left unsutured, the midwife or doctor must discuss the implications with the woman and obtain her informed consent. Details regarding the discussion and consent must be fully documented in the woman's case notes.

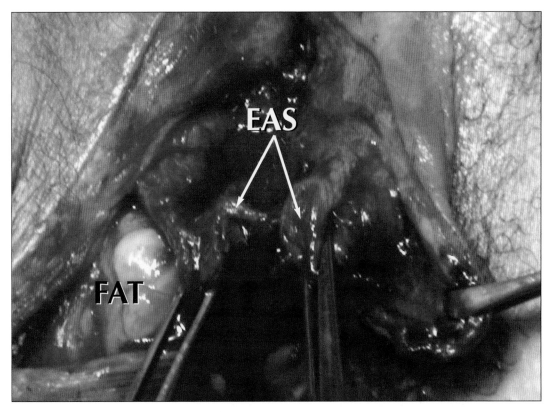

Figure A.1 Third degree tear (Grade 3b) with the external anal sphincter (EAS) grasped by Allis forceps. The ischioanal fat is lateral to the EAS

Repair of episiotomy and second-degree tears

It is not necessary to use lithotomy poles to support the woman's legs during the procedure unless she has a working epidural or spinal anaesthesia. This, apart from being uncomfortable for the woman, may make the trauma difficult for the operator to realign and suture.

It is not essential to use a tampon, as this may obscure visualisation of the apex of the vaginal trauma. Excessive uterine bleeding should be managed appropriately prior to commencing the perineal suturing.

Ensure that the wound is adequately anaesthetised prior to commencing the repair by injecting 10–20 ml 1% lignocaine evenly into the perineal wound (unless there is an epidural in place).

The continuous suturing technique

Current research suggests that perineal trauma should be repaired using the continuous non-locking technique to reapproximate all layers (vagina, perineal muscles and skin) with absorbable polyglactin 910 material (Vicryl rapide®). The steps involved are demonstrated in Figure A.3 and outlined below.

Step 1: suture the vagina

■ Identify the apex and check whether the trauma is unilateral or bilateral.

■ The first stitch is inserted 5–10 mm above the apex of vaginal trauma to secure any bleeding points that may not be visible.

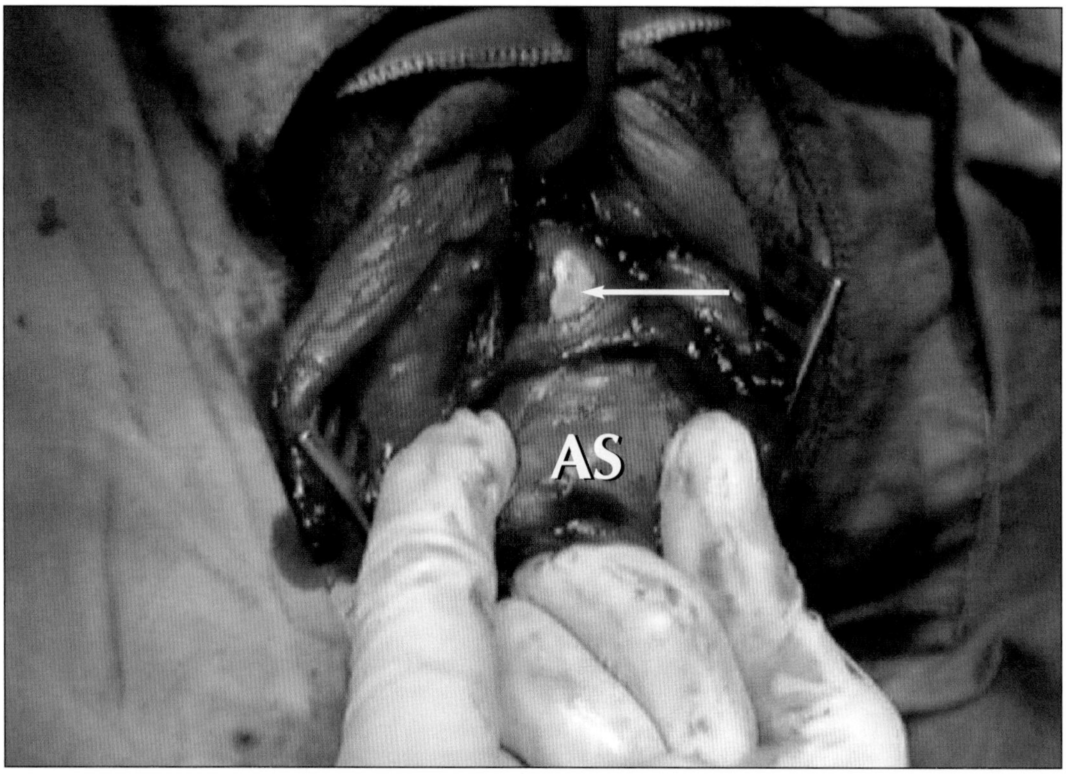

Figure A.2 Arrow demonstrating a buttonhole tear (arrow) in the rectum with an intact anal sphincter (AS)

- Close the vaginal trauma with a loose continuous non-locking stitch.

- Continue to suture down to the hymenal remnants.

- Insert the needle through the skin at the fourchette to emerge in the centre of the perineal muscle trauma.

Step 2: suture the muscle layer

- Check the depth of the trauma.

- Close the perineal muscle (deep and superficial) with continuous non-locking stitches.

- If the trauma is deep, the perineal muscles can be closed using two layers of continuous stitches.

- Realign the muscle so that the skin edges can be reapproximated without tension.

- Ensure that the stitches are not inserted through the rectum or anal canal.

Step 3: suture the perineal skin

- At the inferior end of the wound, bring the needle out just under the skin surface reversing the stitching direction.

- The skin sutures are placed below the skin surface in the subcutaneous tissue thus avoiding the profusion of nerve endings.

- Continue to take bites of tissue from each side of the wound edges until the hymenal remnants are reached.

- Secure the finished repair with a loop or Aberdeen knot placed in the vagina behind the hymenal remnants.

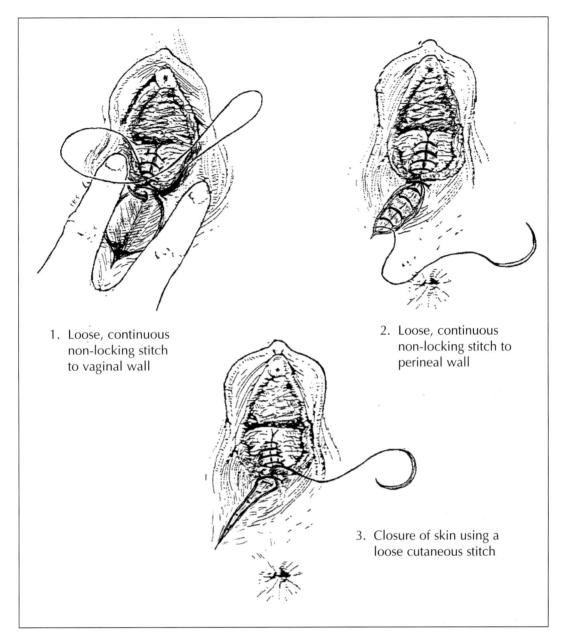

1. Loose, continuous non-locking stitch to vaginal wall

2. Loose, continuous non-locking stitch to perineal wall

3. Closure of skin using a loose cutaneous stitch

Figure A.3 Diagram illustrating continuous suturing technique

Step 4: final check

■ Check that the finished repair is anatomically correct and complete haemostasis is achieved.

■ Perform a vaginal examination and check that the vagina is not stitched too tight.

■ A rectal examination should be performed after completing the repair to ensure that suture material has not been accidentally inserted through the rectal mucosa.

■ Check that all swabs, needles and instruments are correct.

■ Following completion of the repair, the extent of the injury sustained, the suture technique and materials used must be documented in the case notes in black ink. It is also useful to include a diagram to illustrate the extent of the trauma.

Instruments	**Sutures**
■ Weitlander Retractor (or Gilpin retractor)	■ Anal epithelium *Ethicon Vicryl 3-0, 26-mm round-bodied needle W9120*
■ Tooth forceps (fine and strong)	
■ Needle holder (small and large)	■ Internal anal sphincter *Ethicon PDS 3-0, 26-mm round-bodied needle W9124T*
■ Allis forceps (4)	
■ Artery forceps (6)	■ External anal sphincter *Ethicon PDS 3-0, 26-mm round-bodied needle W9124T*
■ McIndoe scissors	
■ Stitch cutting scissors	■ Perineal muscles *Ethicon Vicryl rapide 2-0, 35-mm tapercut needle W9124*
■ Sims speculum Deep vaginal side wall retractors	
■ Sponge holding forceps (4)	■ Perineal skin *Ethicon Vicryl rapide 2-0, 35-mm tapercut needle W9124*
■ Tampon	
■ Large swabs	
■ Diathermy	

Figure A.4 Instruments and sutures used for repair of anal sphincter trauma

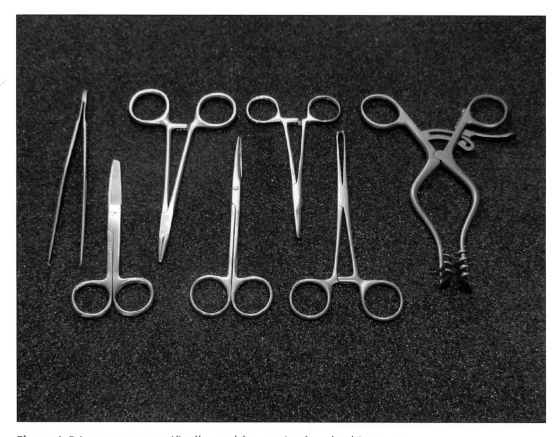

Figure A.5 Instruments specifically used for repair of anal sphincter trauma
From left to right: Tooth forceps, Stitch cutting scissors, Needle holder, McIndoe's scissors, Artery forceps, Allis forceps, Weislander retractor

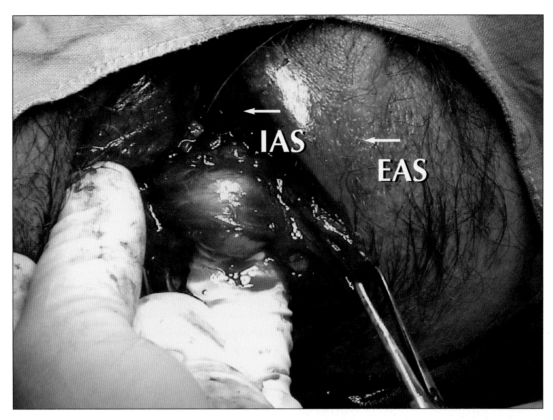

Figure A.6 Third degree tear (Grade 3b) demonstrating intact internal sphincter (IAS) and torn ends of external sphincter (EAS)

Repair of third and fourth degree tears

A repair should be performed only by a doctor experienced in anal sphincter repair or by a trainee under supervision. If in any doubt about diagnosis, it would be prudent to inform the consultant and await a second opinion.

Repair should be conducted in the operating theatre where there is access to good lighting, appropriate equipment and aseptic conditions. The perineal repair pack should contain appropriate instruments (demonstrated in Figures A.4 and A.5).

General or regional (spinal/epidural) anaesthesia is an important prerequisite, particularly for overlap repair, as the inherent tone of the sphincter muscle can cause the torn muscle ends to retract within the sheath. Muscle relaxation is necessary to retrieve the ends especially if it is intended to overlap the muscles without tension.

The full extent of the injury should be evaluated by a careful vaginal and rectal examination in lithotomy and graded according to the classification above.

Step 1: suturing the anal epithelium

In the presence of a fourth-degree tear, the torn anal epithelium is repaired with interrupted polyglactin 3/0 (Vicryl®, Ethicon, Edinburgh, UK) sutures with the knots tied in the anal lumen. A subcuticular repair of the anal epithelium using 3/0 PDS (polydioxanone sulphate) via the transvaginal approach has also been described.

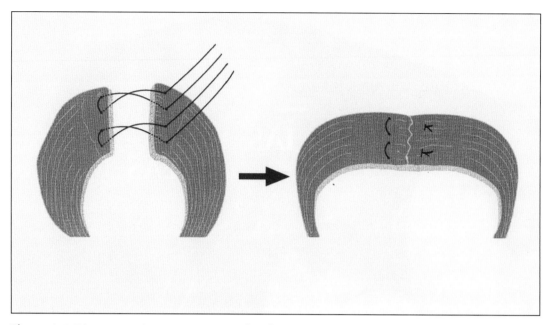

Figure A.7 Diagrammatic representation of end-to-end repair with figure of eight sutures

Step 2: suturing the anal sphincter

The sphincter muscles are repaired with 3/0 PDS dyed sutures. Compared with a braided suture, monofilamentous sutures are believed to be less likely to precipitate infection, non-absorbable monofilament sutures such as Nylon or Prolene (polypropylene) are preferred by some colorectal surgeons and can be equally effective. However, they can cause stitch abscesses and the sharp ends of the suture can cause discomfort, necessitating removal.

The internal anal sphincter should be identified and any tear should be repaired separately from the external sphincter. The internal anal sphincter lies between the external sphincter and the anal epithelium. It is paler than the striated external sphincter (Figure A.6) and the muscle fibres run in a circular fashion. The appearances of internal sphincter can be described as being analogous to the flesh of raw fish as opposed to the red meat appearance of the external sphincter. The ends of the torn muscle are grasped with Allis forceps and an end-to-end repair is performed with interrupted or mattress 3/0 PDS sutures. A torn internal sphincter should be approximated with interrupted sutures as overlapping can be technically difficult.

For repair of a torn external anal sphincter, evidence to date indicates that there is no significant difference in short-term outcome with the end-to-end (Figure A.7) or overlap (Figure A.8) technique and either technique can be used. If less than 50% of the external anal sphincter thickness is torn (3a tear) an end-to-end repair should be performed with mattress sutures to approximate the muscle ends. When more than 50% of the sphincter thickness is torn, one can perform an end-to-end repair but if an overlap repair is going to be performed it would necessitate complete division of the external anal sphincter and therefore an end-to-end is preferable.

The torn ends of the external anal sphincter are identified and grasped with Allis tissue forceps. In order to perform an overlap, the muscle may need mobilisation by dissection with a pair of McIndoe scissors separating it from the ischioanal fat laterally (Figure A.1). If the overlap technique is preferred then the external sphincter should be grasped with Allis forceps and pulled across to overlap in a 'double-breast' fashion. The torn ends of the external sphincter can then be overlapped as shown in using PDS 3/0 sutures. It is important that the full length of the external sphincter is identified to ensure complete approximation or overlap.

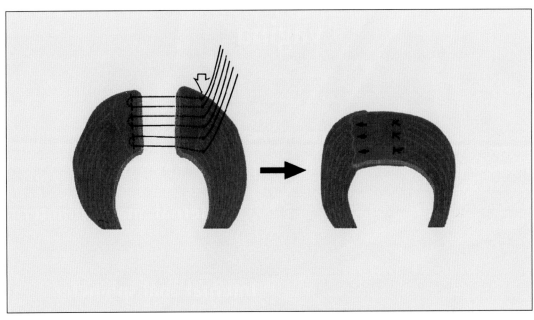

Figure A.8 Diagramatic representation of overlap repair of external anal sphincter

The vaginal skin is then sutured, the muscles of the perineal body are reconstructed and the perineal skin approximated (follow steps 1, 2 and 3 as for repair of episiotomy and second degree tears). Great care should be exercised in reconstructing the perineal muscles to provide support to the sphincter repair and burying the PDS sutures to avoid migration. A short deficient perineum would make the anal sphincter more vulnerable to trauma during a subsequent vaginal delivery.

Step 3

- Follow all steps as for second-degree tears and episiotomy.

- A rectovaginal examination should be performed to confirm complete repair and ensure that all tampons or swabs have been removed.

- Intravenous antibiotics (cefuroxime 1.5 g and metronidazole 500 mg) should be commenced intraoperatively and continued orally for 5–7 days. Although there are no randomised trials to substantiate benefit of this practice, the development of infection could jeopardise repair and lead to incontinence or fistula formation.

- Severe perineal discomfort, particularly following instrumental delivery, is a known cause of urinary retention and following regional anaesthesia it can take up to 12 hours before bladder sensation returns. A Foley catheter should be inserted for about 24 hours unless midwifery staff can ensure that spontaneous voiding occurs at least every 3 hours.

- Good note keeping of the findings and repair techniques is essential. A pictorial representation of the tears may prove to be useful when notes are being reviewed following complications, audit or litigation.

- As passage of a large bolus of hard stool may disrupt the repair, a stool softener (Lactulose 15 ml twice daily) and a bulking agent such as ispaghula husk (Fybogel®), 1 sachet twice daily should be prescribed for 10–14 days postoperatively. The woman must be made to understand the extent of the tear and advised how to seek help if symptoms of infection or incontinence develop.

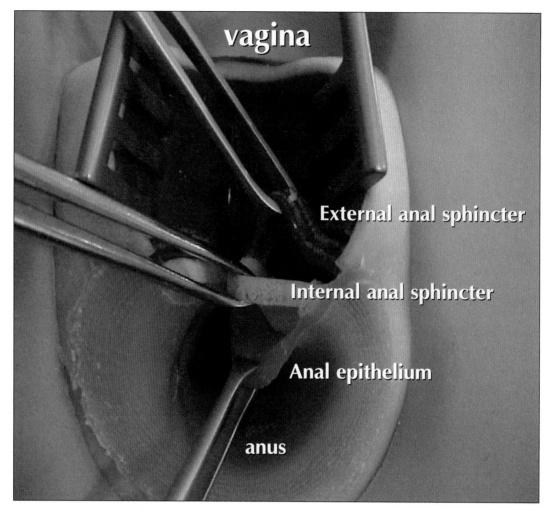

Figure A.9 Purpose built teaching model demonstrating anal sphincter anatomy (www.perineum.net)

Risk management

To minimise litigation, accurate documentation is important. Health professionals must ensure that the instrument and swab counts are correct after completion of suturing.

If a woman declines suturing, she should be given an opportunity to discuss this with the health professional responsible for her care. It is important to inform the woman of the possible risks associated with not suturing and potential problems that may occur if trauma to the anal sphincters is not detected or repaired following birth.

Women should be encouraged to seek help if problems occur in the postpartum period. Many centres now have dedicated perineal clinics to manage problems associated with perineal trauma following childbirth.

More focused and intensive training is required to improve recognition of anal sphincter trauma. This can be facilitated by establishing hands-on workshops using purpose built models (Figure A.9) and fresh animal anal sphincters (www.perineum.net).

Regular audit of perineal repair would help in ensuring higher standards of care.

Suggested further reading

Andrews V, Sultan AH, Thakar R, Jones PW. Occult anal sphincter injuries – myth or reality. *BJOG* 2006;113:195–200.

Andrews V, Thakar R, Sultan AH, Jones PW. Are mediolateral episiotomies actually mediolateral? *BJOG* 2005;112:1156–8.

Carroli G, Belizan J. Episiotomy for vaginal birth. *Cochrane Database Syst Rev* 2004;(1):CD000081.

Kettle C, Hills RK, Jones P, Darby L, Gray R, Johanson R. Continuous versus interrupted perineal repair with standard or rapidly absorbed sutures after spontaneous vaginal birth: a randomised controlled trial. *Lancet* 2002:359;2217–23.

Norton C, Christiansen J, Butler U, Harari D, Nelson RL, Pemberton J, *et al*. Anal incontinence. In: Abrams P, Cardozo L, Khoury, Wein A, editors. *Incontinence*. 2nd ed. Plymouth: Health Publication; 2002. p. 985–1044.

Royal College of Obstetricians and Gynaecologists. *Management of Third and Fourth Degree Perineal Tears Following Vaginal Delivery*. Guideline No. 29. London: RCOG Press; 2001.

Sultan AH, Kamm MA, Hudson CN, Thomas JM, Bartram CI. Anal sphincter disruption during vaginal delivery. *New Engl J Med* 1993;329:1905–11.

Sultan AH, Monga AK, Kumar D, Stanton SL. Primary repair of obstetric anal sphincter rupture using the overlap technique. *Br J Obstet Gynaecol* 1999;106:318–23.

Sultan AH, Thakar R. Lower genital tract and anal sphincter trauma. *Best Pract Res Clin Obstet Gynaecol* 2002;16(1):99–116.

Thakar R, Sultan AH. Management of obstetric anal sphincter injury. *The Obstetrician and Gynaecologist* 2003;5:72–8.

Appendix B

Consent issues

When is consent required?

Consent is required before any treatment, investigation or physical contact with a patient is undertaken. Consent is also required before involving patients in research, teaching or disclosure of confidential information, (which may be written, pictorial or auditory).

In England and Wales there is no statute, as in some countries, stating the principles of consent. Failure to obtain informed consent may give rise to civil or criminal proceedings as any touching of the person no matter how well intentioned is a trespass. However, to protect against a claim of battery, consent only in the broadest terms has to be obtained.

In contrast, a much more demanding obligation to obtain informed consent arises from a duty of care to the patient by the health professional.

Failure to provide sufficient information may deprive a patient of the ability to make an informed choice. If as a result, the patient agrees to a procedure she would have refused had she been fully informed and harm arises as a result, there may be grounds for a claim of negligence (even if the harm is a recognised hazard of the procedure rather than the product of poor management).

The case of Chester versus Afshar suggests that merely failing to provide relevant information to a patient may be found to constitute negligence.[1] In this case, the patient developed cauda equina syndrome following discectomy (a recognised complication of this procedure). She claimed that her surgeon had not warned her of this complication. The court accepted this. She admitted that it was likely that she would have chosen to undergo surgery by the same surgeon, even if she had known, but she had been deprived of the ability to make an informed choice in the matter. The majority view, when this case was appealed in the House of Lords, was that being denied the opportunity to make a properly informed decision about whether to undergo surgery constituted the injury. The implications for English case law as a result of this ruling are profound and the NHS Litigation Authority has issued an alert on this subject.[2]

Whenever possible, consent should be sought well in advance of a procedure and the doctor should recheck immediately prior to the procedure that the patient still consents. In obstetrics, information about any possible complications and the possible treatment options should be made available in the antenatal period. It is recognised that this will not be possible in the emergency situation and that those most at risk are not accessible antenatally.[3]

Why is consent required? The legal and ethical considerations

The need for valid consent is not just a legal requirement but also an ethical principle that reflects respect for an individual's autonomy and is a fundamental part of good practice. This is the view of both the Department of Health[4] and the General Medical Council.[5]

The traditional model of consent is the 'harm avoidance model', in which the patient is informed of the risks of a procedure, described in very general terms, but is otherwise excluded from the decision making process. The doctor in their professional wisdom, decides what the patient should be told; the paternalistic approach. The patient is dealt with 'in an authoritarian but benevolent way, (e.g. by supplying all their needs but regulating their conduct'.[6] This was considered acceptable in the case of Sidaway v Board of Governors of the Bethlehem Royal Hospital. As the judge put it: 'When telling a patient about an operation, the doctor has to decide what ought to be said and how it should be said'.[7]

An increasing emphasis on the rights of individuals in association with concerns, (particularly in the wake of the conviction of the general practitioner, Harold Shipman, for multiple murder of his patients), about whether doctors can be relied upon to 'help or at least do no harm,' has led to the requirement for a more demanding form of consent. This is so called 'autonomy enhancing model of consent', in which the patient must be given all the information they require to make their own fully informed decision about a proposed course of action.

In their 1998 publication,[5] the GMC suggests that obtaining informed consent is a process not an isolated event. It suggests that 'when providing information you must do your best to find out about patients' individual needs and priorities. You should respond honestly to any questions the patient raises'. A whole section is devoted to withholding information: 'You should not withhold information necessary for decision making unless you judge that disclosure of some relevant information would cause the patient serious harm. In this context serious harm does not mean the patient would become upset, or decide to refuse treatment'.

Consent may be implied or express. Implied consent is usually adequate for many episodes of physical contact between patient and doctor. An example of implied consent is the action of a patient holding out an arm for venepuncture to be performed. Such implied consent would usually protect against a charge of battery.

Express consent is required for a procedure carrying a 'material' risk (see below). The validity of consent does not depend on the form in which it is given: a signature on a form will not necessarily make consent valid. Equally, if consent has been validly given, the absence of a signed consent form is no bar to treatment. Written consent is considered advisable when the procedure involved is complex or risky, research or screening rather than clinical care is involved or there may be 'significant consequences for the patient's employment, social or personal life'.[5] It is a legal requirement for some treatments specified in the Human Fertilisation and Human Embryology Act 1990 and The Mental Health Act 1993.

What makes consent valid?

- The patient must have sufficient information.
- The patient must have the capacity to make a decision.
- The patient must be allowed to make the decision voluntarily.
- Consent is obtained by a suitably qualified and trained individual.

Sufficient information

This is an area of uncertainty with considerable changes occurring over time and between countries. Only the case in the UK will be discussed in detail.

In the UK in 1957, in the case of Bolam v Frien Hospital it was established that a doctor's practice would be judged against that of his medical peers – the Bolam principle or 'reasonable doctor test' – and this was specifically applied to what information to give a patient.[8] This was challenged in 1985 in the case of Sidaway. Although the Bolam principle was upheld, it was opined that there might be occasions when information about a particular risk was so obviously necessary that the court would decide that its omission was negligent even if this was not the opinion of a 'responsible body of medical opinion'.[9] By the late 1990s, the Bolam principle was overturned. In the cases of Bolitho and Pearce, the courts made it clear that the court itself would be the final arbiter of what was a reasonable amount of information to give a patient and not the medical profession. The reasonable doctor has been replaced by what the reasonable patient would expect to be told.[10] The situation is different in the USA, where in some states the policy of 'full disclosure' is advocated (the patient is told as much as possible).

Material risk is a risk to which a person in the patient's position would be likely to attach significance. A risk cannot be judged material on the basis of frequency alone.[11] The severity must be taken into account. The individual circumstances of the patient are also pertinent. For example, the risk of infertility following a procedure will be more significant to the primiparous woman than one who has completed her family. The type of information that patients should be told includes a description of the procedure and the incidence and severity of the risks involved (which should be mentioned even if they have not occurred in the practice of the particular doctor involved). There should be discussion on the likely or possible outcome of following or declining to follow a particular course of action and what the alternatives are (if any exist).[5]

The Association of Anaesthetists suggests that factors that might influence what the patient is told might include 'the estimated capacity' (see below) 'of the patient to want to know and to be able to understand the risks' and 'the degree of urgency of the proposed treatment'.[12]

Occasionally, a patient might wish to know very little or request that a relative make decisions for them (commonly the partner in obstetrics). In law, no one may make decisions on behalf of an adult. In this situation, the GMC suggests trying to explain the importance of knowing what is happening to the patient and the Department of Health considers it 'good practice' to record in the notes if information is offered but declined. A relative of an adult cannot choose to withhold information – the patient must be consulted.

In obstetrics, the problem of how much to tell the patient can be particularly demanding. Obstetric patients are usually young and fit. Younger patients want more information.[13] Women and their partners are often highly motivated to become informed: in the UK, over 70% of the population is estimated to have internet access and the number of sites providing information relating to obstetrics run into the thousands. The quality of information is very variable. Several studies show that obstetric patients want more information then they are receiving.[14–16] There is evidence to suggest that providing more information does not increase anxiety levels, in contrast to a common concern amongst the medical profession.[17]

Adversely influencing the opportunity to provide information that women want is lack of time: the majority of medical interventions in childbirth are unplanned, such as augmentation of labour, assisted vaginal delivery, episiotomy or manual removal of the placenta. Two-thirds of caesarean section operations are non-elective. In a 2001 national audit, 16% of caesarean sections were considered to be category 1: when there is immediate threat to the life of the woman and her fetus and delivery within 30 minutes is considered mandatory.[18] When trauma is involved, time is invariably at a premium. Most authorities suggest that women are given information about all the obstetric complications that might arise in the antenatal period to try to circumvent this problem, although some organisations are concerned that this promotes the medicalisation of childbirth. A combination of printed material with face to face question and answer sessions appear to be the most effective way of informing patients.[19]

Capacity

For a patient to have capacity (to be competent) to make a decision concerning medical treatment the following criteria must be met:

■ the patient must be capable of comprehending and retaining information

■ they must be able weigh the information in the balance (evaluate it).

These are known as the Eastman criteria as first stated in Re C.[20]

In the UK, anyone over the age of 18 years is assumed to be competent to chose or refuse treatment, unless shown not to be. This is 'not a question of the degree of intelligence or education of the adult concerned'.[21] In order for a patient to be able to comprehend information, that information must be presented in a form comprehensible to that patient (e.g. in a language they can understand or avoiding written material in the case of illiteracy). The Department of Health warns not to underestimate the capacity to consent by a patient with learning disabilities. Extra effort should be made to present information in a form comprehensible to such patients. Furthermore, the patient need not come to a decision that is seen as rational by others: 'The patient's right of choice exists whether the reasons for making that choice are rational, irrational, unknown or even non-existent (Lord Donaldson in Re T).[21]

No other person can consent to treatment on behalf of any adult, including incompetent ones.

Since 1969, 16- and 17-year-olds are entitled to consent to medical intervention (Section 8, Family Law Reform Act 1969). Unlike adults, however, their refusal of medical treatment may sometimes be overturned by an adult with parental responsibility. The power to overrule is based on the paramount importance of the welfare of the child and should be limited to occasions when the child is at risk of grave and irreversible physical or mental harm. Refusal of treatment by a child or those with parental responsibility can be overruled by a court in the interests of the child's welfare. This has obvious implications in the case of children of Jehovah's Witnesses (this is not the case in Scotland, where a competent child's refusal cannot be overturned).

Children under the age of 16 years may have the capacity to consent to medical treatment if they are judged to be 'Gillick competent' by their doctor. This standard was established in a decision in the House of Lords in 1986, in a case where it was ruled legal to prescribe contraceptives to girls under the age of 16 years without parental consent. The right of a parent to consent to treatment on behalf of a child ends when that child has sufficient intelligence and understanding to consent to the treatment herself.

In the case of obstetrics, it is worth noting that, in the UK in 2000, over 41 000 girls under the age of 18 years became pregnant, of whom 8000 were under 16 years old. A high proportion of young girls seek to terminate their pregnancy. In such circumstances there is potential for conflict between parents and children over whether to terminate the pregnancy and it is vital to establish whether the girl is Gillick competent.

Lack of consent: incompetence

The range of ability among patients follows a continuum from incompetence through to competence.[22] Patients may be competent to consent to some procedures and not others, depending on the complexity and importance of the case. Incapacity may be permanent, temporary or fluctuating.

Where capacity is absent, so that valid consent cannot be obtained, the underlying principle guiding treatment is that of the person's best interests (the 'welfare of the child' in the case of minors). Treatment can and should be given on the legal grounds of necessity. The best interests of an individual do not refer only to their physical health but must depend on:

■ the risks and benefits of available options

■ whether the patient had been previously competent, evidence of previously held views, e.g. advance statement (see below)

■ knowledge of the patient's views or beliefs

■ views of the patient's preferences given by a third party

■ the treatment option that gives the patient most chance of choice in the future.

If incapacity is likely to be temporary (e.g. the patient is anaesthetised or unconscious following an accident), intervention should be limited to that which is in the patient's immediate best interest. This includes routine procedures such as washing, dressing and so on. Any treatment that can be delayed should be, until competence is regained.

If capacity is likely to fluctuate, it is necessary to try to determine a patient's views on possible treatment during periods when they have capacity. These should be recorded.

Under the safeguards of the Mental Health Act 1983, patients who are mentally incapacitated may be treated compulsorily but only for the mental disorder from which they are suffering. In 1996, a parturient with schizophrenia was forced to undergo a caesarean section against her will on the grounds that the caesarean formed part of the treatment for her schizophrenia not because it would save her life or that of her child.[23] The judge was of the opinion that delivery would halt further deterioration to the patient's psychiatric state; psychiatric opinion was that a live birth was necessary to make schizophrenia treatment successful and finally that the patient could not be given strong enough medication until after delivery as it might harm the fetus (but see section on rights of the unborn child).

In the case of the incompetent child, the Children Act 1989 sets out who can assume parental responsibility. These include:

■ the children's parents if married at the time of birth or conception

■ the child's mother if unmarried but not the father, unless they subsequently marry or he is granted parental responsibility by a court

■ a legally appointed guardian

■ a person in whose favour a court has made a residence order for the child

■ a local authority if the child in under its care

■ a local authority or authorised person holding an emergency protection order for the child.

One person with parental responsibility may give consent to essential treatment, in the face of refusal by another, although if practical, such decisions should be referred to a court. In an emergency an incompetent child may be treated without consent from the person with parental responsibility.

The question of capacity and temporary incapacity is a particular dilemma in obstetrics. This has been highlighted by a series of cases in which applications were made to courts to allow emergency caesarean section to be performed against the will of the woman. In the case of CH, mentioned above, the surgery was allowed under the mental Health Act 1983, because the surgery itself was deemed to be an essential part of the treatment of the mental illness. In subsequent cases, the decision whether to allow surgery was based on the question of capacity of the labouring woman, with reference to the Eastman criteria. In one case, the 'pain and acute emotional stress' of labour combined with the patient's history of mental illness (she did not believe she was pregnant) were the grounds on which the judge concluded that she was incapable of weighing up the information presented to her.[24] However, in a second case, later the same day, the same judge concluded that the patient was 'unable to make any valid decision about anything of even the most trivial kind' due to the emotional stress and pain of labour. This was a woman whose obstetrician considered her to be competent and she had no history of mental illness.[25]

A third case involved a patient with a severe needle phobia who required section for breech presentation. In this case it was judged that the woman's capacity was temporarily diminished by the panic and fear induced by her needle phobia.

Factors that may temporarily erode capacity include shock, confusion, fatigue, pain and drugs. All these may be pertinent when considering the capacity of a woman in labour.

Following the case of MB, the court of appeal laid down procedures to be followed when doctors wish to seek declarations from the courts. An application is only likely to be considered if the woman's capacity is in question and it should be the High Court that considers issues of competence. Potential problems should be identified as early as possible and legal procedure to be followed set out in detail.

The Human Rights Act 1998 incorporates the European Convention on Human Rights into UK law. Although early days, it is considered possible that it will serve to strengthen protection of individuals against treatment they refuse (Article 3, prohibition of torture; Article 5, right to liberty and security; Article 6, right to a fair trial) and emphasise their right to be fully informed (Article 8, right to private and family life).[26]

Status of the fetus

The Abortion Act 1967 gave statutory status to the principle that the fetus does not have a legal right to life. The Act sets out clearly the circumstances when termination of pregnancy is allowable, which extends far beyond the physical wellbeing of the woman. A pregnancy may only be terminated if two registered medical practitioners are of the opinion, formed in good faith that an abortion is justified within the terms of the Act, in the light of their clinical judgement of all the particular circumstances of the individual case. The grounds for an abortion are:

(a)   that the pregnancy has not exceeded its 24th week and that the continuance of the pregnancy would involve risk, greater than if the pregnancy were terminated, of injury to the physical or mental health of the pregnant woman or any existing children of her family; or

(b)   that the termination is necessary to prevent grave permanent injury to the physical or mental health of the pregnant woman; or

(c)   that the continuance of the pregnancy would involve risk to the life of the pregnant woman, greater than if the pregnancy were terminated; or

(d)   that there is a substantial risk that if the child were born it would suffer from such physical or mental abnormalities as to be seriously handicapped.

There is no time limit for (b) to (d). The Act goes on to state that 'in determining whether the continuance of pregnancy would involve such risk of injury to health as is mentioned in paragraph (a) or (b)..., account may be taken of the pregnant woman's actual or reasonably foreseeable environment'.

If 'the termination is immediately necessary to save the life or to prevent grave permanent injury to the physical or mental health of the pregnant woman', the pregnancy may be terminated if one registered medical practitioner is of the opinion, formed in good faith that an abortion is justified within the terms of the Act.

The fetus's lack of legal right was demonstrated in a case in which a man unsuccessfully sought an injunction preventing his wife from having an abortion.[27] This case was taken to the European Commission on Human Rights under Article 2 (right to life) but was rejected.

The Court of Appeal's ruling on the case of MB highlights not just issues of competence but also the legal status of the unborn child in relation to its mother's rights. In the judgement of the Court of Appeal, it was categorically stated that the right of a competent woman to agree to or refuse treatment takes precedent over the welfare of the fetus.[28] In a subsequent case, the Court of Appeal concluded: 'Although human, and protected by the law in a number of different ways ... an unborn child is not a separate person from its mother. Its need for medical assistance does not prevail over her rights. She is entitled not to be forced to submit to an invasion of her body against her will, whether her own life or that of her unborn child depends on it. Her right is not reduced or diminished merely because her decision to exercise it may appear morally repugnant'.[29]

Voluntarily given consent

Consent will only be valid if given freely. The GMC starts the section entitled 'Ensuring voluntary decision making', by stating 'it is for the patient not the doctor, to determine what is in the patient's best interests'.[5] However, it accepts that the doctor may want to recommend a particular treatment. This should be acceptable if evidence-based information is presented in a dispassionate manner. It is good practice to document the discussion.

The woman's partner and sometimes other relatives, any of whom may hold strong views about her management, often accompany the obstetric patient. When considering outside influence, 'the will of the patient and the relationship of the person trying to impose their will, must be considered' (Lord Donaldson in Re T).[21] The same factors that may erode capacity may also undermine the woman's ability to withstand coercion (fatigue, pain, stress, etc.). Cultural factors characterising relationships between the sexes may also be a factor. In the not uncommon situation where a woman states 'I will do as my husband decides' it is important to try to establish the woman's wishes, preferably in the absence of the partner. The same may apply to parents, especially in the case of younger girls. In Re T, the Court of Appeal judge upheld the decision to allow a blood transfusion to a patient who was not a Jehovah's Witness but who declined blood, on the grounds that her mother who was a Jehovah's Witness had unduly influenced her.[21]

It should be reiterated that no one can consent to or refuse treatment on behalf of another adult, whether competent or not. Thus, the partner who says 'my wife would have wanted/not have wanted a particular intervention' has no right to impose his view. However, such a statement may alert the doctor to the existence of an advance directive that does have legal weight (see below).

Who can obtain consent?

The person providing treatment is responsible for obtaining consent. The GMC guidance states that this task can be delegated, provided that the person to whom the task is delegated is suitably trained and qualified, obtains consent in an appropriate manner and has sufficient knowledge about the proposed procedure.[5] In GKC v Hammersmith & Queen Charlotte's Special Health Authority, a junior doctor was judged not to have explained that a screening test for Down syndrome (the Bart's test) was predictive rather than diagnostic (as is amniocentesis). The patient subsequently delivered an affected baby and the health authority was found to be negligent. The explanation and description of risk is complex.[30] A doctor who may be in possession of the scientific facts involved may not be trained to communicate such matters.

Advance directives

A patient may use an advance directive to indicate how they would wish to be treated in the case of future incapacity. Such directives are legally binding if:

■ the individual was competent when drawing up the directive. The directive expresses refusal of a treatment (a doctor is not obliged to undertake any particular course of action and cannot be required to undertake an illegal course of action). The circumstances in which the question of treatment arises are those anticipated by the patient when drawing up the directive

■ there is no evidence that the patient may have changed her mind.

An advance directive does not have to be a written statement or formally witnessed.

A doctor cannot choose to ignore a valid advance directive on terms of conscience or belief.

Examples of advance directives include refusal of heroic surgery or resuscitative measures in the case of progressive, debilitating disease and statements that Jehovah's Witnesses may carry, refusing the use of blood or blood products. In the case of obstetrics, the birth plan may fulfil the criteria of an advance directive. In such circumstances, what is paramount is to determine if the patient had anticipated the circumstances (e.g. more severe pain than ever previously experienced), if she had changed her mind and whether the present circumstances have rendered her currently incompetent.

If there are concerns about the validity of an advance directive, it may be necessary to consult the courts. Article 9 of the Human Rights Act 1998 (freedom of thought, conscience and religion) may have an impact in this area in the future.

Summary

- Without basic consent, any physical contact with patients constitutes trespass and could result in a charge of battery or assault.

- Doctors have a duty of care to ensure that their patients give informed consent to procedures. Failure to do may constitute negligence, especially if harm ensues.

- Where informed consent cannot be obtained, doctors may legally provide care based on the principle of necessity, the basis of which is the treatment is in the best interests of the patient.

- While children under the age of 16 years may have the right to consent to treatment independently of their parents, if they are 'Gillick competent', they may not have the right to refuse treatment.

- The fetus has no legal right to life. A pregnant or labouring woman's rights are paramount, even in the face of fetal demise.

- Advance directives, of which birth plans are examples, if valid, are legally binding.

- In general the obstetric population wants and requires more information to inform their treatment decisions.

References

1. Chester v Afshar [2004] UKHL 41.
2. NHS Litigation Authority. NHSLA Risk Alert, Issue 4, (November 2004).
3. Lewis G, editor. *Why Mothers Die 2000–2002. Sixth Report of the Confidential Enquiries into Maternal Deaths in the United Kingdom.* London: RCOG Press; 2004.
4. Department of Health. *Reference Guide to Consent for Examination or Treatment.* London: DoH; 2001 [www.doh.gov.uk/consent/refguide.htm].
5. General Medical Council. *Seeking Patients' Consent: The Ethical Considerations.* London: GMC; 1998 [www.gmc-uk.org/standards/default.htm].
6. Switankowsky IS. *A New Paradigm for Informed Consent.* Lanham, MD: University Press of America; 1998.
7. Sidaway v Board of Governors of the Bethlehem Royal Hospital and Maudsley Hospital and others [1965] AC 871, HL at 871.
8. Bolam v Frien Hospital Management Committee 1957.
9. Sidaway v Board of Governors of Bethlehem Royal Hospital 1985 AC 871.
10. Bolitho v City & Hackney Health Authority 1997, Pearce v United Bristol Healthcare Trust 1999.
11. Rogers v Whitaker 1992.
12. Association of Anaesthetists of Great Britain and Ireland. Information and Consent for Anaesthesia. London; 1999 [www.aagbi.org].
13. Farnhill D, Inglis S. Patients' desire for information about anaesthesia: Australian attitudes. *Anaesthesia* 1993;48:162–4.
14. Kelly GD, Blunt C, Moore PAS, Lewis M. Consent for regional anaesthesia in the United Kingdom: what is material risk? *Int J Obstet Anesth* 2004;13:71–4.
15. Plaat F, McGlennan A. Women in the 21st century deserve more information: Disclosure of

material risk in obstetric anaesthesia *Int J Obstet Anesth* 2004;13:69–70.

16. Pattee C, Ballantyne M, Milne B. Epidural analgesia for labour and delivery: informed consent issues. *Can J Anaesth* 1997;44:918–23.

17. Inglis S, Farnhill D. The effects of providing preoperative statistical anaesthetic risk information. *Anesth Intensive Care* 1993;21:799–805.

18. Royal College of Obstetricians and Gynaecologists Clinical Effectiveness Support Unit. *The National Sentinel Caesarean Section Audit Report.* London: RCOG Press; 2001.

19. Webber D, Higgins L, Baker V. Enhancing recall of information from a patient education booklet: a trial using cardiomyopathy patients. *Patient Educ Couns* 2001;44:263–70.

20. Re C (Adult: Refusal of treatment) 1994.

21. Re T (Adult: Refusal of treatment) 1993.

22. Maybury M, Maybury J. *Consent in Clinical Practice.* Oxford: Radcliffe Medical Press; 2003.

23. Tameside and Glossop Acute Services Trust v CH.

24. Norfolk and Norwich NHS Trust v W 1996.

25. Rochdale NHS Trust v C 1997.

26. Hewson B. Why the Human Rights Act matters to doctors. *BMJ* 2000;321:780–1.

27. Paton v trustees of British Pregnancy Advisory Services 1979.

28. Re MB adult medical treatment 1997.

29. Re S adult refusal of treatment 1992.

30. Sedgwick P, Hall A. Teaching medical students and doctors how to communicate risk. *BMJ* 2003;327:694–5.

Index

Index